PREVENTIVE AUDIOLOGY

An African perspective

AOSIS

Published by AOSIS Books, an imprint of AOSIS Publishing.

AOSIS Publishing
15 Oxford Street, Durbanville 7550, Cape Town, South Africa
Postnet Suite 110, Private Bag X19, Durbanville, 7551, Cape Town, South Africa
Tel: +27 21 975 2602
Website: https://www.aosis.co.za

Cover image: Original design created with the use of provided image. The image is https://www.freepik.com/free-photo/3d-render-medical-with-close-up-ear-soundwaves_10167253.htm#query=hearing&position=1&from_view=search, released under the appropriate Freepik License terms.

Published in 2022
Impression: 1

ISBN: 978-1-77634-245-7 (print)
ISBN: 978-1-77634-246-4 (epub)
ISBN: 978-1-77634-247-1 (pdf)

DOI: https://doi.org/10.4102/aosis.2022.BK209
How to cite this work: Khoza-Shangase, K (ed.) 2022, *Preventive audiology: An African perspective*, AOSIS Books, Cape Town.

Printed and bound in South Africa.

PREVENTIVE AUDIOLOGY

An African perspective

Edited by

KATIJAH KHOZA-SHANGASE

AOSIS

Peer review declaration

The publisher (AOSIS) endorses the South African 'National Scholarly Book Publishers Forum Best Practice for Peer Review of Scholarly Books'. The manuscript underwent an evaluation to compare the level of originality with other published works and was subjected to rigorous two-step peer review before publication, with the identities of the reviewers not revealed to the editor(s) or author(s). The reviewers were independent of the publisher, editor(s), and author(s). The publisher shared feedback on the similarity report and the reviewers' inputs with the manuscript's editor(s) or author(s) to improve the manuscript. Where the reviewers recommended revision and improvements, the editor(s) or author(s) responded adequately to such recommendations. The reviewers commented positively on the scholarly merits of the manuscript and recommended that the manuscript be published.

Research justification

Preventive health care, where preventive audiology is positioned, contains strategies adopted and implemented for disease and disorder prevention. Hearing function can be negatively impacted by numerous factors, including lifestyle choices, environmental factors, genetic predisposition, the burden of disease and other causes. Frequently, hearing impairment can be prevented and its consequences significantly minimised by preventive measures. Such prevention commands conscientiously deliberate anticipatory actions that can fall under primordial, primary, secondary or tertiary levels of prevention. South Africa, as a resource-constrained low- and middle-income country (LMIC), still has a challenge of high numbers of individuals with preventable hearing impairment from the cradle to the grave. Numerous strategies exist for the prevention of hearing impairment across all ages and in various contexts. *Preventive Audiology: An African Perspective* is an original scholarly book that introduces the concept of preventive audiology, with a specific focus on the African context, which is in line with the South African re-engineered primary health care strategy and the World Health Organization's approach. The book reflects on contextually relevant and responsive evidence-based perspectives, grounded in an African context on preventive audiology, in four major ear-and-hearing burdens of disease within the South African context, namely, (1) early hearing detection and intervention (EHDI), (2) middle ear pathologies, (3) ototoxicity and (4) noise-induced hearing loss (NIHL). The book represents innovative research, seen from both South African and global perspectives. It offers new discourse and argues for a paradigm shift in how audiology is theorised and performed, particularly in LMIC contexts. The goal of this book is to motivate for a paradigm shift in how ear-and-hearing health care is approached within this LMIC context, while also arguing for Afrocentric *best practice* evidence that leads to *next practice*. For *Afrocentric epistemology*, which is a different narrative that is deliberately removed from *Western epistemology*, contributors who responded to the call for chapters and had their abstracts accepted were encouraged to allow their own positionality, Afrocentric views and perspectives, and their own research in the field, as well as context to guide their writing. The authors were also urged to supply evidence that will guide decision-making and planning around policy formulation, training, clinical care and research within the African context – without being overly prescriptive in the recommendations and solutions offered. All of this was done with strict adherence to academic writing protocols such as critical engagement with evidence, assurance of originality, and adherence to consistent referencing. Sufficient evidence exists regarding the economics and quality of life investment benefits of preventive care, hence the focus of this edited book as part of a series of books by Khoza-Shangase on African perspectives. All chapters underwent rigorous independent peer review by experts in the field and independent review via AOSIS. The chapters contain no plagiarism, and the book represents a scholarly discourse. The book's target audience consists of specialists in the field of audiology.

Katijah Khoza-Shangase, Department of Audiology, Faculty of Humanities, School of Human and Community Development, University of the Witwatersrand, Johannesburg, South Africa

Contents

Abbreviations and acronyms, boxes, figures and tables appearing in the text and notes

List of abbreviations and acronyms

4IR	Fourth Industrial Revolution
AAA	American Association of Audiology
AABR	automated auditory brainstem response
ABR	auditory brainstem response
AFMC	Association of Faculties of Medicine of Canada
AI	artificial intelligence
AIDS	acquired immune deficiency syndrome
AMA	American Medical Association
AOM	acute otitis media
AR	aural rehabilitation
ART	antiretroviral treatment
ARV	antiretroviral
ASHA	American Speech-Language-Hearing Association
BANC	basic antenatal care
CBA	cost-benefit analysis
CCA	cost-consequence analysis
CCWs	community care workers
CDC	Centre for Disease Control
CEA	cost-effective analysis
CHARGE	coloboma, heart defects, atresia choanae, growth retardation, genital abnormalities and ear abnormalities
CHW	community health worker
COIDA	*Compensation for Occupational Injuries and Diseases Act of 1993*
COVID-19	coronavirus disease 2019
CSDH	Commission on the Social Determinants of Health
CSOM	chronic suppurative otitis media
CHL	conductive hearing loss
CHOICE	CHOosing Interventions that are Cost-Effective

CIOMS	Council for International Organizations of Medical Sciences
CRPD	Committee on the Rights of Persons with Disabilities
CUA	cost-utility analysis
DALY	disability-adjusted life years
dB	decibel
DMRE	Department of Mineral Resources and Energy of South Africa
DoH	Department of Health
DPOAE	distortion-product otoacoustic emission
EAM	external auditory meatus
ECD	early childhood development
ECI	early childhood intervention
EHDI	early hearing detection and intervention
EHF	extended high frequency
EI	early intervention
EMA	European Medicines Agency
ENT	ear, nose and throat
EPI	Extended Programme on Immunisation of 2007
FBNMM	feedback-based noise monitoring model
FCEI	family-centred early intervention
FDA	Food and Drug Administration of the United States of America
FDC	fixed-dose combination
GD	gradient descent
GDAM	gradient descent with adaptive momentum
GDP	gross domestic product
GRDDC	Global Research on Developmental Disabilities Collaborators
HAART	highly active antiretroviral therapy
HCPs	hearing conservation programmes
HICs	high-income countries
HI HOPES	home intervention–hearing and language opportunities parent education services
HIV	human immunodeficiency virus
HPDs	hearing protection devices
HPCSA	Health Professions Council of South Africa
HRR	high-risk register
Hz	hertz
ICER	incremental cost-effectiveness ratio
ICF	International Classification of Functioning, Disability and Health
ICTs	information and communication technologies

IHME	Institute for Health Metrics and Evaluation
IMCI	integrated management of childhood illness
ISHP	Integrated School Health Policy of 2012
JCIH	Joint Committee on Infant Hearing
KZN	KwaZulu-Natal
LMIC	low- and middle-income country
LMICs	low- and-middle-income countries
LOCHI	longitudinal outcomes of children with hearing impairment
LYG	life-years gained
MCWH&N	Maternal, Child and Women's Health and Nutrition Strategic Plan
MDG	UN Millennium Development Goal of 2000
MDR-TB	multidrug-resistant tuberculosis
MHSC	SA Mine Health and Safety Council
ML	machine learning
MLP	multilayer perceptron
MOU	midwife obstetric unit
NDoH	National Department of Health of South Africa
NDP	National Development Plan of 2012
NHA	*National Health Act of 2003*
NHI	National Health Insurance
NHS	Newborn Hearing Screening
NIHL	noise-induced hearing loss
NIHS	newborn infant hearing screening
NIOSH	National Institute for Occupational Safety and Health
NSDA	Negotiated Service Delivery Agreement
OAEs	otoacoustic emissions
OHCs	outer hair cells
OHL	occupational hearing loss
OHN	occupational health nurse
OHP	occupational health practitioners
ONIHL	occupational noise-induced hearing loss
OM	otitis media
OMP	ototoxicity monitoring programme
OSHA	*Occupational Safety and Health Act of 1993*
PBSLH	Professional Board for Speech, Language and Hearing of South Africa
PDMS	proactive data management system
PHC	primary health care

PLH	percentage loss of hearing
PMTCT	prevention of mother-to-child transmission
PMPs	personal music players
PoPIA	*Protection of Personal Information Act of 2020*
PPE	personal protective equipment
PTS	permanent threshold shift
QALYs	quality-adjusted life years
QoL	quality of life
RF	resonant frequency
RHAP	Rural Health Advocacy Project
RoP	retinopathy of prematurity
RSA	Republic of South Africa
SA	South Africa
SAHPRA	South African Health Products Authority
SANDoH	South African National Department of Health
SASL	South African Sign Language
SASLHA	South African Speech Language and Hearing Association
SDG	Sustainable Development Goal of UNESCO
SDGs	Sustainable Development Goals of UNESCO
SLH	speech-language and hearing
SLP	speech-language pathologist
SMEs	Small and Medium Enterprises
SNHL	sensorineural hearing loss
SONA	State of the Nation Address
SSNHL	sudden sensorineural hearing loss
STMNCWH	Strategic Plan for Maternal, Newborn, Child and Women's Health (MNCW&H) and Nutrition in South Africa
STS	standard threshold shift
SVM	support-vector machine
TB	tuberculosis
TBA	telehealth-based audiology
UAC	Universal Audiology Coverage
UHC	Universal Health Coverage
UHF	ultra high-frequency
UK	United Kingdom
UKHSE	UK Health and Safety Executive
UNAIDS	Joint United Nations Programme on HIV/AIDS
UNHS	universal newborn hearing screening

UN	United Nations
USA	United States of America
WAI	wideband acoustic immittance
WFDB	World Federation of the Deafblind
WHO	World Health Organization
WHA	World Health Assembly
WMA	World Medical Association
WSHC	Workplace Safety Health Council
WT	wideband tympanometry
YLD	years lived with disability

Box list

List of figures

List of tables

Acknowledgements

I would like to acknowledge the chapter contributors for their significant contributions to this book. I wish to also acknowledge my precious family for their unending and unconditional support during the journey of putting this book together. I am also greatly indebted to the following scholars and academics who generously agreed to serve as reviewers for chapters, contributing significantly to the quality assurance of this valuable output:

Prof. S. Dada (Centre for Augmentative & Alternative Communication, University of Pretoria)
Dr S. Govender (Sefako Makgatho Health Sciences University)
Prof. S. Dhar (Northwestern University)
Dr K. Masuku (University of the Witwatersrand)
Dr V. de Andrade (University of the Witwatersrand)
Prof. M. Pillay (University of KwaZulu-Natal)
Prof. N. Moroe (University of the Witwatersrand)
Dr K. Coutts (University of the Witwatersrand)
Mrs A. Casoojee (University of the Witwatersrand)
Mrs N.P. Maluleke (Sefako Makgatho Health Sciences University)
Prof. K. Joubert (University of the Witwatersrand)
Dr S. Moodley (Centre for Deafness Studies, University of the Witwatersrand)
Dr B. Sebothoma (University of the Witwatersrand)
Mrs N.B. Khan (University of KwaZulu-Natal)
Prof. A. Kanji (University of the Witwatersrand)
Mr W. Manning (University of KwaZulu-Natal)
Dr M. Zumbi (Sustainable Communities, Barrick Gold Corporation, Dar es Salaam, Tanzania)
Dr A. Edwards (Africa Health Research Institute)
Prof. J. Neille (University of the Witwatersrand)
Dr S. Adams (University of the Witwatersrand)
Ms N. Nagdee (University of the Witwatersrand)

This publication was made possible through a grant received from the *National Institute for the Humanities and Social Sciences*.

Notes on contributors

Katijah Khoza-Shangase
Department of Audiology, Faculty of Humanities,
School of Human and Community Development, University of the Witwatersrand,
Johannesburg, South Africa
Email: katijah.khoza-shangase@wits.ac.za
ORCID: https://orcid.org/0000-0002-6220-9606

Katijah Khoza-Shangase holds a PhD in Speech and Hearing Therapy from the University of the Witwatersrand and is a professor and the former Head of the Speech Pathology and Audiology Department at the University of the Witwatersrand, Johannesburg, South Africa. She was a finalist in the academic category of the Businesswomen Association of South Africa's Finalist in 2017. She has played an instrumental leadership role in the Health Professions Council of South Africa (HSPCA). Khoza-Shangase has received numerous awards, primarily in the areas of research and research supervision, and for her contributions to the scholarly field of audiology. She has authored multiple publications, including peer-reviewed journal articles, technical and research reports, book chapters, articles in conference proceedings and co-edited books. Published in 2019, *Black Academic Voices: The South African Experience* received the 2020 Humanities and Social Sciences (HSS) Award in the non-fiction category from the National Institute of Humanities and Social Sciences (NIHSS) and is one of her most current contributions to the transformation and decolonisation research project. Khoza-Shangase's edited book *Early Detection and Intervention in Audiology: An African Perspective* by Wits University Press was released in 2021 and nominated for the HSS 2022 Awards. She also co-edited two special issues for the *South African Journal of Communication Disorders* (2020, 2022), titled *Occupational Hearing Loss in Africa: An Interdisciplinary View of the Current Status* and *The impact of COVID-19 on SLH Professions in LMICs: Challenges and Opportunities* Explored. Khoza-Shangase's latest research books, *Occupational Noise-induced hearing loss: An African perspective* and *Complexities and challenges in preventive audiology: An African perspective*, were published in 2022 by AOSIS Books, an imprint of AOSIS Scholarly Books, a division of AOSIS Publishing. The 2022 World Scientist and University Rankings ranked her second at the University of the Witwatersrand, third in South Africa and in Africa, fourth in the BRICS countries, and 97th in the world.

Ben Sebothoma
Department of Audiology, Faculty of Humanities,
School of Human and Community Development, University of the Witwatersrand,
Johannesburg, South Africa
Email: ben.sebothoma@wits.ac.za
ORCID: https://orcid.org/0000-0003-4773-3204

Ben Sebothoma is the first Black African male to obtain a PhD in Audiology on the continent of Africa at the University of the Witwatersrand, focusing on middle ear pathologies in HIV/AIDS. He completed his undergraduate training at the University of Cape Town and his MA in Audiology at the University of the Witwatersrand. He is a clinical audiologist and a lecturer in the Department of Audiology at the University of the Witwatersrand in Johannesburg, South Africa. He has lectured and supervised undergraduate and postgraduate students. He has published several scientific research papers in accredited journals, chapters in peer-reviewed scholarly books, and presentations in local and international conference proceedings. His research areas include prevention, identification and management of middle ear pathologies across the lifespan in low- and middle-income countries.

Samantha Govender
Department of Speech-Language Pathology and Audiology,
Faculty of Health Sciences, School of Healthcare Sciences,
Sefako Makgatho Health Sciences University,
Pretoria, South Africa
Email: samantha.govender@smu.ac.za
ORCID: https://orcid.org/0000-0002-4754-5361

Samantha Govender obtained her PhD with a focus on telehealth from the University of KwaZulu-Natal, South Africa, and is a senior lecturer at the Sefako Makgatho Health Sciences University in Pretoria, South Africa. She is an audiologist with over 14 years of experience. Her research focus is community-based health care, specifically providing school-based audiological services to remote and rural South Africa. She has a research interest in ototoxicity monitoring and paediatric audiology. Govender has published several peer-reviewed articles on providing telehealth-based audiological services within the school context. While writing this book, Govender was working towards establishing a telehealth teaching, learning and clinical training centre to develop context-specific guidelines for the South African context.

Karin Joubert
Department of Audiology, Faculty of Humanities,
School of Human and Community Development,
University of the Witwatersrand,
Johannesburg, South Africa
Email: karin.joubert@wits.ac.za
ORCID: https://orcid.org/0000-0002-2366-8607

Karin Joubert holds a PhD which she was awarded in 2009. Joubert is an associate professor in the Department of Audiology at the University of the Witwatersrand in Johannesburg, South Africa. She completed an undergraduate degree in Speech Therapy and Audiology at the University of Pretoria, South Africa, and Joubert's postgraduate qualifications include a Hons degree in

Psychology and a MA in Early Childhood Intervention. In 2014, she established the Ndlovu Wits Audiology Clinic and Outreach Programme, which offers comprehensive community-based audiology services in the rural areas of the Limpopo province in South Africa. Her research seeks to provide evidence-based information that can be used to implement community-based audiology and preventive audiology services that will improve access to hearing health care for under-resourced communities.

Amisha Kanji
Department of Audiology, Faculty of Humanities,
School of Human and Community Development,
University of the Witwatersrand,
Johannesburg, South Africa
Email: amisha.kanji@wits.ac.za
ORCID: https://orcid.org/0000-0002-9577-4935

Amisha Kanji holds a PhD in Audiology and is an associate professor and former Head of the Discipline of Audiology at the University of the Witwatersrand in Johannesburg, South Africa. She lectures undergraduate audiology courses, is involved in clinical and research supervision of students and is the current departmental postgraduate research coordinator. She has been appointed as the Chair of the School of Human and Community Development's Assessment Portfolio. She was awarded the vice-chancellor's transformation team category award in 2019. Kanji served on the HPCSA task team that developed national guidelines for early hearing detection and intervention. She has also served as a member of HPCSA-appointed evaluation panels for speech-language and hearing training programmes. She has several peer-reviewed publications and has presented at local and international conferences. She co-edited the book *Early Detection and Intervention in Audiology: An African Perspective* by Wits University Press (2021). Kanji has acted as an expert peer reviewer for abstract submissions to audiology conferences and reviews in several South African and international journals.

Nomfundo F. Moroe
Department of Audiology, Faculty of Humanities,
School of Human and Community Development,
University of the Witwatersrand,
Johannesburg, South Africa
Email: nomfundo.moroe@wits.ac.za
ORCID: https://orcid.org/0000-0001-7186-5632

Nomfundo F. Moroe holds a PhD and is a associate professor and the former Head of the Discipline of Audiology at the University of the Witwatersrand in Johannesburg, South Africa. She is part of the Department of Higher Education and Training's (DHET) NGap Programme – a programme that involves the recruitment of competent scholars as new academics against carefully designed and balanced equity considerations and in light of the disciplinary areas of greatest need. Moroe is a passionate researcher interested in occupational audiology, complex interventions, deaf culture and deafblindness. She is a CARTA Fellow (Consortium for Advanced Research Training in Africa), a highly competitive programme that trains young and emerging African researchers, and she was conducting postdoctoral research funded by CARTA during the writing of the chapter. She has published several peer-reviewed articles and book chapters and presented at national and international conferences. She has co-edited a special issue scholarly journal for the *South African Journal of Communication Disorders* (AOSIS Journals 2020) titled *Occupational Hearing Loss in Africa: An Interdisciplinary View of the Current Status*. Moroe's latest publication includes a co-edited book titled *Occupational noise-induced hearing loss: An African perspective* (2022) by AOSIS Books, an imprint of AOSIS Scholarly Books, a division of AOSIS Publishing.

Khetsiwe P. Masuku
Department of Speech Pathology, Faculty of Humanities,
School of Human and Community Development,
University of the Witwatersrand,
Johannesburg, South Africa
Email: Khetsiwe.Masuku@wits.ac.za
ORCID: https://orcid.org/0000-0003-3413-689X

Khetsiwe P. Masuku holds a MA in Public Health, a PhD in Augmentative and Alternative Communication (Severe Disability), and is a lecturer in the Department of Speech Pathology at the University of the Witwatersrand in Johannesburg, South Africa. Masuku lectures and supervises speech pathology students at both undergraduate and postgraduate levels. As a researcher, she is interested in the topic of disability, specifically about access for persons with disabilities and caregivers of persons with disabilities. In addition, she is interested in the implementation of disability policies in the context of the African continent. Her other research interests include research in aphasia and deafblindness. She has published several research articles and chapters in peer-reviewed journals and scholarly books.

Ntsako P. Maluleke
[a]Department of Speech-Language Pathology and Audiology,
Faculty of Health Sciences, School of Healthcare Sciences,
Sefako Makgatho Health Sciences University,
Pretoria, South Africa;
[b]Department of Audiology, Faculty of Humanities,
School of Human and Community Development,
University of the Witwatersrand,
Johannesburg, South Africa
Email: precious.slp@gmail.com
ORCID: https://orcid.org/0000-0003-1206-0011

Ntsako P. Maluleke holds an undergraduate degree in Speech and Hearing Therapy and a MA in Audiology from the University of the Witwatersrand.

She is an audiologist and a former lecturer in the Department of Speech-Language Pathology and Audiology at the Sefako Makgatho Health Sciences University in Ga-Rankuwa in Pretoria, South Africa. Maluleke, as an emerging researcher and scholar, has authored several peer-reviewed articles and scholarly book chapters and presented her research at various conferences. Her research interests include early hearing detection and intervention, childhood and school-age hearing impairment, and family-centred intervention. During the writing of this book, she was a PhD candidate at the University of the Witwatersrand, focusing on 'Family-centred EHDI services in South Africa: Caregivers' experience and evaluation of the process and practices in Gauteng'.

Liepollo Ntlhakana
Department of Audiology, Faculty of Humanities,
School of Human and Community Development,
University of the Witwatersrand,
Johannesburg, South Africa
Email: liepollo.ntlhakana@wits.ac.za
ORCID: https://orcid.org/0000-0002-8632-0616

Liepollo Ntlhakana holds a PhD from the School of Public Health at the University of Witwatersrand with research focusing on 'Noise-induced hearing loss (NIHL) in mine workers in South Africa: Risk assessment explored'. Ntlhakana is a lecturer and Deputy Head of the Department of Audiology at the University of the Witwatersrand in Johannesburg, South Africa. She lectures and supervises both audiology undergraduate and postgraduate students. Besides teaching in the Department of Nursing's Occupational Health Nursing Programme, she is also a guest lecturer for the Audiometry short course. Ntlhakana's keen interest in occupational audiology stems from years of experience as the Occupational Audiology portfolio manager for the South African Association of Audiologists (SAAA). Her postdoctoral work focuses on developing a predictive model for the early identification of occupational noise-induced hearing loss (ONIHL).

Chapter 1

Preventive audiology: Ramping up efforts towards an ear-and-hearing healthy nation

Katijah Khoza-Shangase
Department of Audiology, Faculty of Humanities,
School of Human and Community Development, University of the Witwatersrand,
Johannesburg, South Africa

1.1. Introduction

Preventive health care, where preventive audiology is located, consists of measures taken for disease and disability prevention. The American Speech-Language-Hearing Association (ASHA) (1988) documented the prevention of communication disorders as one of the professions' primary responsibilities, with the acknowledgement that 'prevention of communication disorders requires some adjustment in the traditional focus of professional practice in speech-language pathology and audiology'. This association advances the argument that for the prevention of communication disorders to occur, increased efforts are required towards the elimination of the onset and causes of these disorders, as well as the promotion, development and maintenance of optimal communication.

How to cite: Khoza-Shangase, K 2022, 'Preventive audiology: Ramping up efforts towards an ear and hearing healthy nation', ed. K Khoza-Shangase, *Preventive audiology: An African perspective*, AOSIS Books, Cape Town, pp. 1–20. https://doi.org/10.4102/aosis.2022.BK209.01

Hearing function can be influenced by various factors, including lifestyle choices, environmental factors, genetic predisposition, burden of disease, and other causes (Nieman, Reed & Lin 2018). Most often, hearing impairment can be prevented and its consequences minimised through preventive measures. Such prevention requires carefully deliberated anticipatory actions that can be categorised as primordial, primary, secondary or tertiary prevention. Numerous strategies exist for the prevention of hearing impairment across all ages and in various contexts. This chapter reflects on the concept of preventive audiology within the African context, aligned with the South African re-engineered primary health care strategy where the book is based. Deliberations are also congruent with the World Health Organization's (WHO's) (2021) *Hearing Screening Considerations for Implementation.*

This chapter aims to deliberate on evidence-based perspectives grounded in an African context on preventive audiology, with a specific focus on four major ear and hearing burdens of disease within the South African context: (1) early hearing detection and intervention (EHDI), (2) middle ear pathologies, (3) ototoxicity, and (4) noise-induced hearing loss (NIHL). This is done with a clear understanding that there are other areas in audiology that also require inclusion in a preventive audiology book; however, because of the length limits of a book, they can only be addressed in a future edition. This chapter prepares the reader for the book's ultimate goal, which is to motivate for a paradigm shift in how ear-and-hearing health care is approached within this LMIC context while arguing for Afrocentric *best practice* evidence that leads to *next practice*. Sufficient evidence exists regarding the economics and quality of life investment benefits of preventive care, hence the focus of this chapter and this edited book.

Projections calculated based on the WHO's 2018 prevalence estimates indicate that in 2018, the prevalence of disabling hearing loss globally was high and set to increase (WHO 2018a), and these projections show that the numbers will increase in all regions of the world. Currently, just over 6% of the world's population lives with disabling hearing loss. This translates to 466 million persons globally, of which 432 million (93%) are adults and 34 million (7%) are children. By 2050, the WHO estimates that the numbers will grow to over 900 million people with disabling hearing loss (WHO 2018a).

The distribution of disabling hearing loss across different regions of the world shows that the LMICs are home to the highest number of cases of disabling hearing loss, with high-income countries (HICs) hosting only 9.9% of people with disabling hearing loss. Sub-Saharan Africa, where South Africa is located, is home to 10.6% (49.66 million) of the global population of individuals with disabling hearing loss, with only East Asia (21.6%) and South Asia (28.2%) above it on the ranking (WHO 2018a). This high prevalence of hearing loss has various causes.

Causes of hearing loss vary and include the use of particular drugs that are toxic to the ear, exposure to excessive noise, certain infectious diseases, chronic ear infections, complications at birth, ageing, and genetic causes (Nieman et al. 2018). Most of these causes are preventable, which justifies increasing the focus on preventive audiology, particularly in LMIC contexts where the prevalence of disabling hearing loss is reported to be high. WHO (2018a), for instance, reported that 60% of hearing loss in childhood is because of causes that are preventable in nature and that 1.1 billion young individuals between 12 and 35 years of age are at risk of NIHL because of hazardous noise exposure in recreational settings, a cause that is highly preventable (Martin et al. 2006).

Unidentified and unaddressed hearing loss has serious consequences for the individuals affected, their families, and the State, from the cradle to the grave (Khoza-Shangase 2021). Overall, the cascading deleterious consequences of unidentified and unaddressed hearing impairment on a developing child include a significant negative impact on the language abilities and skills, which may result in language delays of at least 2–4 years (Yoshinaga-Itano 2004). These consequences include social and economic ramifications in areas such as education, employment and integration into society (including family and parent–child interactions), all of which impact the individual's quality of life (Maluleke, Khoza-Shangase & Kanji 2019; Moeller 2000; Olusanya 2005; Olusanya & Newton 2007; Rossetti 2004; Yoshinaga-Itano 2004).

As far as preventive causes of hearing loss such as middle ear infections are concerned, unidentified and unaddressed middle ear pathologies have significant implications for any country's health care, over and above consequences for the affected individual (Sebothoma & Khoza-Shangase 2020). The WHO (2018b) estimated that over 700 million people suffer from middle ear pathologies globally, with over half of this challenge in children. Poor or lacking early identification and ineffective treatment of these middle ear pathologies can lead to serious complications. These complications include the following:

1. Acute otitis media developing into chronic suppurative otitis media (CSOM) (30 million cases), with approximately half of these infections leading to the development of permanent hearing loss (WHO 2018b). Kolo et al. (2012) also reported on an association between CSOM and sensori/neural hearing loss, as CSOM is a severe form of middle ear pathology that can cause permanent hearing loss.
2. The occurrence of middle ear pathologies has also been associated with auditory processing problems (Villa & Zachetta 2014).
3. Prolonged middle ear pathologies can lead to intracranial complications (Sharma et al. 2015) and, to some extent, present as a life-threatening condition (Avnstorp et al. 2016).

These complications, as well as the medical and surgical costs related to them, justify a paradigm shift to a preventive approach within contexts where the prevalence of middle ear pathologies is high. This argument is detailed in Chapter 5 wherein a recommendation of a programmatic approach that is deemed contextually relevant, responsive and sustainable within the South African context is put forward.

Similarly, unidentified and unaddressed hearing loss because of ototoxicity, regardless of the often life-sustaining benefits of the treatments causing it, can have significant negative effects on patients (Guo et al. 2010; Paken et al. 2016; Tsintis & La Mache 2004). While ototoxicity is contended to be non-life-threatening in nature, evidence indicates that the detrimental effects of some drugs on the ear and hearing because of their toxic effects on the ear impact communication and quality of life indicators. These indicators are related to health as they lead to significant educational, occupational and social consequences for the affected individual (Govender & Paken 2015; Khoza-Shangase 2010, 2017). The negative ototoxicity effects also have medical treatment adherence consequences for the patient on treatment (Khoza-Shangase 2020), with equally significant cost implications for the State. In children, ototoxicity, like other forms of hearing loss in this age group, can affect cognitive, speech, language and social development, with consequent negative outcomes for academic performance and psychosocial functioning (Health Professions Council of South Africa [HPCSA] 2018). It is for this reason that Bankaitis and Schountz (1998), as well as Khoza-Shangase and Stirk (2016), argued that it is important for audiologists to become actively involved in the drug development process to facilitate early identification of adverse effects such as ototoxicity and vestibular toxicity. Chapter 6 delves into ototoxicity in more detail with specific recommendations for the African context.

Finally, the absence of effective hearing conservation programs (HCPs) that reduce or eliminate NIHL has significant implications for the individuals affected, their families and communities, the companies they work for, and the State as a whole. Besides the NIHL (Ding, Yan & Liu 2019; Moroe et al. 2018; Ntlhakana, Khoza-Shangase & Nelson 2020a), chronic exposure to noise is also linked to various other negative effects on the affected individual, such as impaired cognitive performance, sleep disturbance and onset of conditions such cardiovascular diseases and hypertension (Dale et al. 2015), over and above annoyance (Lusk et al. 2016). Lusk et al. (2016), in support of Yongbing and Martin (2013), stressed that hazardous noise exposure must be treated as a priority and costly public health concern, particularly in LMICs, further arguing that noise is a public health hazard with a considerable effect on the nation's well-being and economic health. For the company and the State, the legal costs and the compensation costs linked to ONIHL are significant

(Thorne et al. 2008). Sufficient global evidence exists to indicate that NIHL is 100% predictable and preventable if effective HCPs are implemented and if all stakeholders are collaborative in their prevention processes, as well as being fully committed to the process of implementing effective preventive measures timeously (Le et al. 2017; Metidieri et al. 2013; Moroe 2020; Moroe et al. 2018; Ntlhakana, Nelson & Khoza-Shangase 2020b). Chapters 11 and 12 carefully and comprehensively deliberate on NIHL globally, with specific recommendations for LMIC contexts such as South Africa.

The presented negative effects of hearing loss make it justifiable that considerable attention should be directed towards ramping up efforts aimed at prevention, in the form of early identification and intervention, in all contexts, but more so in resource-constrained contexts like Africa. This is because unaddressed hearing loss has been reported to pose an annual global cost of US$750 billion (WHO 2018a). The WHO (2018a, 2021), therefore, strongly argued that interventions to prevent, identify and address hearing loss early are worthwhile and can bring significant financial benefits. The fact that implementing preventive health care for young children is known to offer the greatest likelihood of bettering health and changing a child's course of life (Alexander, Brijnath & Mazza 2015). The fact that the prevalence of disabling hearing loss increases with age to affect the economically active more also adds to the urgency of dealing with this burden of hearing loss. Generally, the prevalence of disabling hearing loss has been reported to be 1.7% in children, equal to or greater than 7.6% in adults aged 15 years and older, precipitously rising to almost one in three in adults over the age of 65 years (WHO 2018a). This prevalence rate warrants careful deliberations around paradigm shifting audiology efforts toward preventive audiology.

■ 1.2. Preventive audiology argued

Preventive audiology consists of measures taken for the prevention of hearing loss and its negative consequences. The numerous documented factors that affect hearing function mostly affect LMICs because of the absence of regular health care monitoring systems or competent management (Zaman & Al Mamun 2017). Most often, hearing impairment can be prevented or its consequences minimised by preventive measures, which require carefully deliberated anticipatory actions. South Africa, as a resource-constrained LMIC, still has a challenge of high numbers of individuals with preventable hearing impairment across their lifespans and needs to identify a portfolio of risk factors for preventive audiology to achieve positive ear and hearing outcomes for the nation, without preventive efforts becoming costly for the State. It is, therefore, important to carefully plan all preventive initiatives so that they can achieve the goals for which they are intended.

Sá et al. (2016, p. 1) argued that technological advancements, the rising number of available preventive health care measures and the 'cultural belief that more is always better and some disease-mongering strategies' have all had negative effects on preventive care. Thus, the probability of preventive care producing more harm than good is rousing great concern (Gérvas, Starfield & Heath 2008; Martins et al. 2013; Moynihan, Doust & Henry 2012; Sackett 2002). The same might apply within the African context, so preventive health care initiatives need to be adopted cautiously, with careful planning that bears in mind the South African context. Supported by Getz, Sigurdsson and Hetlevik (2003), Martins et al. (2013) and Moynihan et al. (2012), Sá et al. (2016) asserted that excessive and unnecessary implementation of preventive measures, e.g., recommendation of medical tests, holds significant economic and ethical implications in contemporary clinical practice, hence the importance of identifying a portfolio of major risk factors for hearing loss within the South African context and targeting these in preventive audiology initiatives. Woolf and Stange (2006) argued that because limited resources make it impracticable to provide all health care services to everyone, it is important for countries to implement judicious methods for establishing priorities. This position is why adopting an approach that allows for targeting of major risk factors and ordering the relative magnitude of effective preventive services bears critical implications for all stakeholders, including the patients, clinicians, policymakers and the general public. Resource constraints in LMICs require these stakeholders to collaborate as a community to maximally benefit from the limited resources they have for the public good, in this case, of preventing hearing impairment.

Numerous strategies exist for the prevention of diseases and disorders, including hearing impairment, across all ages and in various contexts. The WHO (2020) provided an operational definition of disease prevention and health promotion that is useful when planning preventive audiology initiatives in any context. This organisation defines prevention as 'population-based and individual-based interventions for primary and secondary (early detection) prevention, aiming to minimise the burden of diseases and associated risk factors', the very goal of preventive audiology as presented in this book. Although not a major focus of this book and not-withstanding the understanding of the natural history of hearing impairment from exposure to causal agents through its development to final consequences (Association of Faculties of Medicine of Canada - AFMC 2013), prevention begins as early as what is described as primordial prevention (AFMC 2013). It further continues up to quaternary prevention where efforts are aimed at preventing injury or damage caused by preventive measures, such as the utilisation of medical interventions whose efficacy has not been established, while ensuring ethical practice (Pandve 2014).

Primordial prevention has been described as initiatives aimed at changing and addressing health determinants of a population and averting the development of factors (behavioural, social, environmental and economic) documented to escalate the future risk of diseases and disorders (AFMC 2013). Unlike in primary prevention, this level of prevention addresses the health determinants at the systemic level rather than at the personal level. Examples of preventive strategies at primordial prevention include preventive clinical services such as vaccination or post-exposure prophylaxis provision for individuals exposed to communicable diseases and general immunisation of individuals in all age groups (WHO 2020). In preventive audiology, primordial prevention would include preventive initiatives such as:

- advocating prenatal care for conditions known as risk factors for permanent childhood sensorineural hearing loss such as maternal rubella and toxoplasmosis (Fitzgibbons, Beswick & Driscoll 2021; Kanji & Khoza-Shangase 2021)
- childhood immunisation against infections that are risk factors for hearing impairment
- 'buying quiet' in mines and other places known to present high risk for NIHL (Khoza-Shangase, Lecheko & Ntlhakana 2020)
- removing or replacing all ototoxic medications from treatment regimens where feasible, including advocacy for the audiologists getting involved in the drug development processes before ototoxic drugs get approved for human consumption (Khoza-Shangase 2017).

The author believes that LMICs should have this level of prevention as a significant focus and cornerstone of their preventive models, where future possible disorders and disabilities are prioritised before the disorders present themselves, as depicted in Figure 1.1. Furthermore, the author proposes that addressing the burden of disease prevention by improving 'social determinants of health' is another major primordial prevention strategy that LMICs should prioritise for disease and disability prevention. Khoza-Shangase (2021) argued that health challenges and the social determinants of health in the South African context perform an important role in the success or failure of any early intervention programme, where the definition of social determinants of health has been stated as 'the circumstances in which people are born, grow up, live, work and age, and the systems put in place to deal with illness are enhanced' (Commission on the Social Determinants of Health [CSDH] 2008, p. 2). Addressing social determinants of health at this primordial prevention level can then be followed by primary, secondary and tertiary prevention programmes.

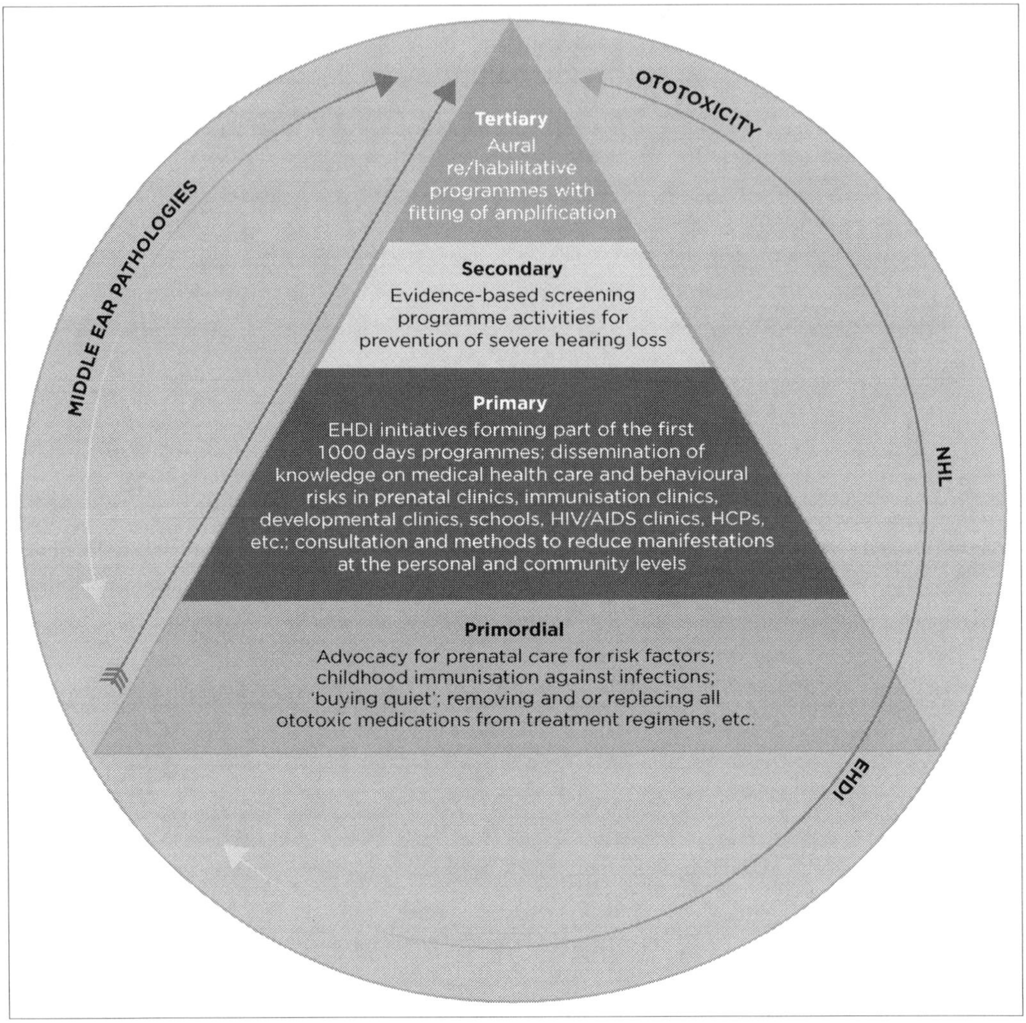

Source: Illustrated by M.R. Shangase, published with permission from M.R. Shangase.
Key: EHDI, early hearing detection and intervention; NIHL, noise-induced hearing loss; HCP, hearing conservation programmes.
FIGURE 1.1: Preventive audiology levels with examples in target areas of South Africa.

Through risk reduction, primary prevention aims to prevent the onset of a specific disease or disorder. This prevention is achieved by altering actions or disease-causing exposures or by growing resistance to the consequences of exposure to the disease agent (AFMC 2013). WHO (2020) stated that primary prevention refers to activities intended to circumvent the appearance of a disease or disorder. In preventive audiology, such activities may include actions to enhance ear-and-hearing health care through transforming the influence of social and economic determinants of health as done in EHDI initiatives that are part of the first 1000 days programmes where nutrition is part of the intervention; the dissemination of knowledge on medical health and behavioural risks in prenatal clinics, immunisation clinics, developmental clinics, schools, HIV/AIDS clinics and HCPs; and in conjunction with consultation and methods to reduce manifestations at the personal and community levels.

Secondary prevention is the level of early detection of the disease or disorder when this prevention advances the likelihood of positive health outcomes (WHO 2020). Procedures to detect and arrest the progression of a disorder before it presents clinically and progresses to levels that lead to deleterious consequences for the sufferer are employed at this level (AFMC 2013). In audiology, this level of prevention (a significant focus of this book) comprises initiatives such as evidence-based screening programmes for the early detection of hearing impairment and ear disease:

- newborn hearing screening [NHS]
- school hearing screening
- community hearing screening
- ototoxicity monitoring
- ONIHL screening and monitoring.

Furthermore, this level can include activities for the prevention of severe hearing loss (e.g. middle ear pathology identification and management), preventive drug therapies, and other efficacious interventions when administered or implemented at an early stage of the disease or disorder (e.g. use of otoprotective agents in ototoxicity and use of personal protection devices in ONIHL). Because secondary prevention refers to the use of measures that may lead to earlier diagnosis and treatment of health conditions, advocacy for mandating such measures (e.g. government mandating of universal NHS) is critical for both initial implementation and sustainability of the programmes. Furthermore, ensuring that sensitive, valid and reliable assessment/screening measures are used in programmes, such as NHS (Kanji & Khoza-Shangase 2018) and HCPs (Moroe et al. 2020; Ntlhakana et al. 2020a, 2020b, 2022); ototoxicity monitoring programmes; use of sensitive measures such as distortion product otoacoustic emissions (DPOAEs); middle ear pathology measures such as video otoscopy and Wideband Absorbance Immittance (Sebothoma & Khoza-Shangase 2018; Sebothoma et al. 2021), is important.

The AFMC (2013) stated that once the disease or disorder has presented itself and treatment provided at the acute phase, tertiary prevention seeks to lessen the impact or the negative consequences of the disease or disorder on the affected individual's function, long life and quality of life. Therefore, tertiary prevention is defined as strategies adopted to reduce or minimise the complications linked with disability from health outcomes (Stucki et al. 2007). In preventive audiology, this includes aural rehabilitative programmes with the fitting of amplification, which, in this book, have been argued to be best presented within a contextually relevant and responsive model of care.

For example, EHDI that is caregiver or family-centred, middle ear pathology prevention programmes that adopt a programmatic approach, HCPs that are collaborative and have the audiologist at the centre of the team, and ototoxicity monitoring programmes that are collaborative, multidisciplinary and standardised. Khoza-Shangase and Kanji (2021) argued that, within the African context, such interventions must be culturally and linguistically sensitive and relevant to the context.

Implementation of preventive health care at the different levels requires strategic planning around resources, including human resources. WHO (2020) highlighted that whereas primary prevention initiatives may be implemented autonomously from capacity building in other health care services, secondary prevention in the form of screening and early detection does require significant training of paraprofessionals if demand versus capacity is a contextual challenge. This position arises because secondary prevention becomes of limited value if the identified disease and disorder cannot receive intervention from other parts of the health care system, which can also be considered unethical (Delatycki 2012; Shickle & Chadwick 1994). Wilson and Jungner (1968) argued that the ability to offer treatment for an identified disease or disorder during prevention initiatives is the most important criterion that primary prevention measures should fulfil. These authors asserted that 'in adhering to the principle of avoiding harm to the patient at all costs (the *primum non nocere* of Hippocrates), treatment must be the first aim' (Wilson & Jungner 1968, p. 27). Therefore, within prevention audiology, volunteers, nurses, audiometricians, teachers' assistants and other middle-level worker cadres can be trained to conduct hearing screening, middle ear pathology screening and ototoxicity monitoring in primary prevention via a task-shifting combined with tele-audiology ear-and-hearing health care delivery model. However, for individuals whose screening result indicates *refer* findings, diagnostic testing and evaluation from audiologists and otorhinolaryngologists must be in place at the secondary prevention level. Chapters 2, 3, 4 and 5 will elaborate on this comprehensively.

Within the South African context, task-shifting and tele-audiology can also form part of health promotion, which WHO (2020) defined as 'the process of empowering people to increase control over their health and its determinants through health literacy efforts and multi-sectoral action to increase healthy behaviours'. This health promotion process is specific to ear-and-hearing health care, which encompasses community-level initiatives or activities for populations at increased risk of hearing impairment because of the identified portfolio of risks. Such activities would include activities such as various media awareness campaigns on calendar days such as Deaf Awareness Month and World Hearing Day, along with others. In these ear-and-hearing health care promotion initiatives, behavioural risk factors such as excessive noise exposure and unsafe ear care, as well as all known risks of hearing impairment, are addressed, with the importance and value of early detection and intervention across the lifespan highlighted.

WHO (2020) highlighted the importance of distinguishing between prevention and promotion, even though these share many goals. Prevention services are characterised as predominantly focused within the health care sector, while promotion services rely on intersectoral initiatives and or are focused on the social determinants of health. This distinction is also applicable to preventive audiology within the South African context. Intersectoral policies and health services interventions to address ear-and-hearing health care; and strategies to promote ear-and-hearing health care, including through education and awareness programmes and increased access to ear-and-hearing health care and communication rehabilitation services are critical aspects of this process. Chapter 4 illustrates this well within the South African context.

This edited book deliberately reviews locally relevant evidence to ground the perspectives presented in an African context to explore preventive audiology within Africa in selected high burdens of ear and hearing disorders within the South African context. The approach adopted allows for an argument of a paradigm shift in how ear-and-hearing health care is approached within this LMIC context.

Chapter 2 strongly argues for increased attention to the implementation of alternative and complimentary service delivery models such as tele-audiology and task-shifting within the African context to resolve challenges regarding demand versus capacity, as far as audiology personnel and the South African population with risk factors for and with hearing impairment are concerned. This chapter's motivation for a paradigm shift in how ear-and-hearing health care is provided within the African context is also supported by the proliferation of emerging technologies to deliver clinical services. The authors argue that taking advantage of these telehealth-supporting technologies will be useful in (1) assisting in providing specialised expertise not otherwise available; (2) enhancing clinicians' productivity; and (3) improving access to quality services in a cost-effective manner – while utilising paraprofessionals during task-shifting. Having considered other contextual challenges within the African context, this chapter offers clear guidelines for increasing access to preventive audiology services while adhering to HPCSA regulated minimum standards and ethical standards.

This chapter explores tele-audiology as one of the strategies that the authors believe is imperative towards upscaling preventive audiology within the African resource-constrained context, with an understanding that other models exist and are possible. The authors of this chapter offer a proposal of how this model of service delivery would work with the use of three big areas of functioning in audiology within the South African context: EHDI, ONIHL and ototoxicity monitoring and management. The authors suggest that this service delivery model must take careful cognisance of policy and regulations challenges with strict adherence to ethics, human rights and medical law. In addition, contextually relevant research must be conducted for any new assessment or intervention strategy to ensure a context-relevant evidence base.

Chapter 3 narrows the focus of tele-audiology to the education sector with the author recommending a PRIME sustainability model for tele-audiology within the South African education sector, following a comprehensive review of identified challenges and barriers to the use of this health care service delivery model. The barriers and challenges include (1) adoption and sustainability challenges, (2) comprehensive service delivery difficulties, (3) guidelines and policy formulation challenges and (4) education and training of health care professionals and ongoing quality improvement. These barriers pose a threat to the adoptability and sustainability of tele-audiology services within the education sector, and careful consideration of these barriers is important for the maximum benefit to be obtained. The PRIME sustainability model presented in this chapter argues to facilitate the growth and maturity of tele-audiology within the African school context and consists of processes including the (1) development, revision and ongoing reviewing of protocols and guidelines; (2) maintaining and evaluation of test reliability and validity, (3) integration and coordination of resources; (4) accessing platforms and funding by key role players so that there is a collaborative response to tele-audiology services within this context; and (5) management and evaluation of programmes and services for quality assurance.

Chapter 4 further deliberates on the health care service delivery models for preventive audiology by delving into more detail on preventive audiology in rural communities in South Africa. Guided by the WHO's (2020) estimates of disabling hearing loss, this chapter advances an argument for action to prevent hearing loss, especially in the rural areas of LMICs such as South Africa. The chapter carefully outlines strategies for hearing loss prevention and deliberates on challenges rural communities face in accessing ear-and-hearing health care services. It contextualises the current status of hearing health services in rural South Africa and proposes an audiology service delivery model that will improve access to affordable, cost-effective, quality hearing health care services in these rural areas. Based on identified health care challenges within rural South Africa, specifically concerning the availability, accessibility and affordability of services, this chapter offers solutions and recommendations for implementing a community-based service model for preventive audiology. The author of this chapter concludes that the community-based service model that is suggested can only be achieved by offering services that (1) are person-centred in their approach, (2) are responsive to patients' needs, (3) are adaptable to changing hearing health care needs, (4) are accountable, and (5) are collaborative.

The aforementioned principles around efficient service delivery models permeate the rest of this book's chapters. Chapter 5 takes the challenge of prevention of middle ear pathologies further, as these pathologies are persistently high in African countries because of multiple risk factors that are predominant in these regions (DeAntonio et al. 2016; Sebothoma & Khoza-Shangase 2018; Tshifularo et al. 2013; Vajpayee, Negi & Kurapati 2013). While middle ear pathologies can be cured if identified early, the prolongation of these pathologies within the middle ear cavity can increase their severity, cause permanent hearing loss, and penetrate and damage other adjacent auditory organs (Minovi & Dazert 2014). Consequently, costly specialised services that are predominantly offered by otorhinolaryngologists may be required to deal with the sequelae. However, the extreme shortage of otorhinolaryngologists and the high levels of poverty in South Africa may restrict access to these services. Therefore, preventive measures become crucial. Although the chapter focuses specifically on the prevention of middle ear pathologies, which have been reported to be increasing in prevalence in LMICs, the recommendation of a programmatic approach to the delivery of preventive initiatives can be applied more widely in preventive audiology.

The authors of this chapter argue that one of the key reasons why traditional models of service delivery do not yield positive preventive outcomes within the South African context is that these models of service delivery function in 'silos' within limited resources contexts, outside of contextually conceived health care programmes that are burden-of-disease and priority-list driven. This chapter, therefore, suggests the alignment of preventive audiology initiatives to the SADoH's programmatic health care approach, which is located within the re-engineered primary health care model. This chapter correctly argues that this programmatic approach may provide an alternative way to prevent middle ear pathologies (and general ear and hearing impairments) by enabling a wider coverage of cases which would not ordinarily be seen under traditional approaches, including those at a greater risk of developing these pathologies and impairments. This chapter also recommends that existing programmes should incorporate current technologies (such as asynchronous tele-audiology) and sensitive measures to increase access and coverage within an ear-and-hearing health care model that includes task-shifting and telepractice as a human resource strategy.

The chapter concludes by suggesting that a programmatic approach to preventive audiology aligns well with the goal of universal health coverage, as it forces health professionals and policymakers to begin deliberating on new approaches to health care delivery and ways of increasing coverage, improving access and achieving early identification, thereby allowing for early intervention. Within already existing programmes in South Africa, the authors propose that audiologists and otorhinolaryngologists do not need to conceive additional programmes but can be incorporated and collaborate within the existing ones. Authors of this chapter caution that while a programmatic approach may be beneficial, careful planning, implementation and monitoring are required to ensure that existing programmes are not strained and that health care providers such as paraprofessionals are not overwhelmed with the expansion of their current scope of function. These are important considerations, particularly in contexts, such as rural communities, where the limited numbers of health care professionals must function far beyond their scopes of practice because of capacity versus demand challenges.

The principle of programmatic approach to preventive audiology continues to be illustrated in Chapter 6. This chapter addresses another burden of ear and hearing disease within the South African context, ototoxicity and the perceived role and value of preventive audiology. Because of the reality of the high prevalence of conditions such as tuberculosis, cancer, HIV and AIDS in the South African context (Khoza-Shangase & Masondo 2020), ototoxicity is one condition requiring careful preventive measures as it is preventable, and or its degree and effects are significantly minimisable if early detection and intervention protocols are followed. This chapter deliberates on contextually relevant evidence based on ototoxicity, with a careful look at the implementation of and adherence to guidelines as per the HPCSA's (2018) national guidelines on the assessment and management of patients receiving ototoxic medications. The chapter calls for standardisation and systematisation of ototoxicity monitoring protocols for clinical sites where ototoxic medications are prescribed and advocates for a clear and centrally located role of audiologists as part of the treatment team to eliminate and or minimise ototoxicity within the South African context. The author provides evidence that supports a pharmaco-audiology vigilance strategy within the South African context that will facilitate accurate, cost-effective, well-organised and dependable comparisons of data within and between patients, treatments and treatment sites. This chapter argues for pharmaco-vigilance as one of the key preventive audiology strategies requiring careful consideration within resource-constrained contexts. Risk-benefit deliberations are presented, with recommended solutions, including the role of task-shifting and tele-audiology in the implementation of preventive measures including ototoxicity monitoring. The chapter concludes that considerations of contextual realities when it comes to pharmacological treatments and their potential role in causing hearing loss will ensure contextual relevance and responsiveness of protocols and programmes adopted.

This principle of programmatic approaches to preventive audiology is seen again in Chapter 7 where EHDI is conceptualised as a cost-effective and risk-reducing programme, which can be firmly located within preventive health care. This chapter comprehensively illustrates how three levels of prevention (primary, secondary and tertiary) are vital for EHDI, particularly as each level addresses an aspect within the continuum of care for all newborns and infants. The author argues that secondary prevention and tertiary prevention entail more involvement from the audiologist and demonstrates how. Because of human resources in health care being a significant and documented challenge within the South African context, the chapter calls for creative solutions to address this challenge and ensure widespread implementation of NHS programmes – the initial, first step to any EHDI programme. The author of this chapter believes that the South African government's plans regarding re-engineering primary health care and universal health coverage may form a good platform for integrating preventive audiology but, more specifically, secondary prevention. Solutions that have been echoed in other chapters with regard to the resource-constrained context of South Africa are offered, including task-shifting, tele-audiology application and considerations for mHealth technology as a means of data management and tracking. An effective data management system that is not naïve to the reality that South Africa has a migration-influenced health care system is critical for preventive audiology initiatives to succeed, because continuity of care is an important aspect as well (Khoza-Shangase 2021). The continuity of care as far as EHDI is concerned raises the importance of holistic patient care in this population, which involves family-centred/caregiver-centred interventions.

This philosophy of family-centred EHDI is deliberated in detail in Chapter 8. In this chapter, the author asserts that, within the South African context, the benefits of early detection of hearing impairment ensued by an effective and timely intervention programme for hearing-impaired children are only possible if caregivers are viewed and treated as key co-drivers of EHDI programmes. The argument presented in the chapter is that such early intervention programmes need to involve all relevant disciplines, be in alignment with current ICT advancements and, most importantly, be in tune with the specific context (family, community, country) in which the child functions, hence the strong argument for a caregiver-centred approach. This argument is presented following the exploration of published evidence on the role of caregivers within families in EHDI programmes while arguing for caregiver-centred (family-centred early intervention [FCEI]) approaches to all EHDI processes within the South African context. The author concludes that being caregiver-centred, therefore FCEI, is key to positive outcomes for children with hearing impairment and that this is particularly true for South Africa, with contextual challenges of an LMIC that is culturally, linguistically and socio-politically diverse. The author strongly argues that FCEI should drive all clinical care initiatives, as the principles in which FCEI is based on embracing the Afrocentric ethos of *ubuntu* as asserted by Khoza-Shangase (2019, p. 77).

Caregivers' involvement in the entire EHDI process throughout their child's development journey is influenced by several factors, and this chapter discusses these factors for practitioners to be well prepared for them when planning, implementing and monitoring EHDI services that involve caregivers. The author acknowledges that while there is generally not one factor that caregivers isolate as the cause of their lack of and or suboptimal involvement in the EHDI process, but instead an interaction of factors over time, one predominant theme is evident from the evidence reviewed in this chapter. At the core of EHDI success is caregiver involvement and routine adoption of family-community-centred approaches by clinicians. The evidence reviewed in this chapter also raises implications for research, teaching and clinical service provision that puts caregivers at the centre of all EHDI initiatives, including all preventive efforts from prenatal care to intervention where negative sequelae of hearing impairment are minimised or eliminated.

Because hearing impairment in children is complex and can occur in the presence of other conditions (Ehn et al. 2019), minimisation of the impact of hearing impairment needs to happen in all these populations as well. Chapter 9 explores challenges with early intervention in the deaf-blind child – an umbrella term denoting any degree of combined vision and hearing impairment. Within this rather neglected area in audiology because of the argued small incidence of children in this population, the chapter argues for increased focus on this neglected sub-population in preventive audiology, through health promotion and prevention or minimisation of the impact of disability-related sequelae on the deaf-blind child. The authors deliberate on the different prevention interventions (primary, secondary and tertiary) for deaf-blind children while providing recommendations on enhancing their quality of life. While acknowledging that deafblindness as a disability cannot be completely eradicated, the authors believe that its incidence can be significantly reduced, thus alleviating the burden of disease in countries already facing challenges in terms of accessing health care services and hence their recommendation for the audiology community to advocate for more primary and secondary prevention methods in the management of deaf-blind children. They argue that preventive audiology initiatives, particularly EHDI, have a significant role to play in potentially preventing deafblindness and minimising its deleterious consequences. They assert that in primary prevention, preventive audiology can contribute through campaign drives highlighting the risk factors associated with deafblindness in developing children and that in secondary prevention, early detection and intervention of deaf-blind children can occur as part of EHDI programmes. Finally, in tertiary prevention, the authors suggest that preventive audiology interventions can focus on providing aural habilitative services, reasonable accommodation access to information and resources for the child and their families, within a collaborative programmatic approach to early intervention provision to prevent the negative sequelae on development and quality of life.

The negative sequelae of EHDI programmes include economic consequences, which can be detrimental to the programme if sufficient and comprehensive economic evaluations are not conducted. Chapter 10 weighs in on this negative outcome of EHDI in more detail. The chapter is premised on the reality that, even with the most outstanding preventive health care strategy, because of causes such as genetic factors, hearing impairment will always be present, albeit in smaller numbers. Based on the HPCSA's (2018) position that EHDI services must ensure optimum, cost-effective solutions, this chapter discusses the need for cost-effectiveness analysis of EHDI programmes for the purpose of developing robust evidence of the positive outcomes associated with these programmes in the South African context, with the aim of placing EHDI programmes on the political advocacy and resource allocation agenda of the South African government. The author discusses cost-effectiveness of EHDI programmes with due recognition of the South African resource-constrained health care system, sustainable development goals (SDGs) and universal health care coverage. This chapter also outlines cost-effectiveness frameworks and provides a discussion of studies conducted in the field of audiology using these frameworks, with a specific focus on the cost-effective analysis (CEA) framework. Recommendations are made on the use of CEA to give EHDI programmes the political and funding support they need within the South African context. The chapter concludes that, within the African context, for EHDI to garner support from policy and legislature as well as budget allocation, cost-effectiveness needs to be established, and therefore, audiologists need to increase their understanding and use of CEA in the field of audiology to advocate for change. The WHO (2014) maintained that measurable economic returns are gained by investing in health in general, not only by the health sector but also by other sectors, as well as the wider economy of the country, and this chapter demonstrates this well with EHDI as a case study within the South African context.

In Chapter 11, the author deliberates on noise as an occupational and environmental hazard. This chapter explores various ways of preventing NIHL at the different levels of prevention to achieve the key objective of HCPs, which is to eliminate the presence of noise as a risk factor, thereby preventing the development of NIHL in people exposed to hazardous noise. The author argues that the principles underpinning HCPs are aligned to health promotion and disease prevention interventions; hence, this chapter seeks to demonstrate how disease prevention interventions complement the HCP pillars and the hierarchy of noise control. The author bases the arguments presented in the chapter on the philosophy that 'prevention is better than cure' and that timely interventions can be less costly and more effective than providing services later in life (Borysiewicz 2009; Khoza-Shangase & Moroe 2020) and makes recommendations aimed at mitigating against factors that negatively contribute towards the success of effective health promotion and prevention of environmental and ONIHL, particularly in South Africa. These recommendations are geared towards specific stakeholders at national and at occupational levels. Nationally, after placing audiologists on the agenda of public health initiatives, one of the key recommendations put forward is raising awareness about the impact of noise on the quality of life and the well-being of the community at large, as well as increasing awareness about the need to include hearing acuity when other medical screenings are undertaken nationally. Occupationally, the author suggests that HCPs implemented in the workplace be responsive to the needs of the population exposed to excessive noise and that these are implemented accordingly.

Chapter 12 narrows the focus of the impact of noise to occupational exposure, with the author arguing for increased efforts towards the development of contextually relevant and responsive evidence in ONIHL and HCPs as part of preventive audiology initiatives within the African context. This chapter has gathered and compiled current evidence in identified areas in occupational audiology and contextualised this within the African context. The author describes and discusses findings while highlighting implications for the field of audiology, engineering and occupational audiology. This chapter is premised on the reality that the prevalence of occupational hearing loss (OHL) remains high in LMICs such as South Africa (Ntlhakana et al. 2020b). The author believes that this is a severe condemnation to occupational health as hearing loss is recognised to be a heavier burden in LMICs than in HICs, particularly in a country like South Africa with significant socio-economic inequality, where OHL can become a barrier to employment prospects and opportunities for the individual affected (Thorne 2006). The author emphasises that determining the status of OHL and its management in LMICs is vital if tactical planning around it is to be systematic and successful and recommends that LMICs learn from HICs, but for Africa, ensuring Afrocentric application of available evidence is key to successful implementation and monitoring of preventive audiology measures in ONIHL to achieve zero ear harm.

Ensuring zero ear harm, while learning from HICs, lastly, Chapter 13 continues on this NIHL vein but focusing more on data capturing and analysis methods utilised in HCPs and how these, if used properly, can lead to successful preventive audiology outcomes in ONIHL. The complex nature of ONIHL, with the additional complexity brought by the diverse nature of the occupational exposures specific to the South African mines, mostly different types of noises emitted by various mining equipment, at different exposure levels, calls for interventions that are based on comprehensive, valid and reliable data (Ntlhakana et al. 2020a, 2022). The authors argue that ways of managing miners at risk for ONIHL must be reimagined and predictive tools in preventing ONIHL need to be further explored within the South African context. The design of reliable models to predict ONIHL is discussed, and its reliance on the internal and external validation done by machine learning models deliberated on, all aimed at providing more reliable predictions of ONIHL in larger sample sizes. Application of machine learning models in predicting ONIHL is a new concept in the South African mining industry, and this chapter introduces rationale and opportunities for these models for the prevention and early identification of ONIHL. The authors conclude that because of the high prevalence rates of ONIHL recorded in South African mines, availability of the mines' HCP electronic data and availability of the miners' electronic medical audiometry records, there is a need to explore machine learning analysis methods as part of efforts towards preventing ONIHL in this context.

1.3. Conclusion

The role and value of preventive audiology cannot be underestimated, particularly in resource-constrained contexts such as LMICs. The availability of international evidence and guidelines does not automatically solve challenges related to ear and hearing problems in all contexts because of feasibility difficulties encountered and contextual challenges confronted in various contexts. The differences in influencing factors, risk registers (and portfolios of risks) across the lifespan, protocols adopted, availability of resources (including capacity versus demand ratios) and others call for contextualised solutions to the provision of ear and hearing services. Specifically, these differences call for assessment and intervention modifications that are responsive and relevant to the context, research that is local needs driven for local benefit and clinical focus that will facilitate the emergence of 'next practice' and not just adopts 'best practice' within this context. Within the South African context, establishing contextually relevant best/next practice requires adherence to principles reflected in the National Health Insurance (NHI) Plan, as well as assessment and intervention that takes careful cognisance of epidemiological data and linguistic and cultural diversity data that are evidence-based and context-driven. Heightened contextual awareness facilitates vigilance-driven services (e.g. pharmaco-vigilance, noise vigilance, burden of disease vigilance, risk factors vigilance and concomitant or synergistic factors vigilance) that ensure context responsiveness, context relevance and context responsibility in all preventive audiology initiatives. Where assessment and intervention strategies call for changes, such as task-shifting and training of paraprofessionals, national deliberations around minimum standards of training, regulations of practice and resource allocations around this model of care should occur.

This book is a research-driven introduction of preventive audiology as a paradigm of ear-and-hearing health care within the African context. It is aimed at providing current, contextually relevant and responsive evidence related to preventive audiology in LMICs, with a very specific focus on the African context using South Africa as a case study. The book, which is the first volume, comprehensively covers preventive audiology in four ear and hearing burdens of disease, with careful consideration of solutions and recommendations that are contextually relevant. The recommendations and solutions provided have considered the risks versus benefits of all the audiology clinical initiatives/interventions/programmes presented in accordance with contextual relevance, contextual responsiveness and contextual responsibility/accountability. The interventions/programmes explored are systematic and comprehensive, have a strategic plan behind them and involve ear and hearing practitioners in the conceptualisation, development and monitoring, with creative solutions for the implementation aspect to meet the South African demand versus capacity challenge. However, what is presented in this book may be applicable to other LMICs, similar to the South African context, where preventive audiology forms part of ramping up efforts towards ear-and-hearing-healthy nations.

Chapter 2

Tele-audiology and preventive audiology: A capacity versus demand challenge imperative in South Africa

Katijah Khoza-Shangase
Department of Audiology, Faculty of Humanities,
School of Human and Community Development, University of the Witwatersrand,
Johannesburg, South Africa

Ben Sebothoma
Department of Audiology, Faculty of Humanities,
School of Human and Community Development, University of the Witwatersrand,
Johannesburg, South Africa

2.1. Introduction

The well-documented challenges regarding capacity versus demand in audiology human resources and the South African population at risk of and with hearing impairment call for a paradigm shift in how ear-and-hearing health care is provided within this context. One key shift in thinking involves using different service delivery models and task-shifting in preventive

How to cite: Khoza-Shangase, K & Sebothoma, B 2022, 'Tele-audiology and preventive audiology: A capacity versus demand challenge imperative in South Africa', ed. K Khoza-Shangase, *Preventive audiology: An African perspective*, AOSIS Books, Cape Town, pp. 21–40. https://doi.org/10.4102/aosis.2022.BK209.02

audiology service provision. The practical use of existing and emerging technology to provide clinical services can assist in providing specialised expertise not otherwise available, enhance clinicians' productivity and expand access to quality services in a cost-effective way while utilising paraprofessionals in task-shifting. Successful, ethical and safe task-shifting of services within the audiologists' scope of practice requires effective and efficient management by practicing audiologists and is a model of service delivery that has not been widely utilised within the South African audiology community (Khoza-Shangase 2022).

In LMICs such as South Africa, the provision of preventive audiology at all levels (detailed in ch. 1) is confronted by numerous factors, with capacity versus demand challenges being one of the key difficulties. Tele-audiology is an opportunity requiring thoughtful consideration within preventive audiology in these contexts, with the advent of coronavirus disease 2019 (COVID-19) highlighting this opportunity even more. Its use within these contexts is at its infancy, with limited evidence in the field of preventive audiology. This chapter explores tele-audiology as one of the strategies, which the authors believe is imperative to upscaling preventive audiology within the African resource-constrained context. The chapter provides deliberations around preventive audiology in South Africa, with an exploration of challenges faced by audiologists within this context. This discussion is carried out to raise a need for consideration of telehealth and task-shifting as a strategy to bridge some of the identified barriers to service delivery of audiology care within this context. A definition of tele-audiology, a proposal of how it would work, an argument for its importance in preventive audiology within the South African context and a description of how it can be applied within this context are provided. Three key areas of functioning in audiology are given as case examples:

- EHDI
- ONIHL
- ototoxicity monitoring and management.

An inclusive approach has been adopted in this chapter, which includes asynchronous tele-audiology, remote patient monitoring and real-time tele-audiology. The chapter ends by identifying tele-audiology challenges with implementation and providing solutions within preventive audiology.

Globally, WHO (2018) estimated that greater than 6.1% of the global population lives with disabling hearing loss. This constitutes approximately 466 million persons, with 93% (432 million) being adults, one-third over the age of 65 years and 7% (34 million) children. The WHO estimates that the number of people with disabling hearing loss will increase over the years, with estimates of up to 630 million people by 2030 and over 900 million people by 2050. Closer to home, the prevalence of hearing impairment is reported to be higher in sub-Saharan Africa than in other regions of the world (Mulwafu,

Kuper & Ensink 2016; Wonkam Tingang et al. 2020). It is argued that these numbers will increase over the coming decades, with presbycusis and hearing loss related to the burden of diseases, such as tuberculosis (TB) and human immunodeficiency virus (HIV), most prevalent in this context (Christopher et al. 2013; Khoza-Shangase 2010, 2017; Tshifularo, Govender & Monama 2013) and influencing the numbers. Farmer et al. (2010) also predicted that 70% of cancers will be reported in LMICs by 2030, including cancers of the ear, nose and throat. The implications of cancer treatments on hearing function are also a concern in these contexts. All these factors indicate a strong need for the consideration of more innovative models of ear-and-hearing health care service provision in sub-Saharan Africa and other similar LMIC contexts.

The Speech, Language and Hearing (SLH) Professions Board of the HPCSA strongly advocates for best-practice-guided assessment and intervention services within service delivery models that are contextually, linguistically and culturally congruent with the South African context and population (Khoza-Shangase 2020). This best practice includes the use of telehealth and mobile practice in rendering clinical services. Despite this call and the demands raised by the COVID-19 pandemic, not much has been achieved to align the use of telehealth in audiology with service delivery models within the South African context. The literature on tele-audiology in South Africa has focused primarily on reaching many people who live in underserved areas (Dawood et al. 2020; Sandström et al. 2020; Van Wyk, Mahomed-Asmail & Swanepoel 2019). Given that South African audiological practice is still based on Euro-Western epistemology and ideology (Khoza-Shangase & Mophosho 2018, 2021), there is a need for careful consideration and deliberation around the delivery of audiological services through telehealth systems. The authors of this chapter believe that if these deliberations and considerations are not carefully conducted, telehealth may continue to perpetuate the colonial audiological service delivery that is not culturally appropriate nor adhere to the *Health Professions Act of 1974* as well as to the South African constitution.

Khoza-Shangase (2020) argued that SLH services must consider all the contextual attributes to respond appropriately and optimally to those who receive the services. This allows for innovation that leads to *next practice*, while observing health priorities and the burden of disease within the South African context. Consequently, this author asserts that SLH services that are naïve of context run the risk of being irrelevant and costly for the patient, the State and the SLH professions. Such services are bound to be less or non-efficacious. Within a resource-constrained context such as South Africa, such services are also bound to be inaccessible to the majority who need them.

Audiology, as one of the health care services, also falls under the WHO's call for universal health coverage (UHC), which can be termed universal audiology coverage (UAC). The WHO's Director-General, Dr Tedros Adhanom

Ghebreyesus, asserts that 'all roads lead to universal health coverage', while acknowledging that countries 'take different paths – using either public or private providers' (Ghebreyesus 2017). However, this Director-General also highlights that countries 'will need to know where they stand on universal health coverage, benchmarked against others'. Furthermore, he emphasises that UHC is not an end in itself but supports the realisation of the additional health-related UNESCO sustainable development goals (SDGs). The African audiology profession needs to respond to this call and ensure that UAC is also achieved.

In South Africa, UAC, similar to UHC, is nowhere near being achieved. The SADoH aims to achieve UHC in the near future by implementing the NHI to tackle the stark divide in health care between the rich and the poor (Keeton 2010; National Health Insurance Bill 2019). Currently, numerous challenges have been identified towards the achievement of UHC in South Africa, hence the passing of the NHI bill (2019). Health financing is one of the key challenges facing the South African government, which leads to cascading other barriers toward UHC (and consequently barriers to UAC). The capacity versus demand challenge emanates from these financing difficulties and rages on as one large obstruction to the delivery of health care services, particularly in the public health care sector, which provides for the underprivileged who constitute approximately 80% of the South African population.

Fagan and Jacobs (2009) reported in their survey conducted in sub-Saharan countries that there is an extreme shortage of hearing health professionals such as audiologists, speech-language pathologists and otorhinolaryngologists, and this remained the same in the later survey (Mulwafu et al. 2017). Mulwafu et al. (2017), in their review of the 2015 survey of otorhinolaryngology services in sub-Saharan Africa, found that otorhinolaryngology, audiology and speech therapy services and training opportunities in sub-Saharan Africa have remained stagnant over the years. Specifically, this study found that between 2009 and 2015, the number of otorhinolaryngologists had risen by 43%, audiologists by 2.5%, and speech therapists by 30%. When considering the size of the population, these findings indicated that the number of these professionals had decreased per 100,000 people in four countries. This is because the population surveyed also increased from 486 million to 600 million. For example, in 2015, there were 444 audiologists in a population of 55.4 million, which represented less than one audiologist per 100,000 people. In a South African study, Pillay et al. (2020) found that available hearing health professionals registered with the HPCSA are located mainly in three provinces, namely, Western Cape, Gauteng and KwaZulu-Natal. These professionals are reported to provide services primarily in private practices, making accessibility to the majority of the population challenging. It is even more concerning that in a population of approximately 80% black Africans (StatsSA 2019), only 15.2% of the SLH professionals are black Africans (Pillay et al. 2020). Implications of this are significant when considering the documented impact of language and culture in clinical health care service provision (Flood & Rohloff 2018). Mulwafu et al. (2017) argued that this clear capacity-to-demand challenge can be overcome through increased collaboration with private organisations and HICs, the development of new and improved current training programmes in Africa, and task-shifting some services to primary health workers. Task-shifting has been successfully implemented in mental health and other areas of health care practice and medicine (Bolton 2019; Magidson et al. 2017) but to a lesser degree in audiology, particularly in South Africa.

Section 27 of the *South African Bill of Rights* in the Constitution guarantees every citizen access to health services. The South African health care system comprises the public sector (managed by the government) and the private sector, which is privately financed and requires ownership of medical aid (medical insurance) to access primary health care services. The public health services have three main levels of care (primary, secondary and tertiary) that exist under and are administered by the nine provincial departments of health. South Africans can access health care services in either of these two sectors; however, financial standing determines the ability to access private health care. As a result of the socio-economic inequalities in South Africa, a majority of the population access health care in the public sector, where the primary health care (PHC) approach is the preferred government approach. Within the private health sector, individual health care practitioners who run private practices or surgeries independently or within private hospitals provide health care services. These private health care services are mainly found in urban areas, which implies a lack of access for the 64.7% of the population who are reported to reside in provinces that are largely rural in nature (Gordon et al. 2020; Mahlathi & Dlamini 2015). Naidoo (2012) reported that only 16% of the population access private health care, with 84% requiring public health care, and this inequality in access does not seem to change (Gordon et al. 2020; Mhlanga & Garidzirai 2020).

With the aforementioned health care distribution wherein over 80% of the South African population depend entirely on public health facilities, the fact that only 30% of specialists in the country work in the public sector and fewer than two out of 10 SLH practitioners working in public facilities (Khoza-Shangase 2019), clear capacity versus demand challenges are evident. Khoza-Shangase and Moroe (2020) argued that this capacity versus demand challenge becomes far pronounced in settings less viewed as conventional spaces of practice for audiologists in South Africa, such as in occupational audiology settings. Current statistics indicate negligible numbers of SLH professionals registered with the HPCSA by January of 2020, for the size of the South African population of over 55 million. Explicitly, only 1612 speech therapists and audiologists, 788 audiologists and 164 hearing-aid acousticians were registered for this whole population, for provision of ear-and-hearing health care services in both the public and private health care sectors. In provinces where mining is mainly found as an industry, including North West (7), Limpopo (23), Mpumalanga (47) and Northern Cape (11), an even lesser number of audiologists are found. These negligible numbers of SLH professionals clearly illustrate the capacity versus demand challenge in the country (Khoza-Shangase 2019), with obvious implications for the implementation and monitoring of preventive audiology initiatives such as HCPs, ototoxicity monitoring and management and EHDI, to name a few. Within the available health spending, this capacity versus demand challenge underlines the value of investigating tele-audiology for preventive audiology within this context.

Health spending in South Africa has been reported to be challenging during low economic growth and fiscal constraint, with health-focused expenditure transpiring in over 10 years of little national economic growth and increasing input costs (Blecher et al. 2017), and the recent grading of the economy to 'junk' status (Wallace 2020). Ratings agency Moody's Investors Service shifted South Africa's credit ranking to 'junk' status on 27 March 2020 because of the country's slowdown in economic growth and increasing debt burden (Wallace 2020). Wasserman (2020) argued that this poor economic status will deteriorate during the COVID-19 pandemic, as South Africa will lose billions in tax income during the lockdown while having to inject more money into a recessionary economy, money the country does not have. The South African government would need to pay extra in interest, which has negative implications for the allocation of money for services, such as health care, education and so on, and less infrastructure investments. This economic challenge has led and will continue to steer the health sector to respond in various ways, which raises serious implications for UHC as well as UAC and audiology service delivery within the South African context. The numbers of health care personnel and practitioners have been significantly reduced, with a number of posts getting frozen when vacated. There has been a focus on greater savings on medicine tenders, the establishment of ministerial 'non-negotiable' budget items, budget cuts on administration and expenditure as well as on buildings and medical equipment, budget cuts on capital projects and equipment purchases, with increased emphasis on PHC (Blecher et al. 2017; Nyasulu & Pandya 2020), and most recently prioritising COVID-19 management - arguably - at the expense of other burdens of disease (Wallace 2020). The staff crisis, particularly in the public sector, compromises the quality of care and leaves the existing staff overworked. Khoza-Shangase (2020) argued that all these challenges affect any health care initiative, particularly those initiatives seen not to be targeting 'life-threatening' conditions and are therefore less priority, such as SLH services, and most rehabilitation services, under which audiology falls.

Provision of preventive audiology services, therefore, becomes a significant challenge to implement within the South African context where it has to vie for attention with the life-threatening burdens of disease that are highly prevalent, such as HIV, AIDS and TB. Audiology services within this context, which are contextually relevant and responsive, can only succeed if innovative service delivery models within programmatic approaches to health care are adopted. For example, incorporation of audiology in the three major audiology areas that are the focus of this chapter (EHDI, ONIHL, and ototoxicity monitoring and management) may be facilitated in national health care programmes, such as MomConnect, First 1000 days, Striving for zero-harm, and TB/HIV Collaborative Programme, respectively. Task-shifting and the use of tele-audiology within such programmes would be one of the innovative ways of addressing access within this capacity versus demand-challenged context. Chapters 3, 4 and 5 delve into such programmatic approaches for preventive audiology within the South African context.

■ 2.2. Task-shifting and tele-audiology

Task-shifting is a process of delegation in a resource-constrained context, where tasks not requiring specialisation are moved, where appropriate, to less specialised personnel (WHO 2008). The WHO (2008) argued that by reorganising the workforce in this manner, this process offers a practicable answer for improving health care coverage by efficiently utilising the already available human resources and by rapidly expanding capacity while training and retention programmes are increased. Task-shifting was encouraged by the international consensus that recognised an urgent need for advancements in the functioning of health systems, including meaningful bolstering of human resources for health, to be able to achieve UHC. This is why this process is imperative for the South African audiology community where significant capacity versus demand challenges exist. Authors of this chapter believe that task-shifting, coupled with tele-audiology to maintain quality of care, is an innovative way of exploiting and converging both the already available financial and the human resources and resources that can be procured for the size of the population requiring preventive audiology services in the African context.

Task-shifting has been adopted in several countries for years to address capacity versus demand challenges because of the shortage of higher-skilled health care workers (Fulton et al. 2011; WHO 2017). As useful as it can be to increase access to services, particularly in LMICs, task-shifting has its weaknesses and challenges, specifically in the absence of regulations and monitoring. In Ghana, Baine, Kasangaki and Baine (2018), in a study on *Task-shifting in health service delivery from a decision- and policymakers' perspective*, found that since 1918 in that country, task-shifting had been applied with least compliance to the WHO (2008) recommendations and guidelines. They also found that the country had no national policies and guidelines on the implementation of this process and that a majority of policymakers and decision-makers in that country were not in support of task-shifting because of their perception that the less-skilled health workers were incompetent.

Within the field of SLH in South Africa, attempts at task-shifting failed significantly in the past with the negative experience of mid-level workers in the form of a former 2-year Speech and Hearing Therapy (Community Work) Diploma training that was offered by the University of the Witwatersrand in 1984, motivated for by the South African Speech Language and Hearing Association (SASLHA), with the goal of expediting the training of black people in the SLH field (Aron 1984, 1986, 1987, 1989). With the conceptualisation of this task-shifting initiative not being sound, the documented motivation being racially grounded, the scope of work ill-defined and non-regulated, uncertainties and poor control around the type of practice (independent versus supervised practice), as well as training challenges, were documented. Tshule (1994) investigated the experiences of the students and staff who were part of this diploma programme and found extreme dissatisfaction with the programme, not only from students but also from staff involved in training. Students found the diploma not to be challenging. It was not appropriate for the job they were supposed to perform, it did not allow them to be gainfully employed, and it did not offer them any career progression opportunities. That is beside the fact that it failed to meet the minimum expectations of students and its objectives were deemed inappropriate by the training staff.

To prevent a repeat of this negative experience for the SLH professions, the HPCSA has set up a scope of practice, a training curriculum and regulations for mid-level workers. Should the concept of task-shifting be embraced by the DoH, these cadres would need to be employed in that sector under supervised practice, which implies a need for strong political will around the DoH's human resource strategy that is more responsive to the contextual needs. As part of task-shifting initiatives, Pillay et al. (2020) strongly argued for mid-level worker role development as a key strategy to address the South African SLH workforce challenge in a cost-effective and pragmatic manner in order to increase access to SLH services currently and in the future.

Baine et al. (2018) recommended that task-shifting be used only:

1. in the presence of supervision and education systems that are sufficiently resourced, effective, supportive and ongoing
2. in the context where qualified health care workers continue to be trained and increased in the human resource strategy (where task-shifting is not used to replace qualified personnel)
3. where conditions of service are conducive for human resource motivation and retention
4. where all this is guided and supported by the country's national policy and frameworks to underpin implementation.

Lehmann et al. (2009) earlier shared similar sentiments about task-shifting as an answer to the human resources crisis in Africa. These authors argued that any long-term task-shifting success depends entirely on the sitting government's strong political will and fiscal commitments. These authors asserted that this process requires (1) an integrated and comprehensive reconfiguration of health teams, (2) adapted regulatory frameworks and scopes of practice, (3) improved training infrastructure and (4) access to dependable medium- to long-term funding (Lehmann et al. 2009, p. 1), which within the South African context, the authors believe can be done within the envisioned NHI.

The importance of enabling national-level governance that ensures availability and implementation of an appropriate facilitatory regulatory framework, as well as relevant policies, governance that influences and supports training institutions and ensures the availability of sufficient resources, and governance that reins in the cooperation of the various stakeholders is highlighted by these authors. These facilitators are key for task-shifting to be efficient and effective and significantly contribute toward developing relevant, effective, equitable and sustainable health care systems. The authors of this chapter support these recommendations around facilitators for successful implementation of task-shifting and suggest that in the South African context, telehealth (tele-audiology) can be utilised as a service delivery model to ensure that access through task-shifting occurs within programmes that will maintain minimum standards as prescribed by the HPCSA.

Although task-shifting and tele-audiology offer promise to deliver service to marginalised communities, there is a need to re-imagine how it would work in the context of South Africa and other LMICs. Khoza-Shangase, Moroe and Neille (2021a) advanced significant benefits of telepractice within the South African context under five themes:

1. training and preparation yield favourable outcomes
2. use of telepractice within a hybrid model that includes task-shifting is best
3. telepractice allowing for cost-effectiveness of the service delivery
4. access to service provision and supervision that could be external to the South African borders (internationalisation)
5. modality outcomes that yield similar outcomes and are comparable.

In re-imagining the use of tele-audiology and task-shifting within the African context, widespread use of task-shifting and tele-audiology should be carefully done in a manner that does not perpetuate an arguably colonial-based service. Therefore, there is a need for serious deliberation around the implementation of this shift in paradigm. One such deliberation is with regard to individuals who are responsible for planning and implementation. This means that task-shifting and tele-audiology may need to take a bottom-up approach, where various individuals, including those with hearing disability, are involved in all phases of planning, implementation and monitoring.

Conventionally, community health workers (CHWs) and volunteers have been shown to play a critical role in audiology task-shifting through tele-audiology (O'Donovan et al. 2019). Biagio et al. (2013) showed that facilitators (i.e. volunteers) can provide a platform for asynchronous tele-audiology, while Hussein et al. (2018) later showed that CHWs can be trained to use smartphone hearing screening using the mHealth system. Although South African nurses may be overworked (Oosthuizen & Ehlers 2007), nurses may be ideal to ensure that universal newborn hearing screening is successfully implemented within birthing facilities across the country. Khan, Joseph and Adhikari (2018) and Khoza-Shangase et al. (2017) emphasised that nurses should be capacitated to conduct hearing screening because they are the most accessible health care personnel at all levels of health care. Fulton et al. (2011) recommended the use of technology with task-shifting and viewed this as a policy option that has the potential to raise the practical and creative efficiency of health care delivery, expanding the number of quality services offered cost-effectively.

Mundeva et al. (2018) raised critical ethical issues that need consideration in task-shifting. These authors highlighted challenges that cadres engaging in task-shifting encounter, such as (1) performing emotionally and physically arduous responsibilities with frequently unsatisfactory training, (2) absence of supervision and payment and (3) working in contexts where they are inadequately incorporated into health systems, which has negative effects on the quality of care provided and on promotions prospects (career progression) and lead to employee disempowerment, feelings of being exploited and taken for granted. These authors believe that these issues can be addressed if a number of ethical principles are prioritised, which include beneficence, justice, respect for persons, cultural humility and proportionality. Consequently, these authors stress the importance of policymakers and programme implementers prioritising ethical principles in planning and implementing such programmes – a sentiment, along with concerted political will, strongly shared by the authors of this chapter.

Suen et al. (2019) presented arguments for the use of CHWs in collaboration with professional health care workers under their direct supervision to overcome the capacity versus demand challenges in LMICs, in the field of audiology. These authors lament that if such service delivery models are not explored, little progress will be attained in challenging the global burden of hearing loss, despite all existing evidence for the effects of untreated hearing impairment and the availability of evidence-based interventions. They reiterate calls that have been made to confront hearing loss as a public health challenge, while highlighting that prospects exist to rely on public health approaches to deal with hearing care at the population level, as raised by Olusanya, Neumann and Saunders (2014), the National Academies of Sciences Engineering and Medicine (2016) and The Lancet (2016). Suen et al. (2019) suggested that these public health approaches include the utilisation of public and community health assistants, peer counsellors and health promoters. In the case of audiology, these approaches may also include PHC nurses, teacher assistants and trained volunteers. All these cadres, if trained and regulated as per the HPCSA's minimum standards, regulations and scope of practice and supervised by audiologists, can through the use of tele-audiology be valuable in innovative approaches to increasing access to ear-and-hearing health care within the African context.

Four factors that support developing tele-audiology clinical practice include (1) shortage of audiologists, (2) largely PC-based testing equipment that allows audiologists to operate diagnostic equipment located at a distance site from the desktop PC using remote control software, (3) availability of videoconferencing facilities for real-time tele-audiology applications and (4) availability of guidelines (AAA 2008; ASLHA 2005; Hayes 2012). Although these are international, while the HPCSA is still developing local guidelines, consideration of these factors by the South African audiology community is useful for establishing contextual responsiveness. Tele-audiology, in conjunction with task-shifting, could increase access while also addressing employment opportunity challenges that South Africa is grappling with.

Tele-audiology, as a subset of telehealth, has become a more practical, feasible and logical approach to delivering hearing care, particularly in resource-constrained contexts; although this has not been readily adopted nor widely practised in countries such as South Africa – even in the context of COVID-19 the regulations of which were pushing for it (Sebothoma et al. 2021). This model of service delivery was established in the mid-1990s, primarily to deliver audiological care in regions with inadequate access to health care because of a shortage of resources, as in the South African context. Telehealth (i.e. tele-audiology) has been defined as the utilisation of telecommunication technologies to reach patients, lessen obstacles to best health care in underserved communities, enhance patient approval and accessibility to health care practitioners, reduce professional seclusion in remote rural areas, aid practitioners enlarge their practice reach and spare patients from having to migrate long distances to obtain high-quality care (Krupinski 2015). Within the South African context, where there is an obvious capacity versus demand challenge with audiological services and limited rehabilitation resources for the hearing-impaired, where a case for preventive health care has been made, tele-audiology may serve the very basic function of access to preventive care. An apparent benefit of tele-audiology is that it may facilitate overcoming universal barriers to accessing hearing care, such as distance from service providers and associated costs (Schweitzer et al. 1999). Within the South African context, tele-audiology can also allow for continuity of care where patients identified within the health care sector can continue to receive intervention within other sectors such as the education sector (EHDI)

(Khoza-Shangase et al. 2021b) and the occupational sector or industry (including ONIHL) (Khoza-Shangase & Moroe 2020), where currently there are very limited, if any, audiology services.

The authors provide adequate motivation to make use of the opportunities from the COVID-19 pandemic and increase the use of tele-audiology. They, additionally, recommend manufacturing of highly computerised assessment and intervention technology resources for preventive audiology in LMIC contexts with expanded access to web cameras and access to affordable government-subsidised broadband connectivity. Within the South African context, the increased efforts by the government toward information and communication technologies (ICTs) and the Fourth Industrial Revolution (4IR) make this an opportune time to carefully deliberate on this (State of the Nation Address [SONA] 2020). Recent evidence from contexts similar to South Africa, such as India, also supports this approach as a cost-effective delivery model. Ramkumar et al.'s (2018) study indicates better cost outcomes when:

- broadband Internet for tele-diagnostics is utilised
- economical human resources and equipment with consequent lowest cost per patient screened
- maximised follow-up expenses with the cost per patient being reduced substantially for diagnostic audiology assessment and for the cost per patient identified when tele-audiology is used.

Krumm and Syms (2011) reported that hybrid delivery, where both asynchronous and synchronous tele-audiology modes of delivery are utilised, has been used for various audiological scopes of practice. The authors also recommend hybrid delivery for preventive audiology within the African context, where asynchronous (store-and-forward remote monitoring) and synchronous (live interaction and mobile health) are combined. Even though the health care professional (audiologist) might not present at the time of the consultation, synchronous tele-audiology involves the health care professional being present during the consultation. This includes examples such as videoconferencing, remote programming of hearing technologies such as hearing aids and cochlear implants (Hughes, Sevier & Choi 2018; Krumm & Syms 2011), and remote conduction of electrophysiological testing, to name a few. While a synchronous tele-audiology approach has been documented to be beneficial, its implementation may not be practicable yet within the South African context. As a result of an insufficient number of audiologists, this anticipated implementation challenge is made more challenging by network connectivity challenges in South Africa. Steuerward et al. (2018) emphasised that the synchronous telehealth technique needs the audiologist to be present during remote assessment with broadband network connectivity. The proposed telehealth treatment might be challenging, but if network connectivity difficulties can be overcome, it can serve as the next viable intervention option for a health care professional who lives far from patients requiring services, primarily if task-shifting cadres are implemented.

However, the asynchronous telehealth approach can be utilised in the absence of the audiologist, where paraprofessionals or site facilitators can be trained to perform certain audiological tests, save the findings, and forward them to the audiologist later for analysis and intervention planning (Fabry 2010). This application is one of the motivations for why tele-audiology would be ideal for the human resource-constrained South African primary preventive hearing care setup. Research has illustrated the accuracy of asynchronous tele-audiology when compared with traditional face-to-face diagnosis by qualified professionals (Biagio et al. 2013, 2014).

Further evidence indicates that tele-audiology is suitable for hearing loss prevention programmes such as:

- ototoxicity monitoring and ONIHL monitoring (Folmer et al. 2012; Saunders & Griest 2009)
- performance of otoscopy and video otoscopy, immittance and NHS (Krumm & Syms 2011)
- measurements of otoacoustic emissions
- pure-tone audiometry
- programming cochlear implants via neural response or telemetry assessment (Krumm & Vento 2013).

Swanepoel et al. (2010) believed that the asynchronous method is more feasible for the South African context, especially in school settings. These authors further provided a scope of application of possibilities for tele-audiology within LMIC contexts, which needs to be fully explored for preventive audiology to increase access to hearing care for the majority of the currently underserved populations in South Africa. Khoza-Shangase and Moroe (2020) demonstrated how, for example, within specific scopes of practice in audiology, structured, systematic and sustainable implementation of tele-audiology can be adopted by recommending a tele-hearing conservation programme model that covers all pillars of HCPs, as illustrated in Figure 2.1.

As a result of the shortage of resources, and also with the advent of the COVID-19 pandemic, the tele-HCP model can be very useful. Khoza-Shangase and Moroe (2020) proposed that tele-hearing conservation can use a variety of advancements in tele-audiology, including wireless and booth-less technology for hearing testing, mobile technology for booth-less audiometry, pure-tone audiometry through earphone attenuation and hearing screening via smartphone applications. Benson (2020) further reported that audiological assessment during COVID-19 should include video otoscopy, tympanometry and pure-tone audiometry, which can all be conducted through real-time

TELE-Hearing conservation programme (TELE-HCP)

Pillar	Periodic noise exposure measurement/ monitoring	Engineering controls	Administrative controls	Personal hearing protection	Employee/ management education, motivation and training	Risk-based medical examination, medical surveillance and audiometric evaluations	Record-keeping
Synchronous	• Real-time noise exposure measurements/ monitoring via videoconferencing and application sharing • Quality control of noise exposure measurements/ monitoring via interactive videoconferencing	• Real-time videoconference-based engineering controls and quality control. Examples: Monitoring equipment or machinery maintenance, equipment replacement, isolating or enclosing noise source, and treating the room. • Interactive videoconferencing recommendations to reduce workers' exposure to noise in real-time, including modifications or replacements of equipment and physical changes to reduce noise levels	• Provide employers with real-time interactive videoconference presentations to reduce workplace noise exposure • Mentor and guide rotating workers in excessively noisy jobs (creating work pattern where employees are not exposed to an eight-hour, time-weighted average [TWA] over 90 dB), resulting in increased distance between workers and noise source	• Real-time interactive videoconference presentations and demonstrations on PHPs (selection, use, and maintenance) • Interactive videoconferencing for tele-monitoring and cutom fitting PHPs guided by an audiologist • Counselling and troubleshooting PHPs and their use via interactive videoconferencing	• Real-time interactive videoconference presentations • Tele-mentoring and guidance during assessments or procedures • Discussing difficult result/cases with experienced clinicians • Ward rounds involving diagnostic paper assessments, medical surveillance, and potential claims	• Real-time screening and/or diagnostic assessment via videoconferencing and application sharing • Quality control of screening and/or diagnostic assessment via interactive videoconferencing • Assessments and examinations conducted in real-time through videoconferencing and sharing of applications • Audiology directed by an audiologist – case history, video-otoscopy, immittance, OAE, pure tone audiometry, AEPs, etc. • Quality control of the medical examination via interactive videoconferencing	• Real-time record-keeping of all components of HCPs via videoconferencing and application sharing • Quality control of all records via interactive videoconferencing • Real-time proactive use of data for effective HCP implementation

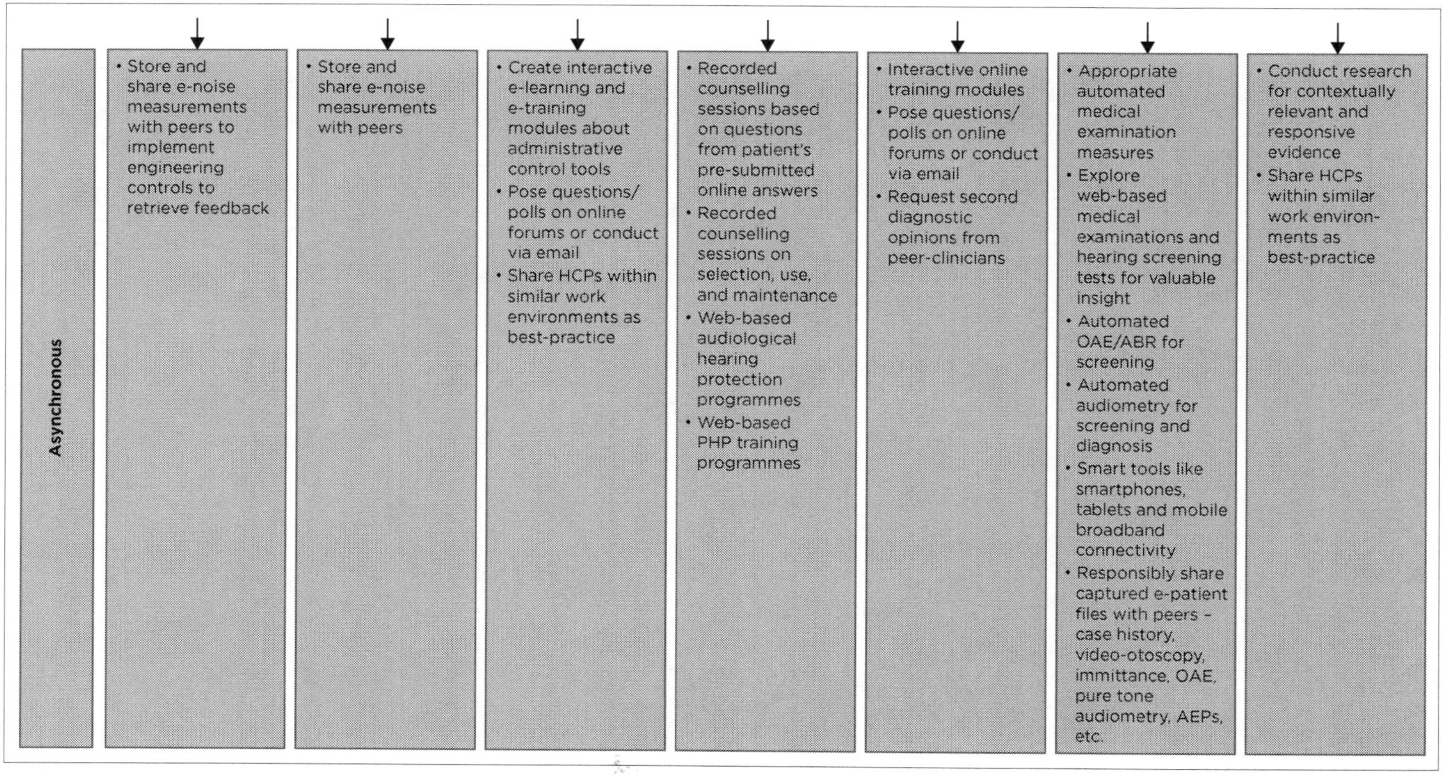

Source: Khoza-Shangase and Moroe (2020).
Key: HCP, hearing conservation programme.

FIGURE 2.1: Possibilities of tele-audiology use in hearing conservation programmes for all pillars (tele-hearing conservation programmes).

synchronous and asynchronously tele-audiology (Coco 2020; Khoza-Shangase & Moroe 2020; Sebothoma et al. 2021). To ensure that assessments are completed successfully and all seven pillars are implemented, paraprofessionals such as CHWs must be trained (Dawood et al. 2020).

The potential purpose and feasible impact of tele-audiology within the African preventive audiology context are significant. The South African audiology community needs to engage in a tele-audiology mapping exercise, incorporating task-shifting training to develop this delivery model to increase access to services not only to South African audiologists but also to volunteer audiologists from across the world. Swanepoel et al. (2010) recommended this strategy and suggested exploring the use of the tele-audiology network[1] for this very purpose. The authors, however, highlighted the importance of strict adherence to the South African regulations governing health care during this process.

■ 2.3. Considerations around tele-audiology for preventive audiology

Sufficient evidence has been presented supporting the use of tele-audiology to improve access to hearing care and reach, particularly in resource-constrained contexts. Furthermore, enough supported arguments have been presented for the application of task-shifting as a service delivery model to facilitate UAC. The application of these methods remains challenging and presents certain concerns, particularly where contextual regulations and policies governing their implementation do not yet exist, where political will may be lacking, and where resource allocation has not prioritised this model as part of the HR strategy, equipment procurement and cadre training. Such concerns require careful deliberation:

1. Numerous challenges are envisaged in the implementation of tele-audiology for preventive audiology within the South African context, although pronouncements at national government levels promise plans that can facilitate the resolution of these challenges (SONA 2020). The challenges include (1) computer literacy and competence of potential users (Carter, Horrigan & Hudyma 2010), (2) the availability of a network connection (Grogan-Johnson et al. 2015), (3) the ability to understand and follow ethical and legal prescriptive guidelines and standards governing direct practice (Grogan-Johnson et al. 2015; Grol & Grimshaw 2003). As a fourth concern, the management of data transmission, retrieval, and storage online (Grogan-Johnson et al. 2015); and, last but not least, linguistic and cultural diversity impacts on using it (Khoza-Shangase & Mophosho 2018, 2021;

1. See www.teleaudiology.org.

Khoza-Shangase et al. 2021a). Careful deliberations and planning around these challenges are key to the successful implementation of telehealth to facilitate preventive audiology in the South African context.

2. The fact that in the 2017 South African Health Review, Siegfried, Wilkinson and Hofman (2017) reported that no precise provision is made in the National Health Act and that health technology assessment is narrowly and incompletely defined is another concern that requires careful consideration before tele-audiology can be comprehensively rolled out for preventive audiology within the South African context. In the same report, a need to improve telehealth capacity building is identified and highlighted, with the acknowledgement that training opportunities in telehealth are inadequate; however, government has goals to stimulate this training through education and research, with universities identified as key stakeholders to expediate this capacity development process. Universities are tasked with the development of well-structured education and training courses and adhering to minimum standards to offer the academic and practical skills needed for implementing clinical and educational services via a telehealth model, as well as developing appropriate ICT infrastructure support specific to telehealth. By implementing tele-audiology within primary preventive health care, efficient, ethically, and well-resourced telehealth models can establish evidence bases that are context-relevant and contextually responsive. This goes hand in hand with the availability of national policies and regulations, as well as training around task-shifting, with adherence to WHO guidelines, national guidelines, scopes of practice and minimum standards under careful supervision and monitoring. The aforementioned policy and regulation considerations are over and above the need to ensure firm adherence to ethics, human rights and medical law surrounding the use of task-shifting and tele-audiology. In their quest to increase access to preventive audiological services through this service delivery model, audiologists must take heed of the six ethical challenges identified by Naudé and Bornman (2021) to be relevant in tele-audiology. These six challenges, consisting of competence, informed consent, privacy and confidentiality, licensure, reimbursement for services, and effectiveness of services and programme validation, are essential for well-organised, successful and ethical implementation of tele-audiology and task-shifting.
3. Without sufficient training and education of audiology students in the use and implementation of telehealth (Edirippulige, Armfield & Smith 2012; Govender & Mars 2018; Khoza-Shangase et al. 2021a), and without collaboration with paraprofessionals in task-shifting, recommendations made in this chapter are less likely to succeed. Limited inclusion of telehealth training in African education and training programmes because of the lack of standards and regulations surrounding ethical practice around this model of delivery has been documented (Edirippulige et al. 2012; Govender & Mars 2018; Khoza-Shangase et al. 2021a). Edirippulige et al. (2012)

recommended the introduction of telehealth at all graduate levels in higher education for health care professionals so that they can provide clinical care through this model of health care delivery, while Khoza-Shangase et al. (2021a) argued that clinical educators should also be equipped in using this modality for teletraining and telesupervision. This approach includes the HPCSA SLH Board development of a task team to develop guidelines for telepractice in SLH programmes in order to guide the professionals and protect the public. The use of short courses and mandatory CPD training for continued professional development is an additional strategy to reach those not within the formal education and training programmes but who require the knowledge and skills to provide services.

4. There appears to be limited collaborative and synergistic functioning between the various South African departments, such as Health, Labour and Education, in as far as assessment and management of patients with hearing impairment or those at risk of developing one, thus not only impacting identification but also the continuity of care for patients in these sectors. Although the South African health care acts and policies are progressively acknowledging the importance of ICT in health care, particularly within the 4IR, and they advocate for the utilisation of technology and telehealth applications within the health care service delivery model (Govender & Mars 2018), this recognition has not been extended to occupational health and safety in the form of HCPs and the school health care programmes currently in place. The recognition of ICT in health led to the development of the National Digital Strategy 2012–2016 (DoH 2012), with the most recent 2019–2024 National Digital Health Strategy (DoH 2019). All these endeavours from the DoH need to be extended to the other sectors where preventive audiology can be implemented.
5. The evidence in the use of tele-audiology for identification of auditory pathologies such as hearing impairment and middle ear disorders, and on the implementation of appropriate management such as hearing aid fitting, forms an important part of efforts aimed at alleviating barriers to successful preventive audiology care. However, tele-audiology can also be used as part of preventive and promotive education measures for both task-shifting cadres and patients (e.g. education awareness in HCPs). Awareness programmes around some of the causes of auditory pathologies that are preventable excessive exposure to noise in children listening to mp3's on portable media player devices, such as iPods (WHO 2015), the use of hearing protection devices in HCPs (Ntlhakana et al. 2015) and the importance of early intervention for middle ear pathologies in this population (Sebothoma 2020), the importance of ototoxicity monitoring (Khoza-Shangase 2010, 2013; Khoza-Shangase & Stirk 2016), and contextual risk factors for hearing impairment in infants (Fitzgibbons, Beswick & Driscoll 2021; Kanji & Khoza-Shangase 2019) – remain one of the key

benefits of tele-audiology in primary prevention of hearing impairment in LMIC contexts. Such awareness campaigns can efficiently be carried out by task-shifting cadres with coordination and supervision by audiologists through hybrid tele-audiology delivery. These campaigns would be best conducted and sustained through programmatic initiatives, such as those listed earlier (First 1000 days, Striving for zero-harm and TB/HIV Collaborative Programme).

6. Connectivity and Internet access for the majority of the South African population remains a challenge, although significant progress has been made. The rush of boosted Internet access within South Africa has reportedly reached new high levels, with the surge expected to increase in the future. According to the Electronic Communications Network, it is anticipated that in 2020 the Internet of Things and Machine-to-Machine's installed bases will have accessed 35 million users for the South African market, with a positive impact on the country including increased accessibility to health care initiatives such as hearing care (if capitalised). The partnering of the South African government with the World Economic Forum in an initiative 'Internet for All' in 2017, which aimed to facilitate universal access to Internet by 2020 as stated by the South African Government News Agency, has not materialised, and this could present challenges for tele-audiology. Nonetheless, the General Household Survey (2018) revealed that '64.7% of South African households had at least one member who had access to, or used the Internet either at home, work, place of study or Internet cafés', providing contextual data that need to be considered in planning tele-audiology for this context.
7. Through asynchronous tele-audiology, middle ear pathologies and hearing impairments, as well as auditory processing disorders, have a more extensive evidence base from resource-constrained settings such as communities, mines, and schools (Olusanya et al. 2004; Potgieter et al. 2018; Swanepoel et al. 2014), yet tele-audiology is still in its infancy, despite receiving significant attention. There also remains even more limited contextually relevant evidence that has considered the linguistic and cultural diversity of the South African context, as well as the incongruence between professionals and patients in terms of this diversity, which requires attention.

■ 2.4. Conclusion

Tele-audiology and task-shifting is a relatively new service delivery model, which is particularly useful in resource-constrained settings. Because of the significant capacity versus demand challenges in LMIC contexts and the need for scaling up audiology professionals' goal of preventing hearing impairment under their scope of practice, careful consideration of this platform and strategy for UAC is required. Because of the documented increasing prevalence of hearing impairment in these contexts, alternative strategies to implement and monitor hearing care programmes, such as the use of tele-audiology and task-shifting, become critical. Failure to deliberate on such models of service delivery will indicate a lost opportunity to improve access to audiological services for these populations, particularly with the documented evidence of technological advancements in ICT and audiology. Technological advances increase opportunities for alternative service delivery models that are contextually responsive, patient centred, and that take into account linguistic and cultural diversity and, most recently, social distancing linked to pandemics such as the novel COVID-19. The use of tele-audiology facilitates developments such as:

- hearing screening using smartphone applications
- wireless and booth-less technology for hearing testing
- diagnostic pure-tone audiometry without a sound-treated environment
- pure-tone audiometry outside a sound booth using earphone attenuation
- integrated noise monitoring
- automation, which substantially boost the audiology community's capacity to offer ear and hearing services to distant and isolated resource-constrained contexts, such as the South African mining context.

The use of hybrid tele-audiology delivery alongside task-shifting presents the immense possibility for preventive audiology.

These service delivery models must consider policy and regulations challenges and must adhere to ethics, human rights and medical law, with full political will from the government. Furthermore, like any new assessment or intervention strategy, significant contextually relevant research would need to be conducted to ensure a contextually relevant evidence base that will allow for best practice, which has taken contextual issues such as linguistic and cultural diversity into consideration.

Chapter 3

Tele-audiology within the African school context: Opportunities, challenges and proposed solutions

Samantha Govender
Department of Speech-Language Pathology and Audiology,
Faculty of Health Sciences, School of Healthcare Sciences,
Sefako Makgatho Health Sciences University,
Pretoria, South Africa

3.1. Introduction

A high prevalence of hearing impairment exists among school-going children in LMICs, particularly within the African continent. Sufficient evidence has established that undiagnosed hearing impairment has negative consequences for the overall development of the hearing-impaired child. Efforts towards early identification and intervention of hearing impairment within the African context have been compromised by numerous factors, including a lack of financial, technical and human resources, as well as poor infrastructure and poor follow-up. These challenges are observed within the health care sector and within the education sector. Telehealth-based audiology (TBA) programmes have the potential to resolve a number of

How to cite: Govender, S 2022, 'Tele-audiology within the African school context: Opportunities, challenges and proposed solutions', ed. K Khoza-Shangase, *Preventive audiology: An African perspective*, AOSIS Books, Cape Town, pp. 41–63. https://doi.org/10.4102/aosis.2022.BK209.03

these challenges and achieve a reduction in the burden and impact of hearing impairment among school-aged children, as both screening and diagnostic and intervention services can be delivered within the school context to ensure comprehensive service delivery (Khoza-Shangase 2021). Telehealth-based audiology services have been proven to have the potential to address such service delivery challenges, particularly to rural and remotely located schools, and their validity and reliability are well established. A comprehensive audiology service delivery package from hearing screening to aural rehabilitation services can be provided via tele-audiology. However, several barriers within the African context pose a threat to the adoptability and sustainability of these services, and careful consideration of these barriers is important for the maximum benefit to be obtained from them. This chapter deliberates on audiological care within the African school context and explores TBA as a model of service delivery, with a careful exploration of the challenges and barriers to the adoption and implementation of TBA within this context. The chapter also provides plausible solutions and offers a sustainability model to support the growth of TBA within the African school context.

Audiology services are only as strong as the health care system within which they function. The African health care system is challenged by the increasing burden of disease, poor prevention and detection programmes, as well as poor health intervention strategies. Health care on the continent is further influenced by financial, social and political factors. It is, therefore, necessary to first understand the factors impacting the African health care system to contextualise the challenges facing audiology service delivery and the impetus for TBA services. Chapters 1 and 2 comprehensively discuss these challenges while arguing for preventive audiology as a strategy to ramp up efforts toward an ear and hearing healthy nation.

Amidst Africa's political and economic instability lies the burdensome issues surrounding poverty and endemic communicable and non-communicable diseases. Africa holds countries such as South Africa, Kenya and Nigeria that have had unfortunate historical injustices and socio-economic inequalities that compromised health, wealth and well-being, and these countries are still redressing these inequalities of the past (Chukwudozie 2015; Ilinca et al. 2019; Maphumulo & Bhengu 2019). Inequalities in resource distribution, education and income levels persist. Reports emerging from various African countries reveal that the Gini coefficient, which is a measure of income inequality, has increased over the years, implying that the economic gap between those that are affluent and those that are poor has intensified, with countries like South Africa, Namibia and Botswana demonstrating the most inequality (Gini > 0.60) (The World Bank 2017; UN 2017). The intergenerational progression of poverty has ensured that the income divide remains, and this has direct implications for childcare.

There are distinct and glaring differences in health, education and quality of life (QoL) between children from rich and poor households globally (Wimer et al. 2016). The UN, through its SDGs, has tried to close this inequality gap that exists between the rich and poor (UN 2015). SDG 3 speaks to ensuring healthy lives and promoting the well-being of all children. However, the health, well-being and QoL of children in Africa remain a concern because of financial constraints and under-resourced health care systems (Bigna & Noubiap 2019; Khoza-Shangase 2021; Roberton et al. 2020; Roelen et al. 2017).

The health care systems of the majority of African countries comprise the state-owned and privately owned health care sectors. In South Africa, for example, the public health care sector services a larger proportion of the population (approximately 86%) than the private sector does, but paradoxically the private health care sector has greater access to specialised health care services, a larger workforce and better-equipped hospitals (Jobson 2015; WHO 2017). Adding to the above challenges faced by the public health care sector is the increasing and changing patterns of disease burden among the population residing in rural and remote locations (Mayosi & Benatar 2014). It is stated that the African continent only has 3% of the world's health care workers yet presents with 24% of the global burden of disease (Scott & Mars 2015). In addition, Africa has the largest child population globally (UN Department of Economic and Social Affairs, Population Division 2017), and this has implications for resource distribution and adequate financial resources steered towards childcare. The demand for childcare has placed a strain on the functioning of the public health care system in the continent.

Retention of health care workers in Africa has also become a problem as professionals either undergo urbanisation, move into the private sector or emigrate to earn more lucrative salaries and work in better-functioning health care systems (Merugumala, Pothula & Cooper 2017; Centre for Development and Enterprise 2011). According to Mayosi and Benatar (2014), lack of trained health care professionals, disparities in wealth, education and health care are core issues affecting the African population. In addition to this, the translation of health care policy and the development of programmes into practice has been slow, and evidence of this has been documented in audiology within the South African context (Khoza-Shangase & Masondo 2020, 2021).

Taking South Africa as an example, since its shift to democracy in 1994, the South African government has initiated several programmes and services. These include free health care for women and children, introducing primary health care (PHC) services in the health care system and the improvement thereof with the re-engineering of PHC, the Integrated School Health Programme (ISHP) (2012) and the recent plans around the NHI. The NHI is reported to be aimed at stabilising the fragmentation that exists between the private and public health care sectors; however, the progress of its implementation has been slow, although the NHI bill has been passed. The ISHP (2012), one of the other intended programmes, has also faced technical and resource challenges and has therefore not been comprehensively implemented nationwide (Khoza-Shangase, Sebothoma & Moroe 2021). The failure to successfully implement these health care programmes has led to poor health outcomes and increased mortality rates among African children (WHO 2020).

The WHO (2020) reported high levels of mortality and the burden of disease in children across the world. In 2017, almost 5.4 million children under five-years-old died from preventable causes including malnutrition, malaria and diarrhoea (WHO 2019), mainly because of malnutrition, malaria and birth complications (WHO 2019). The WHO further stated that children in Africa are 14 times more likely to lose their lives than their counterparts residing in high-income regions. Alongside the staggering mortality rate lies the concerns arising from various disabilities, including sensory deficits (Naipal & Rampersad 2018). The prevalence of sensory deficits, primarily vision and hearing loss, among children in Africa has debilitating effects and far-reaching consequences across all developmental spheres (Mulwafu, Kuper & Ensink 2016; Naipal & Rampersad 2018). Chapter 9 will further explore early detection and intervention of the combination of these two sensory deficits: deafblindness. This chapter focuses on hearing loss in Africa.

The global prevalence of childhood hearing loss is estimated to be around 34 million, and Africa makes up 5% of this global prevalence (Adedeji et al. 2015; Al-Rowaily et al. 2012; Tian et al. 2015; WHO 2017). In a study conducted by Desalew and colleagues (2020), hearing loss prevalence among children in sub-Saharan Africa was reported to be 10%. In addition, the study reported the prevalence of hearing impairment for community or school-based children to be 6%, with the prevalence for children with comorbidities (HIV and TB) at 23%. The causes of childhood hearing impairment contributing to these prevalence rates are diverse.

Globally, genetic-related causes constitute 24%–39% of congenital hearing impairment in children (Adedayo & Olawale 2014). According to Birkeland and Lesperance (2016), genetic-related causes of hearing loss are likely to remain high as medical advances contribute toward decreasing the acquired causes of hearing problems. Acquired hearing loss can be caused by conditions such as head injuries, measles and mumps, ototoxic medications or infections (Adedeji et al. 2015; Butler 2012).

Otitis media (OM) is one of the major causes contributing to acquired hearing loss among children (Adedeji et al. 2015). It is estimated that approximately 80% of children will experience acute OM by their third birthday, with at least 50% of these children going on to develop hearing impairment (Vos et al. 2015). This is largely because of the lack of access to early detection and intervention programmes during those early years of life. Chapter 5 comprehensively discusses preventing middle ear pathologies in a South African context and proposes a programmatic approach to prevent these pathologies as a clinical framework.

According to the WHO (2017), almost 60% of childhood hearing loss, such as OM-related hearing loss, can be prevented with appropriate management, thus emphasising the role of preventive audiology within this age group. However, unfortunately, this model of ear-and-hearing health care is largely curtailed by the absence of adequate and standardised audiological care throughout African countries, thereby negatively impacting hearing-impaired children's development. If the hearing loss goes undetected for years, detection and intervention programmes within the formal schooling environment could at least provide an opportunity for management, albeit late.

The optimisation of development in children with hearing impairment must be prioritised. To ensure that these children reach their full potential in terms of academic, speech and language, as well as vocational and socio-emotional development, early intervention and timeous management must occur (Maluleke, Chiwutsi & Khoza-Shangase 2021). This can only be achieved if there is adequate access to health care services. School health services provide an opportunity for school-going children to be monitored within the school context so that health barriers to learning can be identified and managed (Khoza-Shangase et al. 2021). The school environment is an ideal context in which to deliver health care services; however, because of the lack of technical, human and financial resources, audiology service delivery in schools has been stagnant (Khoza-Shangase 2021; Peer & Fagan 2015). Audiologists have therefore been exploring the use of TBA services to provide both screening and diagnostic services to facilitate early detection and intervention efforts for school-aged children.

The use of TBA services within the school context presents many benefits to ensuring the prevention of hearing impairment, as well as the identification and management of hearing deficits. Telehealth-based audiology services could help remedy the shortfalls associated with the current health care service delivery model, particularly in remote and rural areas where travelling and accessibility to high-quality services are lacking. The health care system within the continent largely comprises three layers, namely primary, secondary and tertiary prevention (Kisling & Das 2021). The aim of these structures is to ensure that early detection and intervention take place to avoid or reduce the full impact that a disease or condition has on a person. Telehealth applications are well suited to support all three layers of prevention, and its utility has the potential to reduce the burden of disease. Telehealth applications allow for the provision of health care services via one of three models (Krumm 2007). The synchronous model of hearing testing is conducted in real-time, where the patient is tested via live streaming through videoconferencing facilities. The patient is, therefore, set up and prepared for testing by a trained assistant, while the test is conducted by a qualified health professional anywhere in the world (Krumm 2007). Asynchronous testing is conducted in a store-and-forward manner, where testing is conducted by a trained assistant, and the results are stored and can be sent later via email or to a secure website for interpretation by a qualified health care professional (Krumm 2007). The hybrid model refers to the combination of both models (synchronous and asynchronous). All these models of service delivery require a laptop computer or tablet personal computer with Internet connectivity, specialised noise monitoring headphones that replace the soundproof booth, and trained personnel in order to provide services.

Telehealth has been seen as a solution to resolving inequalities that exist in health care service delivery between rural and urban areas, the rich and poor, as well as between low and high socio-economic countries (Govender & Mars 2018a; Swanepoel et al. 2010). The integration of telehealth into the PHC service delivery model provides an opportunity for better access to experts and specialists, thereby reducing the intransigent problems linked to travelling, as well as eliminating unnecessary referrals. The WHO (2013) emphasised that telehealth, within the various contexts, particularly the school context, could improve detection and intervention rates of disabling conditions such as hearing loss. However, this model of service delivery is constrained by many barriers to its successful and sustained implementation. These barriers are immense within the current African health care context. Although this chapter focuses on computer-based telehealth applications, it is also worth mentioning that the more recent mobile health innovations have seen increased coverage in screening and diagnostic services within schools (Chu et al. 2019; Yousuf Hussein et al. 2018).

This chapter, therefore, aims to firstly provide an overview of prevention, identification and management of hearing impairments, sharply focusing on the current challenges to early detection of hearing loss within the school context. The chapter then describes the benefits of TBA services within the school context and the related barriers to its implementation. The chapter then offers proposed solutions within the framework of a developmental model.

3.2. Prevention, identification and management of hearing impairment and associated implications for tele-audiology-based services

3.2.1. Challenges with prevention, identification and management of hearing impairment within the African context

Nestled within the compromised African health care systems is the lack of adequate early detection and intervention services. Based on the prevalence of hearing impairment, particularly within the African context, early detection and intervention services should make up a routine and mandatory service. Early identification of hearing impairment has proven highly beneficial for optimal childhood development (Ching et al. 2017), and this is likely to occur if a hearing impairment is identified while the child is still within the critical period of development (Nada, Khater & Saeed 2014). Early intervention and detection of hearing impairment should be available at birth and during the early school years for acquired losses to avoid the deleterious effects on the child and their family. Ching et al. (2017) reported a strong relationship between the age of identification of hearing impairment and language, speech, social-emotional and cognitive development. Newton (2013) provided a review of studies outlining the beneficial outcomes associated with early detection and intervention of childhood hearing loss, such as optimal language development, increased vocational opportunities and healthy social-emotional development. Unfortunately, current health funding models continue to under-service early detection and intervention programmes for hearing loss because of their focus on more life-threatening conditions such as HIV, AIDS and TB, which have demanded the countries' health resources. Appropriate and timeous management of hearing impairment is fundamental to optimal social, emotional, behavioural and academic development (Mahomed, Swanepoel & Ayieko 2014; Mulwafu et al. 2016; Warner-Czyz et al. 2015). Within the South African context, Chapter 2 of this book suggests careful deliberation of prioritisation of health resources, with a specific focus on the use of tele-audiology and task-shifting to address the capacity versus demand challenges within the South African context.

It is reported that less than 10% of children with disabilities receive some type of education, with only 2% of these children receiving formal classroom education. Furthermore, a significant number of children with disabilities tend to drop out of school because of the lack of infrastructure, resources and assistive devices to facilitate and support learning (African Report on Children with Disabilities 2014; Khoza-Shangase et al. 2021). In the South African White

Paper on Special Needs Education (DoBE 2001), inclusive education is emphasised as an important aspect in ensuring that children with disabilities obtain the necessary competencies and skills that will enable them to have successful, independent and fulfilling lives. This is in keeping with the UN Convention on the Rights of a Child Article 23 which speaks to the rights of children with disabilities, emphasising that governments must ensure that appropriate support is provided to such children within the home, educational setting and societal spheres. This is largely because of the understanding that teaching and learning are facilitated through an auditory-verbal approach. Studies by Bess and Tharpe (2008) on 60 school-aged children with unilateral hearing loss, found that 37% of them failed at least one grade, and a further 13% required additional academic support than their normal-hearing peers. They further state that more than 30% of children, particularly those with mild unilateral hearing loss continue to struggle academically despite the increased awareness about the condition and increased evidence to promote early identification and intervention services. Hearing problems, be they unilateral or bilateral, can result in limited vocabulary acquisition and can negatively influence a child's development of reading skills (Mpofu & Chimhenga 2013).

Regarding social and emotional development, it is well-documented that children with disabilities and their families face discrimination and marginalisation as society views their differences as inadequacies (Janardhana et al. 2015). They also face the emotional burden of not receiving timeous and efficient management because of the lack of adequately trained professionals, unstable economies that are unable to support funding of the health sector, as well as physical limitations and barriers such as inefficient transport systems to health care facilities. These conditions are made worse by poor implementation of government legislation and ineffective policies, creating an unfavourable climate for a child with disabilities to thrive.

The WHO (2001) developed the International Classification of Functioning, Disability and Health (ICF) framework that promotes the integration of individuals with disabilities into society without stigmatisation. This framework largely correlates with the South African constitution, in particular the Bill of Rights. The Bill of Rights emphasises the child's legal and constitutional right of access to education, resources, health care and dignity without fear of prejudice. Despite these efforts, children with hearing impairment continue to experience socio-emotional problems (Stevenson et al. 2015), speech and language delays (Fulcher et al. 2015; Tharpe 2008), vocational limitations (Punch, Hyde & Creed 2004) and barriers to social integration (Bush, Kaufman & McNulty 2017; Theunissen et al. 2014). Such challenges contribute to poor QoL for the hearing-impaired child.

It is reported that children with hearing impairment face increased anxiety within the classroom context because of the constant fear of misunderstanding or missing the verbal content taught by the teacher (Mpofu & Chimhenga 2013). This creates social isolation as the child develops fears about interaction and socialisation. Bess and Tharpe (2008) found that behavioural problems were more prevalent in children with hearing loss than those with normal hearing. This is because of their frustration with communication and socialisation. Both these academic and social challenges could ultimately impact vocational opportunities for these children.

The *Employment Equity Act* (1998) and the *White Paper on an Integrated National Disability Strategy* (South Africa, 1997) for South Africa outline guiding principles for employers regarding equal employment opportunities for persons with disabilities. These documents support fair opportunity and non-discrimination for such employees. The ICF further describes functioning in relation to disability and highlights the importance of ensuring that individuals with disability enjoy the same social, environmental, vocational and personal opportunities as those without disabilities. Unfortunately, despite all the policies and guidelines, hearing-impaired individuals are still marginalised because of their impairment, which is viewed negatively by employers because of its perceived negative impact on productivity and profit margins. A study based on students with severe-to-profound hearing loss that completed high school was conducted by the Centre of Assessment and Demographic Studies at Gallaudet University in the United States (Rawlings 1994). Almost two-thirds of the learners went on to pursue postgraduate studies. However, 72% acquired minimal wage jobs with no promise of growth within their jobs. This situation is even more significant in Africa as most hearing-impaired children either do not finish formal schooling or have limited access to tertiary education and training, thus further limiting their vocational opportunities (Muwaniki & Muvirimi 2017).

Because of the above-mentioned academic, social, emotional and vocational implications, most countries and health constituents favour the philosophy of Universal Newborn Hearing Screening (UNHS) to facilitate the early identification of hearing impairment. Unfortunately, most African countries lack legislation regarding mandatory NHS largely because of the over-burdened and constrained health care system (Khoza-Shangase & Kanji 2021; Mahomed-Asmail et al. 2016a). Therefore, school-based hearing screening becomes especially important for preschool and school-aged children so that a hearing impairment can be identified and managed timeously, thus reducing its impact on development (HPCSA 2019). In addition, through education and awareness, the prevention of auditory impairment can be emphasised. The provision of health services within the school contexts aims to reduce the burden of disease among learners, increase awareness and improve the early identification of health conditions as well as provide access to health care services. However, the provision of early detection and intervention audiology services in Africa continues to be an arduous task because of multiple factors (Govender et al. 2015).

One of these factors relates to the low audiologist to high patient ratio, particularly within the LMIC context, making equal and adequate distribution of services unattainable (Khoza-Shangase & Mophosho 2018). Almost 80% of the global population of those with moderate to profound hearing loss live within LMICs (WHO 2017). Furthermore, there remains a high rural population density in Africa, with an almost 2% growth in 2018 in the rural population across the sub-Saharan Africa (Macrotrends 2020). This, however, has not corresponded with a subsequent increase of growth in the number of health care workers situated within these areas. A case in point is South Africa, which has 46% of its population living in rural areas and only 12% of health care workers servicing these areas (Mburu & George 2017; WHO 2017). The urban and rural divide presents its own set of challenges. The extension of health care services to children residing within rural areas remains a concern. Therefore, school health nurses have been tasked with the responsibility of hearing screening; however, because of inadequate equipment, training and transport limitations, school-based hearing screening has not been successfully implemented (ISHP 2012). Additionally, having a child screened without the necessary follow-up is of little benefit. Screening services without established referral systems have serious ethical implications. Chapter 4 of this book delves into these rurality-associated challenges when recommending community-based audiology services as an effective strategy for the prevention of hearing loss in rural communities.

Another challenge with audiological service delivery relates to dependency and reliance on equipment and infrastructure, especially for diagnostic testing, as it is insufficient only to provide screening services to children. Conventional audiology services are largely dependent on equipment and infrastructure, limiting their application in under-resourced areas. These minimum requirements for conducting audiological testing are a soundproof or sound-treated booth or a quiet environment in the case of screening, an audiometer (either diagnostic or screening, depending on the need), an otoscope, a middle ear analyser and accessories for testing, which includes headphones and a bone conduction vibrator. Because of the nature of current audiological methods of testing, often referred to as conventional audiological methods, only one person at a time can be assessed in a quiet or noise-controlled environment, as in the case of diagnostic testing. Because of reliance on strict environmental controls, diagnostic audiological testing is often non-transferable outside the context of an audiology clinical setting.

The aforementioned discussion outlines the harsh reality of a child with hearing impairment within the African context. The factors impacting early detection, intervention and management of childhood hearing impairment in LMICs should actuate the continent's consciousness in the provision of optimal hearing health care. The challenges associated with current service delivery within schools must awaken the continent to leverage all available resources to advance their trajectory towards the attainment of quality child health care, which includes ear-and-hearing health care. Sadly, the response has been passive. To promote the prevention of hearing impairment and scale up early detection and intervention efforts, ICTs (tele-audiology) are being utilised to provide services to children within the rural and remote African context. The validity and reliability of this modality have been confirmed, and its results are congruent with those obtained from conventional methods of audiological testing (Brennan-Jones, Eikelboom & Swanepoel 2017; Govender & Mars 2017; Mahomed et al. 2013; Margolis et al. 2010; Swanepoel et al. 2010). Tele-audiology-based services have been in existence within the profession for a long time. It is a widely accepted method of testing that reduces clinician variability and subjectivity (Brennan-Jones et al. 2017; Mahomed et al. 2013). Tele-audiology-based services can hasten the early detection and prevention of hearing impairment as the testing can be done anywhere at any time, reducing the delays with appointments and transport to well-resourced settings. The review of the literature also highlights the lack of school-based studies that evaluate the telerehabilitation aspect of TBA services such as remote hearing aid fittings and aural rehabilitation. However, several barriers within the African context prevent its sustained implementation.

3.2.2. Telehealth-based audiology services within the African school context: Benefits and challenges

Telehealth services have the potential to improve access to health care, particularly to remote and rural locations (Cason & Cohn 2014). The use of ICT in health care has become a feasible method of service delivery because of the increase in access to Internet connectivity. Audiologists have been exploring the use of telehealth-based services within various contexts, including within the school environment, to improve early detection and intervention services.

The conceptualisation and development of tele-audiology measures were derived from the antecedents of conventional audiology services and comprise a battery of several audiology tests. TBA services were developed to address the challenges associated with conventional testing (Govender & Mars 2018a). Telehealth-based audiology services could potentially address the issue of access to services in remote and rural areas, as such technology does not require the use of a sound-treated facility. Published evidence presents various studies regarding clinical and non-clinical uses of tele-audiology via one or more of the three ways that such services can be delivered, namely asynchronous (store-and-forward), synchronous or a combination of both methods (Brennan-Jones et al. 2017).

Significant advancements have been made in the areas of hearing screening and diagnostic testing using telehealth methods (Kam et al. 2014; Ramkumar et al. 2014). More studies are also emerging on telerehabilitation within the audiology profession (Brennan-Jones et al. 2017; Ferrari & Bernardez-Braga 2009; Govender & Mars 2017; Kuzovkov et al. 2014; Ramos et al. 2009). Tele-audiology services can be used to provide screening, diagnostic and management services. Studies confirm the validity and reliability of the service delivery model and the positive outcomes of such services (Bradford, Caffery & Smith 2015; Brennan-Jones et al. 2017; Govender & Mars 2017).

Existing studies validate the reliability of automated hearing test results (Brennan-Jones et al. 2017; Mahomed-Asmail et al. 2016b). However, only a limited number of diagnostic studies have been conducted (Botasso et al. 2015; Havenga et al., 2017; Mahomed et al. 2014). Remote hearing screening was conducted at a rurally located school on 32 children (Lancaster et al. 2008). Two screening tests were conducted on each participant (one on-site and another remote). The results obtained for both screening procedures were comparable, indicating no significant differences between test results. Similar findings were obtained from remote hearing screening studies conducted within the school context by Monica and colleagues (2016) and Skarzynski and colleagues (2016). These studies do highlight certain challenges relating to technical issues, child-related and school-related variables such as noise levels, concentration levels and connectivity issues.

Regarding diagnostic pure-tone audiometry using tele-audiology, asynchronous testing was conducted on 149 children (an average age of 6.9 years) without a sound-treated environment both within a soundproof booth with conventional audiometry and with a computerised device (Swanepoel et al. 2013). No statistically significant differences were found between thresholds recorded under both test conditions. Similar findings recorded by Mahomed-Asmail and colleagues (2016a) reported no differences between manual and automated air and bone conduction audiometry. Govender and Mars (2018a) found that school-based asynchronous telehealth hearing testing can be used to facilitate the early identification of hearing loss. These studies did mention that protocol revision for telehealth testing, clear instructions for school-aged children and connectivity issues must be addressed to ensure reliable results.

The findings of the above-mentioned studies implied that the telehealth results were reliable and reflected the results of the gold standard for audiology testing (pure-tone audiometry). The survey of literature clearly illustrates that TBA service delivery is a practical and realistic option for hearing testing within the school context, provided that the technical issues such as connectivity, patient set up and appropriate instructions are given to children. However, its widespread utility has been variable. A question therefore raised is whether TBA and its intended usage of servicing the most vulnerable within Africa have materialised. Biehl and Petryna (eds. 2013, p. 4) stated that 'any sustainable (medical) development has to reach and improve the conditions of the poorest and most vulnerable groups carrying the highest burdens of ill health'. This statement speaks to the aspect of sustainable and contextually relevant health care models, including TBA interventions. There appear to be several challenges that impede the implementation of TBA services. To best understand the challenges associated with TBA services within schools, scoping reviews of peer-reviewed studies were conducted by Govender and Mars (2017) and updated by the author in this chapter. The results of the reviews were analysed thematically, and four relevant challenges relating to TBA services were highlighted both globally and specifically within the African school context.

3.2.3. Challenge one: Adoption and sustainability

Adoption of telehealth technology in Africa by Audiologists and patients has been slow. The reasons relate to high telecommunications costs, computer literacy issues, motivation to use technology, lack of an active e-health strategy and instability of electricity provision that greatly impedes the usage of ICT in schools. Several studies performed globally and within the African continent reflect that lack of computer literacy, reluctance towards change and preference towards traditional methods of service delivery pose key barriers to the adoption and sustainability of telehealth (Medhanyie et al. 2015; Schwarz, Ward & Willcock 2014; Scott Kruse et al. 2018).

Scott Kruse et al. (2018) identified 33 barriers to the uptake of telehealth. The identified issues included technically challenged staff (11%), followed by resistance to change (8%), cost (8%), reimbursement issues (5%) and level of education of patients that prevented them from using technology (5%). These findings are congruent with that of Medhanyie et al. (2015), who conducted a study into the success factors contributing to telehealth and mHealth within the SSA context. The study found that technology, user acceptance, short- and long-term funding, organisational factors and political or legislative aspects largely determine the successful outcomes of a telehealth programme.

Rourke, Bromwich and Chan (2014) stated that lack of user acceptance of technology is a primary reason for poor uptake of telehealth and that exposure to and experience with telehealth increases positivity. Telehealth services were never established to replace conventional service delivery methods but were developed to supplement current practices and increase access to services. A mindset shift is cardinal to the sustainability of telehealth services within the African context. A good starting point in addressing this issue is to conduct mass-scale e-readiness evaluations among teachers, CHW, health professionals, parents and learners to gauge the areas that need to be addressed within a telehealth acceptability model. General literacy levels are relatively low in Africa, with e-Literacy rates being even lower (Deen-Swarray 2016). Deen-Swarray (2016) conducted a study on e-literacy rates in Arica and found that both adoption and range of ICT use correlate with increased basic literacy and e-literacy rates. Integrating education, e-learning training and improving e-literacy rates is paramount to the successful uptake of telehealth in Africa. A further barrier to the adoption and sustainability is the lack of adequate infrastructure. The evident digital divide between urban and rural schools across Africa is exacerbated by the lack of stable ICT networks, electricity access and limitations of computers and videoconferencing facilities. While most governments across many African countries, including South Africa, have formulated policies to address the digital divide, there has been a lack of implementation to this point. In a study conducted in several African countries including Nigeria, Uganda and Madagascar, it was found that fewer than 5% of rural primary schools have access to electricity (UNESCO Institute for Statistics 2015). Other countries such as South Africa, Tanzania and Lesotho had comparatively better electricity coverage in rural primary schools of around 20% (UNESCO Institute for Statistics 2015); however, connectivity issues remain a concern. Racial inequalities in the past geographical landscape of the rural areas and the lack of adequate and safe access and entry to some rural and remote areas of Africa are all contributory factors to the lack of adequate infrastructure. Electricity and connectivity are essential components in creating an ICT-enabled environment for tele-audiology services in rural African schools.

3.2.4. Challenge two: Comprehensive service delivery

Most TBA studies conducted in the African school context are based on screening outcomes. It is widely known that access to specialist and diagnostic services within the rural African context is challenging. The realistic approach to holistic management of auditory childhood disorders as well as to ensure prevention and promotion of hearing and ear care would be to introduce a comprehensive audiology programme within the school context, ensuring the identification of hearing impairment is followed up by appropriate intervention and management strategies. This would result in beneficial outcomes across the different facades of a person's life, ultimately contributing to economic benefits for a country. Figure 3.1 displays the long-term positive impact of early detection and intervention.

This implies an integration of all audiology services within a telehealth programme from screening to management. More attention needs to be given to diagnostic and intervention services as most studies conducted on

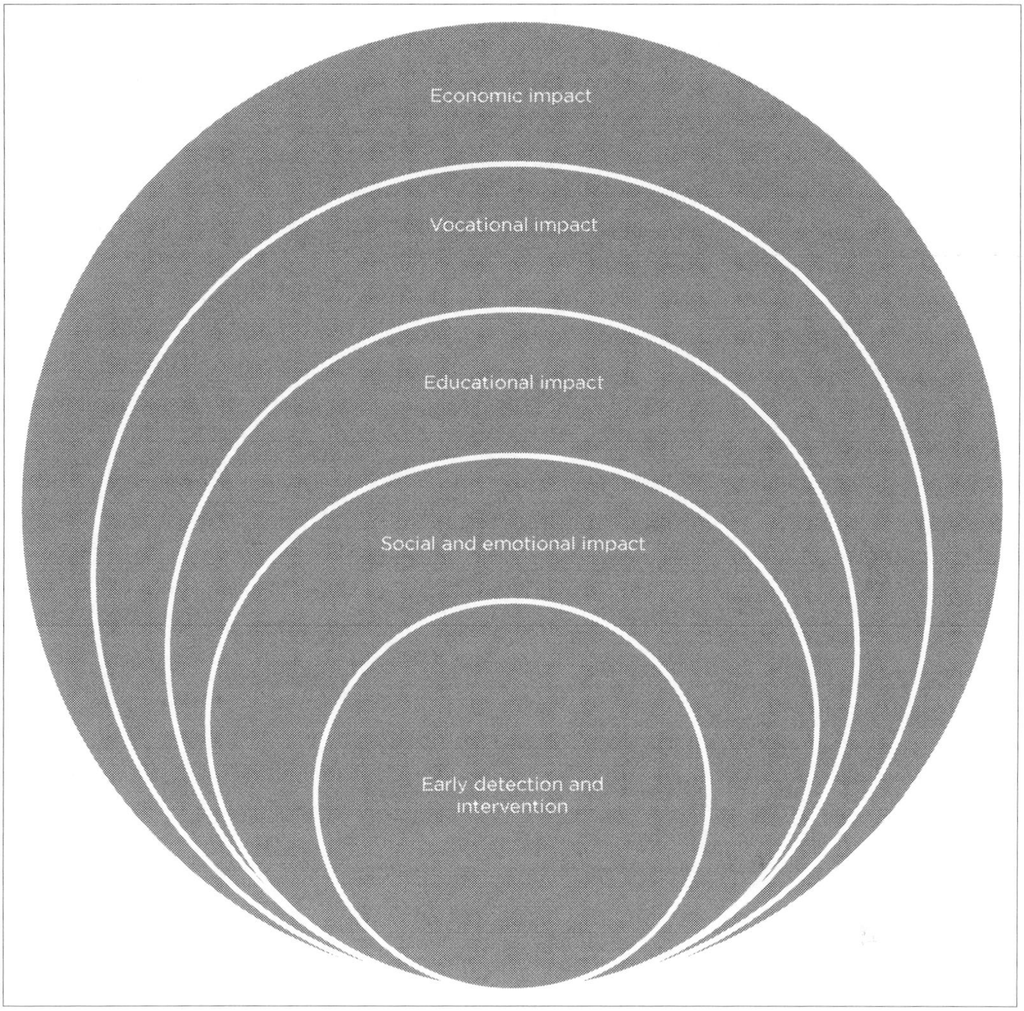

FIGURE 3.1: Depiction of the positive impact of early identification.

telehealth services in schools are based on screening data (Govender & Mars 2017). Screening services are only effective if follow-up diagnostic services are provided. However, the availability of assistive devices after the assessment is completed is constrained by financial issues (Wilson et al. 2017). Studies done in Southern African countries indicate that there is a disproportionate relationship between the availability of assistive devices and the prevalence of disorders, with provision favouring mobility challenges over communication disorders, despite the higher prevalence of communication disorders in relation to other disorders (Matter & Eide 2018).

Contributing to the challenge of delivering comprehensive services is the lack of standardised protocols for TBA. Protocol adaptations are required to provide tele-audiology services to children (Hughes et al. 2012; Khoza-Shangase & Kassner 2013). These include the need for conditioning techniques prior to testing because of the complexity of the equipment, the need for correction factors and the inclusion of other tests such as tympanometry and speech audiometry testing within a telehealth test environment (Botasso et al. 2015; Maclennan-Smith, Swanepoel & Hall 2013). Modifications to conventional protocols should be developed based on evidence-based practice (Hughes et al. 2012).

3.2.5. Challenge three: Guidelines and policy formulation

According to Krupinski and Bernard (2014), developing operational, technical and ethical guidelines and standards is necessary to ensure the effective and safe delivery of quality health care. In addition, the recent reports of the American Medical Association (AMA) (2014, 2016) on coverage and payment of telehealth recommend that for payment to be made, the delivery of telehealth services must follow evidence-based practice guidelines to ensure patient safety, quality of care and positive health outcomes. One of the goals of the guidelines is to ensure that the standard of care provided via telehealth methods is comparable to and as reliable as the conventional methods of conducting such tests (Krupinski & Bernard 2014).

None of the African countries have developed a set of comprehensive, evidence-based practice, clinical or operational guidelines. South Africa provides general Ethical Guidelines for Good Practice in Telemedicine (HPCSA 2014). These guidelines, as well as several other procedural documents available in other African countries, are largely based on European- and American-based guidelines (World Medical Association [WMA] 2009). These available guidelines have some fundamental flaws. The HPCSA Ethical Guidelines, for example, do not speak to clinical guidelines. Clinical guidelines are developed by a team of experts that outline appropriate treatment and care as well as recommendations as well as rehabilitation and follow-up (Kredo et al. 2017). Clinical guidelines inform clinical decision-making for both the practitioner and the patient to ensure quality or process of care and patient outcomes. This would be especially important in documenting how these processes should take place for both an asynchronous and synchronous TBA programme. These are in effect operational and technical guidelines for telemedicine but not clinical guidelines. More importantly, none of the documents speak directly to tele-audiology.

As stated in the various African e-health strategies, clinical, operational, ethical, legal and technical guidelines are required. Of primary importance at present for tele-audiology are clinical and ethical guidelines. It would be difficult to apply generic guidelines within the school context. Using the example of school screening and diagnostic testing, the currently available guidelines in Africa state that it is the duty and responsibility of the consulting practitioner to obtain informed consent for telehealth purposes. The consulting practitioner, in this instance, would not necessarily be a medical practitioner but may be a school principal, or a district health or education official who is conducting the screening programme. Such detail requires careful articulation within school-based tele-audiology guidelines. In addition, the HPCSA guidelines require that a copy of the consent form be kept with the patient's records and a duplicate given to the patient. This has implications for gatekeeper access, confidentiality issues, password encryption, language issues and assurance of follow-up of recommendations; in other words, a good tracking and monitoring electronic system.

The HPCSA telemedicine guidelines further state that patient-initiated telehealth should be restricted to the circumstance in which a prior health care–patient relationship exists, thereby allowing the health care practitioner to obtain sufficient knowledge of the patient's clinical condition before making a diagnosis, treatment or recommendation. This will effectively block most, if not all, tele-audiology screening and diagnostic services in schools. There are also concerns about the validity of consent. Consent should ideally be obtained in the patient's first language, but the lexicons of African languages have failed to keep pace with technology and there are no words for many technical terms. In a study in KwaZulu-Natal, only 7% of patients at a rural hospital understood the sentence, 'I consent to a telemedicine consultation' in their mother tongue, isiZulu (Jack, Hlombe & Mars 2014). If the learner or caregivers cannot comprehend what is required or cannot interpret the terminology appropriately then this may render the informed consent invalid.

Another challenge related to tele-audiology guidelines in Africa is the fragmentation of related policies and guidelines. The sustainability and feasibility of the tele-audiology services within the African school context require a coordinated approach. Health departments, education departments and policymakers need to ensure the alignment of policies and plans. For example, policies relating to targeted screening of risk factors for hearing impairment, eEducation policies, the country's e-health strategy and school health policies should speak to coordinated efforts and joint funding to ensure maximum benefit and responsible usage of resources. There is merit in health and education departments coming together to pool their resources in setting up ICT infrastructure within schools so that such infrastructure can be used both for teaching and learning as well as to conduct medical surveillance.

The absence of guidelines for tele-audiology has been identified as a barrier to its uptake. Guidelines must therefore be developed to protect patients and practitioners and satisfy the concerns of regulators. They must be developed by local experts, be relevant to local needs and conditions, and be evidence or at least experience based. This will not be easy in the absence of broad and prolonged local experience in all aspects of tele-audiology. However, this should not be a deterrent and the work to develop guidelines needs to commence.

3.2.6. Challenge four: Education and training of health care professionals

One of the telehealth promotion strategies (see Govender & Mars 2018b), particularly within developing contexts, is to assimilate telehealth-care approaches into the education and training programmes of health care professionals to improve awareness, utility and sustainability in a variety of health care contexts (cf. Edirippulige, Armfield & Smith 2013). The benefits associated with telehealth provide the impetus for student and professional training across the health care disciplines. Students need to receive their training from institutions that have experienced faculty with relevant content knowledge and research experience in the field. In South Africa, for example, the DoH outlines 10 priorities (10-point plan) within the national service delivery agreement (NSDA), one of which is the need to improve health infrastructure, including the use of ICT and sophisticated technology to advance patient care (SANDoH 2012). One aspect identified within the strategic objectives is the need to improve telehealth capacity building. The strategy notes that educational opportunities in telehealth are limited, and the government therefore aims to promote capacity development in telehealth through education and research. Universities through their academic staff have been identified as key role players to facilitate this process. Related to this is the development of education and training courses that are well structured to provide the theoretical and practical competencies required for administering clinical and educational services via a telehealth model.

Telehealth can improve service delivery to remote and rural areas, reduce health service disparities that exist between socio-economic groups and reduce health costs. Education and training in this area would strengthen the capacity to deliver and sustain these services (Edirippulige et al. 2013). Ehnfors and Grobe (2004) mentioned that lack of technical knowledge is a real challenge facing health care professionals who may find themselves in the future working in a technologically driven health care system without the necessary competencies. This statement provides a strong motivation for education and training and the need for certification programmes for both academics and health care professionals. Frenk et al. (2010) mentioned that the transformation of education for health care professionals is needed to strengthen health systems. It was emphasised that ICT is important for transformative learning by exposing undergraduates to telehealth models of service delivery. In a study conducted by Govender and Mars (2017) on health sciences academics across several higher education institutions, it was found that 59% (n = 66) of academics were unfamiliar with terms such as synchronous and asynchronous services. Eighty per cent of academics felt it necessary to include telehealth into the curriculum. The majority (89%) did not conduct research in telehealth. Seventy-one per cent felt positive that telehealth could benefit their respective professions, and 30% stated that lack of standards creates a negative attitude towards the area and its sustainability. Most participants (77%) felt that their final-year students knew very little about telehealth upon exiting the programme. Table 3.1 below displays some of the findings from the study.

These findings support the view that education and training in TBA services must be accelerated. This is particularly important as countries around the world navigate through the current COVID-19 pandemic. It is fundamental that students be trained to work in a digital world.

In attempting to meet the training needs of students and graduates, Govender and Mars (2017) outlined six key areas that need to be included in a telehealth training programme. These areas are (1) terminology, standards, protocol and guidelines development associated with telehealth services, (2) contextually relevant practice, (3) computer literacy and technological competence, (4) limitations of telehealth services, (5) ethical issues and (6) data management with synchronous and asynchronous services.

Contextual relevance is important within health care, especially when one considers establishing infrastructure and rolling out technology to promote health services. In a context where social determinants of health have contributed to inequitable distribution of health in terms of its resources and

TABLE 3.1: Attitudes of South African academics regarding telehealth (n = 66).

Item	Yes	%
Telehealth can positively impact our profession.	47	71
Lack of standards, guidelines and policy make it difficult to implement such practice.	20	30
Face-to-face contact is central to our professional interaction, making tele-audiology inappropriate.	10	15
Telehealth can address the barriers to services related to access and language between clinician and patient.	47	71
Telehealth can improve health service delivery in SA.	47	71
Telehealth is a promising concept, provided that a structured curriculum is designed to train students appropriately.	50	76
I think that telehealth is sustainable within the SA context.	32	48
Introducing Telehealth into clinical training would not improve learning outcomes by increasing exposure to more diverse patients.	18	27

Source: Govender and Mars (2017).

access (McLaren, Ardington & Leibbrandt 2013), together with redressing the injustices of the past, careful consideration must be taken to ensure that these service delivery models are both feasible and sustainable.

Data management and technological competences are a particularly important part of telehealth services, especially when one considers the intricacies associated with the storage, retrieval and transmission of patient information. Failure to do so adequately could result in malpractice. According to Scott Kruse et al. (2018), understanding technology, together with its advancement and development, is absolutely integral in promoting the progression of the science behind telehealth. They emphasised that it is important to also understand how the patient views technology and its ability to assist them in health care. This understanding is largely developed from the information imparted by a knowledgeable health care provider. Understanding how technology works is important, considering that telehealth technology can range from simple videoconferencing technology to sophisticated computer programmes and virtual environments (Karr 2012). While countries around the world and in Africa have significantly progressed in providing medical technology and information systems to support the health care system, the lack of trained professionals has resulted in its under-utilisation (Jobson 2015). The future of telehealth services depends largely on the pursuit of high-quality training and development, as it is difficult to envisage technological-based health care without transforming the training of health care professionals.

An understanding of legal and ethical issues related to telehealth service delivery is crucial for effective practice (George, Whitehouse & Duquenouy 2013). Ethical practice guides professional behaviour and is central to service delivery. Townsend and Scott (2019) outlined several current ethical challenges facing the implementation of telehealth practices in Africa. These include the fluidity of the doctor-patient relationship, privacy, confidentiality, data protection, accountability, liability, consent, record-keeping, data storage and authentication. It is essential that ethical practice is regulated by professional bodies to ensure equitable, standardised and fair practice. Townsend and Scott (2019) further articulated the need for guidelines to speak to the triangulation of patient protection rights, transformative practice and health care innovation. Recently, Naudé and Bornman (2021) carefully deliberated on ethical challenges relating to EHDI in the context of tele-audiology within the South African context, where they asserted that ethical challenges in this area refer to six concepts; (1) licensure, (2) competence, (3) privacy and confidentiality, (4) informed consent, (5) effectiveness of services and programme validation and (6) reimbursement for services.

3.3. Recommendations and solutions

Several challenges were highlighted in the aforementioned discussion. To advance TBA services in the African context, there needs to be clear articulation from policy to implementation and monitoring. This is important to ensure both sustainability and quality of services provided. In addition, for the sustainability of TBA, consideration must be within the auspices of the current health funding model of countries. As an example, South Africa is currently underway in rolling out its NHI programme (DoH 2019). This programme is intended to pool health funding so that there is equitable and equal distribution of health resources. It is recommended that key stakeholders engage governments to incorporate tele-based programmes into the fiscal policy. This would ensure that the necessary support and prioritisation are given to such programmes. The proposed developmental model for TBA services within the African school context has been developed by the author of this chapter, and this is depicted in Figure 3.2 (PRIME sustainability model for tele-audiology). The PRIME maturity model is proposed to advance the utility and sustainability of telehealth by ensuring the development and usage of protocols and guidelines, ensuring that all audiometric procedures and processes are reliable and valid by applying integration and organisation of resource distribution, particularly within health and education in order to reduce expenditure, to apply effective management solutions over TBA services and finally to ensure education and training of professions, as well as monitoring and evaluation of TBA programmes. A maturity model assists in improving capacity and efficiency by providing structure to implement and sustain a programme. Against the backdrop of the current economic climate and societal health care challenges, sustainability models propose the efficient utility of financial and human resources. In addition, such models can support, maintain and increase the economic benefits of such a model by reducing negative effects, thereby ensuring longevity and future utility of the service.

The PRIME sustainability model is a five-stage process to ensure that the appropriate components are considered when tele-audiology programmes within the school context are considered. Protocols, standards and guidelines are navigational tools needed by all key role players working towards the development and application of tele-audiology programmes in schools. Protocols provide a reasonable sequence of how the service should be delivered and ensures the future service delivery is consistent and offers consensus in practice for all health care professionals. Protocols can be revised and adapted alongside best practice guidelines and clinical discretion. These changes are often first discussed and approved by professional bodies before being adopted. Standards are aligned to regulations within a particular profession or country (ESG 2015). These standards are formulated by various structures and stakeholders. Guidelines ensure reliability and quality assurance

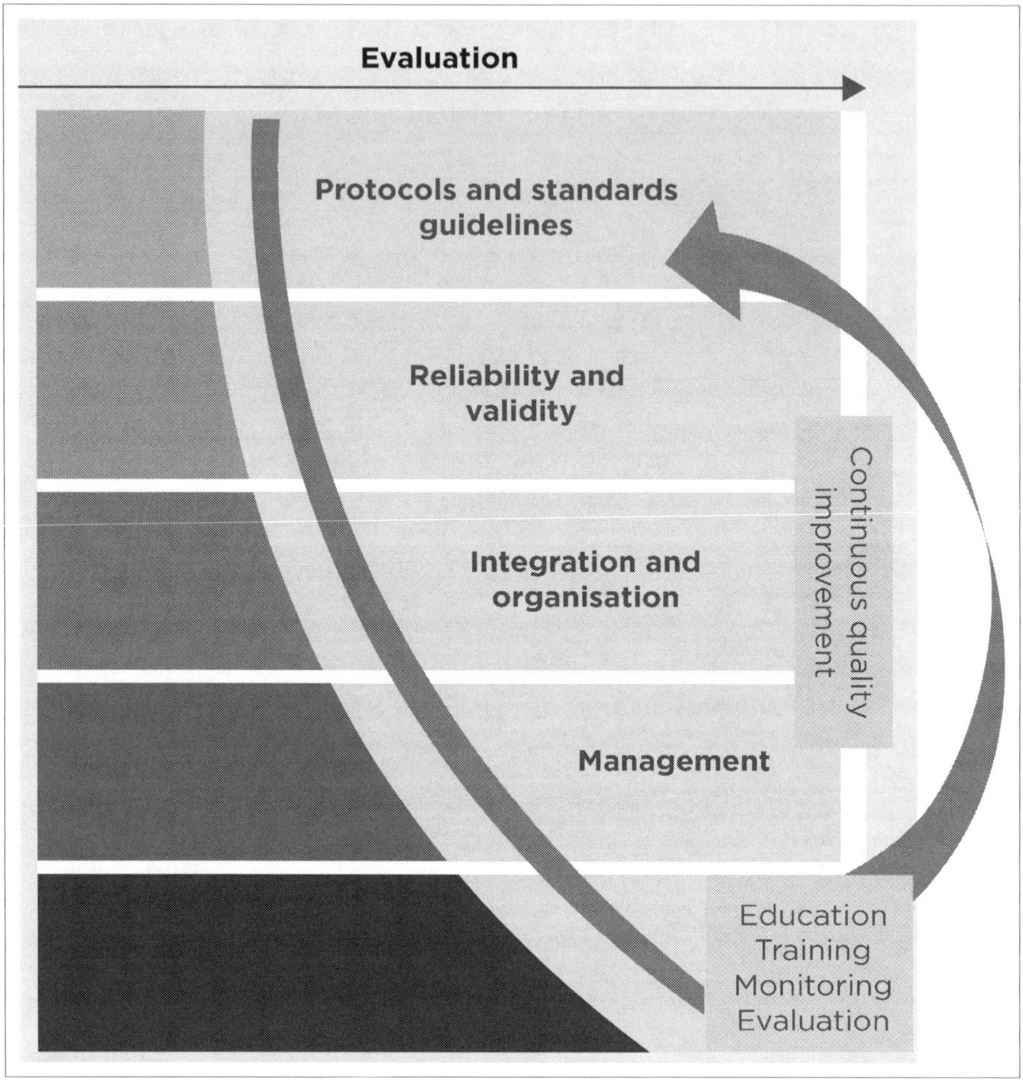

FIGURE 3.2: PRIME sustainability model for tele-audiology.

(ESG 2015). Health care professionals have stated that while they find telehealth to be a practical and resourceful addition to traditional health practices, the lack of guidelines raises concerns in the reliability of test outcomes. Reliability and validity of test equipment and protocols must be an ongoing process and must be extended to diverse populations to ensure generalisability. Integration and organisation are of particular importance within the African context given the constrained resources. The preferred approach would be to integrate TBA into the current audiology service delivery framework. The integration must be seamless and logical.

More importantly, the integration must be evidence-based. An implementation plan that includes coordination between the DoE and DoH would be mutually beneficial, practical and cost-efficient. Management in this model does not only refer to managing the audiological programme within the school context but refers to change management and capacity building through education, training and development. Ongoing and consistent evaluation of health care models and systems is synonymous with quality assurance measures. As depicted in Figure 3.2, this maturity model is not a linear, once-off approach but suggests a feedback loop. This implies that all aspects must continually be considered to improve the quality and standard of health care delivery through TBA services.

■ 3.4. Conclusion

Africa faces numerous challenges when it comes to addressing the health care needs of children. Poverty, burden of disease, limited access to services and under-resourced health care facilities impact on health and QoL outcomes for children. Sensory deficits are prevalent among African children. Hearing impairment can negatively impact the academic, social, emotional and vocational areas of a child's life. Audiology services offered within the school context offer a solution to the reduction in hearing impairment among children; however, this has been met with several challenges, including infrastructure inadequacies, financial and human resource limitations and the lack of a coordinated and sustained approach. Telehealth-based audiology services are feasible and can be useful in identifying hearing impairment for children in rural and remote areas. The widespread utility of TBA services is constrained by four primary key challenges. These include *adoption and sustainability, comprehensive service delivery, guidelines and policy formulation, education and training of health care professionals* and *ongoing quality improvement*. A sustainability model is proposed to facilitate the growth and maturity of tele-audiology within the African school context and consists of processes including the development, revision and ongoing reviewing of protocols and guidelines, maintaining and evaluating test reliability and validity, integration and coordination of resources, platforms and funding by key role players so that there is a collaborative response to TBA services, and finally the management and evaluation of programmes and services to ensure quality assurance.

Chapter 4

Community-based audiology services: An effective strategy for the prevention of hearing loss in rural communities

Karin Joubert
Department of Audiology, Faculty of Humanities,
School of Human and Community Development,
University of the Witwatersrand,
Johannesburg, South Africa

■ 4.1. Introduction

Irrespective of the age of onset, disabling hearing loss is a complex phenomenon with devastating consequences. There is a global concern over the rapid increase of disabling hearing loss, which is mostly because of the corresponding rise and ageing of the global population. It is estimated that by the year 2030, 630 million people will live with disabling hearing loss (WHO 2020b). This staggering projection demands action to prevent hearing loss, especially in the rural areas of LMICs such as South Africa. In this chapter, the author defines health access, outlines strategies for the prevention of hearing

How to cite: Joubert, K 2022, 'Community-based audiology services: An effective strategy for the prevention of hearing loss in rural communities', ed. K Khoza-Shangase, *Preventive audiology: An African perspective*, AOSIS Books, Cape Town, pp. 65–91. https://doi.org/10.4102/aosis.2022.BK209.04

loss and deliberates on challenges faced by rural communities in accessing ear-and-hearing health care, contextualises the current status of hearing health services in rural South Africa, and proposes an audiology service delivery model that will improve access to affordable, cost-effective, quality hearing health services in these areas. All this is carried out to ensure sustainable universal audiology service provision, in line with the WHO's UHC imperative, which the country is aiming for with the new NHI bill.

The right to access ear-and-hearing health care by people who live in rural communities is a global issue, as untreated hearing loss is more prevalent in these communities (Chan et al. 2018; Joubert & Botha 2019). Hearing loss negatively impacts the person with hearing loss and his family (WHO 2020b). The functional impact of untreated hearing loss includes the individuals' ability to communicate with others, as well as the academic performance of children and young adults. The communication challenges lead to social and emotional difficulties, which can cause feelings of frustration, loneliness and isolation, especially in older individuals with hearing loss. The economic impact of untreated hearing loss on the health sector, costs of educational support, loss of productivity and societal costs are significant (WHO 2020b). It has also been found that adults with hearing loss have a higher unemployment rate than those with normal hearing (WHO 2020b). Hearing loss is thus positively correlated with poverty, educational attainment and manual labour - issues that are prominent in rural areas (Chan et al. 2018). Rural communities that already face limited access to hearing health services, with high unemployment and poverty rates, are thus adversely affected by untreated hearing loss (Chan et al. 2018).

4.2. Background

4.2.1. Access to health care

Access to health care is a complicated concept, as is demonstrated in the diversity of interpretations of the concept among researchers (Edusei & Amoah 2014; Levesque, Harris & Russell 2013). Access is defined as a way or means of approach or entry; as the right to approach, reach, enter or make use of something (Collins Dictionary 2020), while it has also been defined as the degree of 'fit' between clients and the system in question (Penchansky & Thomas 1981). Specifically, access to health care refers to '[...] the opportunity to identify health care needs, to seek health care services, to reach, to obtain or use health care services and to actually have the need for services fulfilled' (Levesque et al. 2013, p. 8). For us to understand what access to health care involves, the factors that influence the entry to or use of a given health care system require clarification.

The comprehensive and multifaceted nature of Levesque and colleagues' (2013) definition of access to health care highlights that factors relating to structural features should be considered when assessing access (Edusei & Amoah 2014). Five dimensions that have been identified to influence one's ability and willingness to enter or use a facility or service, as depicted in Figure 4.1, include (1) availability, (2) accessibility, (3) affordability, (4) accommodation and (5) acceptability (Edusei & Amoah 2014).

□ 4.2.1.1. Availability

Availability refers to the opportunities and options people have concerning health care (Edusei & Amoah 2014). It implies that health services (either the physical space or appropriate type of service providers and resources) can be easily reached in a timely manner (Levesque et al. 2013; Peters et al. 2008). Often, the availability of services is measured using indicators such as the

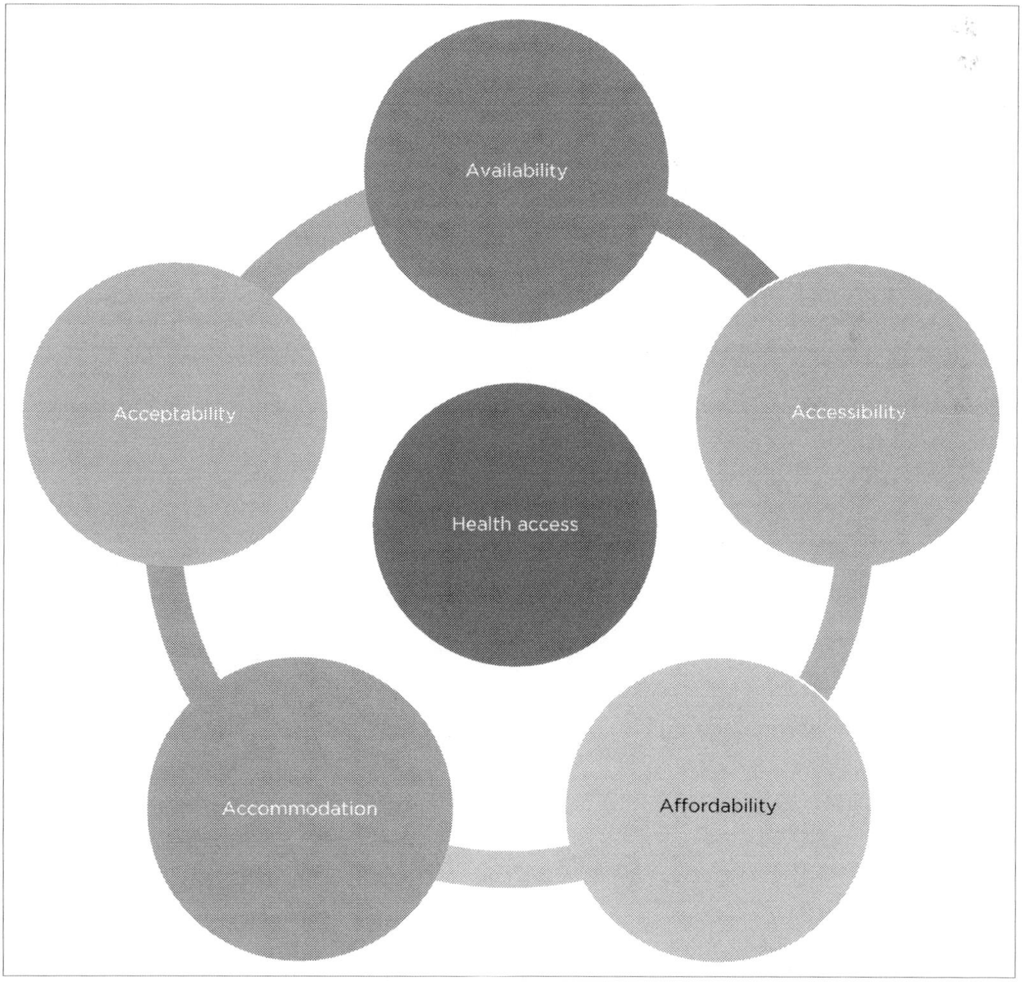

FIGURE 4.1: Dimensions of health access.

number of health care workers (e.g. audiologists) per unit population. The author contends that issues relating to the availability of health services, especially hearing health services, are some of the reasons why rural communities are marginalised, particularly within the African context.

◻ 4.2.1.2. Accessibility

Accessibility denotes the physical distance or travelling time from the location of the user to the service delivery point (Edusei & Amoah 2014; Peters et al. 2008), in this case ear-and-hearing health care facilities. If available resources are unevenly spread around geographical locations and across levels of health care, access is deemed to be restricted. Distance to facilities, travel time, quality of roads and access to transport are important factors in when, where and how people use health care services (Peters et al. 2008).

◻ 4.2.1.3. Affordability

Affordability implies the financial capacity to use resources and time to access relevant health services (Levesque et al. 2013). The financial component is one of the key factors that allow or prevent individuals from using health services of their choice (Edusei & Amoah 2014). The costs of accessing health care include direct user fees (treatment fees), related costs (transport, medication, food and accommodation) and opportunity costs (travel and waiting times) (Peters et al. 2008). The impact of these costs depends on the user's willingness and ability to pay.

◻ 4.2.1.4. Accommodation

Accommodation entails the adequacy of the services, how the services are provided, and the integrated and continuous nature thereof (Edusei & Amoah 2014). The accommodative nature of a given service includes factors such as hours of operation, appointment systems, waiting times, and the technical and interpersonal quality of the services provided (Edusei & Amoah 2014). Some people may be either encouraged or discouraged by the status of one or more of these factors (Peters et al. 2008). Long waiting times, poor queue management or unfriendly and unprofessional staff may, for example, dissuade patients from accessing health services. It is also argued that less educated members of society may have difficulties in accessing health services because of a lack of knowledge and information, illiteracy and ignorance (Edusei & Amoah 2014). In this vein, accommodation is related to potential users' health literacy, self-efficacy and self-management, as well as their capacity to communicate their needs (Levesque et al. 2013).

4.2.1.5. Acceptability

Acceptability is '[...] the match between how responsive health service providers are to the social and cultural expectations of individual users and communities' (Peters et al. 2008, p. 162). Levesque and colleagues (2013) included professional values, norms, gender and culture as factors related to acceptability. It thus represents people's expectations and perceptions regarding the services provided in relation to the factors mentioned (Peters et al. 2008).

In summary, the ability of governments to address health problems is affected by several wide-ranging factors, including the availability of health services, affordability of services, accessibility of the services, the accommodating nature of the available services and how acceptable the available services and facilities are to the user (Edusei & Amoah 2014).

4.2.2. The South African health care system

The South African health care system is divided between the private and public sectors, with most of the population (82.21%) dependent on the public sector for health care (Statistics South Africa [StatsSA] 2017). Since the year 1994, the government has made progress toward the reform and improvement of the public health sector (Burger & Christian 2018). With the expansion of the physical availability of public health facilities, the geographical availability of these services has improved, especially for the poorest and most marginalised (Burger & Christian 2018). Despite the increased geographical availability of health services, the health care system is distressed (Dhai & Mahomed 2018) and fraught with problems, which negatively impacts its service delivery. Identified challenges include ineffective leadership and management (Dhai & Mahomed 2018; Malakoane et al. 2020; Taylor et al. 2018), fragmentation of health services (Malakoane et al. 2020), poor financial management (Dhai & Mahomed 2018; Malakoane et al. 2020), chronic staff shortages (Dhai & Mahomed 2018; Malakoane et al. 2020; Taylor et al. 2018), equipment shortages (Maphumulo & Bhengu 2019) and increased litigation costs (Maphumulo & Bhengu 2019; Taylor et al. 2018).

South Africa's public health care system is built upon the primary health care (PHC) approach. This approach addresses the main health problems in the community by providing promotive, preventive, curative and rehabilitative services (DoH 2017). According to the Alma-Ata Declaration, PHC is the first level of contact for individuals, families and communities with the national health system, which brings health care as close as possible to where people live and work and constitutes the first element of a continuing health care process (WHO 1978, p. 1). However, the concentration of resources and services in hospitals relies on expensive curative services at the expense of early interventions that are aimed at health promotion and prevention of disease. With curative services as the priority, rehabilitation services are also neglected. Curative services remain one of the most significant cost drivers of the public health care system (Eagar, Rensburg & Versteeg-Mojanaga 2013).

In pursuit of UHC, the South African government recently promulgated the NHI bill. *Universal health coverage* means that:

> [*A*]ll individuals and communities receive the health services they need without suffering financial hardship. It includes the full spectrum of essential, quality health services, from health promotion to prevention, treatment, rehabilitation, and palliative care. (WHO 2020a:n.p.)

Three related objectives are represented in this definition: equity in access to health services, quality health services that will improve the health of users and financial risk protection (DoH 2017). The adoption and achievement of UHC will go a long way to help the country achieve SDG Goal 3 (to ensure healthy lives and promote well-being for all at all ages), which was adopted in 2015 by the UN.

The NHI aims to build on the reforms already implemented in the country. Designed as a health financing system, the NHI will pool funds with which services can be purchased to provide all South Africans with universal access to quality, affordable personal health services, regardless of their socio-economic status. Health services that will be covered by the NHI will be free and specific to an individual's need for health care. It is envisaged that the implementation of the NHI will 'address structural imbalances in the health system and reduce the burden of disease' (DoH 2017). As a response to the current challenges in the health care system (such as poor performance and persistent inequalities), the NHI further aims to improve quality, coverage and equity for vulnerable subgroups (Burger & Christian 2018), such as those living in rural communities.

4.2.3. Rurality

Rurality is more than a geographical location as it also refers to the 'structure, state, and QoL of people living in sparsely populated areas' (Duncan, Sherry & Watson 2011, p. 42). These complexities in defining rurality are acknowledged by Watermeyer and Barratt (2013) who defined rural areas as:

> [*R*]emote areas with poor infrastructure, poor basic service provision, low levels of literacy, high levels of unemployment, limited access to health and education services, and high incidence of communicable diseases such as HIV and AIDS. (p. 3)

The Rural Health Advocacy Project (RHAP) uses the term 'rural' more specifically in relation to rural health care access. According to the RHAP definition, 'rural' is typically characterised by six aspects: geographical remoteness and long distances between levels of care, topographical features (e.g. mountainous landscapes) that hinder physical access to health care, low population densities, high cost of service delivery because of lower economies of scale, difficulties in recruiting and retaining health care workers, and a common characterisation by higher levels of deprivation than urban areas (Eagar et al. 2013).

4.3. Prevalence of hearing loss: Current trends

The rates of hearing loss around the globe are set to increase significantly over the next century (WHO 2018). The WHO (2020b) estimated that by the year 2030, nearly 630 million people will have disabling hearing loss. This number will rise even further to 900 million by 2050 if the current demographic trends continue. The extent of this problem is further reflected in the 1.1 billion young people alone who are at risk of hearing loss because of exposure to loud sounds in recreational settings (Chadha, Kamenov & Cieza 2019). The global financial burden of unaddressed hearing loss is significant and is projected at more than US$750bn annually (WHO 2020b). The changing profile of global hearing loss will be more evident in the South Asian, Asia Pacific and sub-Saharan Africa regions, where the prevalence is currently estimated to be nearly four times that of high-income areas (WHO 2018). This calls for careful planning around the prevention of hearing loss by LMICs, such as South Africa.

4.4. Prevention of hearing loss

The alarming rise in the prevalence of hearing loss was recognised at the 70th World Health Assembly (WHA), which adopted resolution WHA 70.13 on the prevention of deafness and hearing loss in 2017 (Box 4.1). South Africa, as an active member state of the WHO, is included in the call to take stronger action to integrate strategies for ear-and-hearing health care within the framework of its health system and to ensure that these services are accessible to those who need them (WHO 2017b). Resolution WHA 70.13 includes nine guidelines that serve as a roadmap to achieving universal hearing care, particularly in LMICs. Adhering to these guidelines will close the gap between the high need for hearing services, low demand because of limited awareness and the low supply of hearing care resources (e.g. workforce, equipment and technology).

Governments, hearing health care professionals and other stakeholders should embrace this high-level global interest in the disability-inclusive development agenda (WHO 2018). This level of interest should be used as the impetus behind taking steps toward active implementation of contextually relevant programmes to stem the upward rise of disabling hearing loss.

BOX 4.1: WHO guidelines for the prevention of deafness and hearing loss.

Member states of the World Health Organization are urged to:
• Integrate strategies for ear-and-hearing health care within the framework of their primary health care systems, under the umbrella of universal health coverage, by such means as raising awareness at all levels and building political commitment and intersectoral collaboration.
• Collect high-quality population-based data on ear diseases and hearing loss to develop evidence-based strategies and policies.
• Establish suitable training programmes for the development of human resources in the field of ear-and-hearing health care.
• Ensure the highest possible vaccination coverage against rubella, measles, mumps and meningitis, in line with the immunisation targets of the Global Vaccine Action Plan 2011–2020, and in accordance with national priorities.
• Develop, implement and monitor screening programmes for early identification of ear diseases, such as chronic suppurative otitis media and hearing loss in high-risk populations, including infants, young children, older adults and individuals exposed to noise in occupational and recreational settings.
• Improve access to affordable, cost-effective, high-quality, assistive hearing technologies and products, including hearing aids, cochlear implants and other assistive devices, as part of universal health care coverage, taking into account the delivery capacity of health care systems equitably and sustainably.
• Develop and implement regulations for the control of noise in occupational settings, at entertainment venues and through personal audio systems, as well as for the control of ototoxic medicines.
• Improve access to a variety of ways of communicating through promoting alternative methods of communication, such as sign language and text captions.
• Actively work towards attaining the goals in UNESCOs 2030 Agenda for Sustainable Development SDG 3 to ensure a healthy lifestyle and to promote well-being for all individuals of all ages. SDG 4 aims to provide inclusive and equitable quality education and promote lifelong learning opportunities for all individuals. These two sustainable development goals (SDGs) have specific reference to individuals experiencing hearing loss.

Source: WHO (2017b, p. 2).

Encouragingly, it is suggested that 50% of all cases of hearing loss can be prevented through public health measures (WHO 2019). In children (0–15 years), it is estimated that 60% of hearing loss may be attributed to preventable causes, such as infections (including cytomegalovirus, chronic OM, measles, meningitis and mumps), complications at the time of birth and use of ototoxic medicines in expecting mothers and babies (WHO 2019). In LMICs, this figure is significantly higher at 75% (WHO 2019).

In support of World Health Assembly resolution WHA 70.13 highlighting the issue of deafness and hearing loss, practical strategies to guide the prevention of deafness and hearing loss have been published (Olusanya, Neumann & Saunders 2014; WHO 2019), which should be adapted to the specific needs for hearing health care of a country. Three levels of prevention are proposed: primary, secondary and tertiary levels, with typical activities outlined for each of the levels (Figure 4.2). These prevention strategies are relevant to all age groups. Specific disorders and risk factors related to deafness and hearing loss are included for each age group.

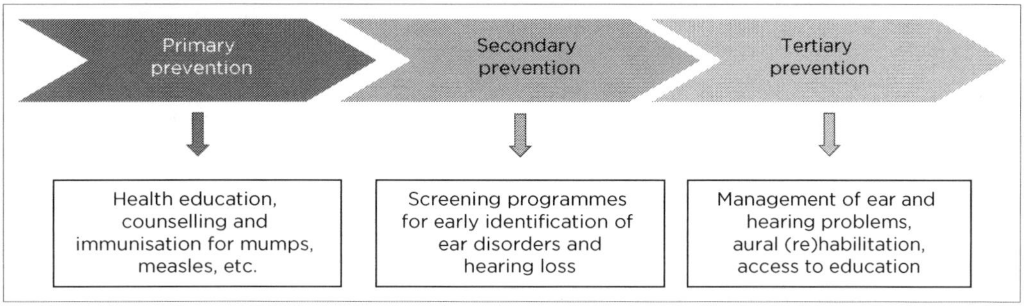

FIGURE 4.2: Hearing loss prevention strategies.

4.4.1. Primary prevention

In LMICs, the primary prevention of deafness and hearing loss must be prioritised. Primary prevention largely involves the promotion of a healthy lifestyle, better nutrition and personal hygiene, health education, counselling and immunisation against diseases such as measles, meningitis, mumps and rubella (WHO 2019). Primary prevention, for the most part, can be integrated within the framework of PHC services. A thorough understanding of the aetiology of and risk factors for hearing loss in a given population is, however, critical before implementation (Olusanya et al. 2014).

With health education being one of the most important primary prevention strategies, health care workers at all levels of care should be empowered with the knowledge to provide appropriate health education and counselling to the public. Specific focus should be placed on (1) the risk factors for hearing loss, (2) practices related to healthy ear care and safe listening and (3) the role of the audiologist in the identification and management of hearing-related problems.

The Extended Programme on Immunisation (EPI), initiated by the 27th WHA in 1974, is an example of the success of primary prevention strategies. In 2014, immunisation against diseases such as measles, meningitis, mumps and rubella protected more than 80% of children across the world from preventable conditions (Davis 2019). It has been found that immunisation remains the most cost-effective public health care intervention (Davis 2019; DoH 2014).

4.4.2. Secondary prevention

The focus of secondary prevention is on the implementation of screening programmes for the early identification of ear diseases (e.g. otitis externa and acute or chronic OM), impacted cerumen, foreign bodies and hearing loss (Olusanya et al. 2014; WHO 2019). These screening programmes should target high-risk populations, such as infants, young children, people exposed to occupational and recreational noise, and older adults (WHO 2017b). Examples of screening programmes include universal neonatal screening and routine screening on formal school-entry. Should ear disease or hearing loss be identified, prompt treatment and management are recommended (Olusanya et al. 2014). Chapters 5, 6, 7, and 11 in this book provide evidence, challenges and solutions for the South African context on secondary-level prevention in early detection of middle ear pathologies, NHS, ototoxicity and early detection of occupational-and environmental noise.

The management of hearing loss throughout the life course is important as events and experiences earlier in life (such as middle ear pathologies, use of ototoxic medication and prolonged exposure to occupational-and recreational noise) may contribute to hearing loss later in life (Davis et al. 2016). According to the life course health development (LCHD) model (Halfon & Hochstein 2002; Halfon et al. 2014), the promotion of healthy hearing is a lifelong process (Davis et al. 2016).

4.4.3. Tertiary prevention

Once hearing loss has been identified, tertiary prevention activities should be implemented to minimise the associated negative consequences of hearing loss. These activities include the fitting of hearing amplification devices (such as hearing aids and cochlear implants), aural habilitation or rehabilitation, sign language training and, most importantly, access to education (Olusanya et al. 2014) and employment.

The afore-presented prevention strategies provide governments, hearing health care professionals and other stakeholders with concrete guidelines on how to arrest the current upward trend in the global burden of hearing impairment. Using the UHC impetus and drive towards implementation of NHI, the prevention of hearing loss must be prioritised by the South African government. This is particularly important as hearing loss has become a major global health concern and is now ranked as the fourth leading contributor of years lived with disability (Wilson et al. 2017).

Increasing awareness of the problem of deafness and hearing loss has resulted in increasing demand for ear and hearing health care services worldwide, including in sub-Saharan Africa.

4.5. Ear-and-hearing health care in sub-Saharan Africa

The prevalence rate of disabling hearing loss globally is 6.12% (Mulwafu et al. 2016). A systematic review of hearing loss in sub-Saharan Africa indicated that the prevalence rate of hearing loss ranged from 7.7% in children and school-based studies to 17% for population-based studies (Mulwafu, Kuper & Ensink 2016). Given the ageing population and other illnesses such as HIV and tuberculosis, Mulwafu et al. (2016) asserted that the burden of hearing loss will likely increase dramatically in sub-Saharan Africa.

Despite the growing demand for ear-and-hearing health care services in sub-Saharan Africa, access to these services is limited. A survey conducted in 22 sub-Saharan African countries provided evidence-based data on the availability of ear-and-hearing health care services in these countries (Mulwafu et al. 2017). The data indicate that across the sample, the ratio of otorhinolaryngologists to the population was 1:1.2 and 1:0.8 million for audiologists (Mulwafu et al. 2017). However, if the numbers of audiologists from Kenya, Sudan and South Africa are excluded, the numbers of audiologists become extremely low (Mulwafu et al. 2017). This practitioner-to-population ratio negatively affects the coverage rate for ear-and-hearing health care services.

To complicate matters further, the availability of relevant equipment and assistive devices to render these services is limited. Most countries included in Mulwafu et al.'s (2017) study (66%–87%) rated the availability of equipment as non-existent or poor. Respondents concurred that the lack of basic equipment is the most significant limitation in providing services (Mulwafu et al. 2017). Another study reported that, overall, in four sub-Saharan countries (South Africa, Namibia, Malawi and Sudan), the provision of assistive technology, such as hearing aids and rehabilitation services, was poor and fragmented (Visagie et al. 2017).

No information was available on the accessibility, affordability, accommodation and acceptability of ear-and-hearing health care services in the sub-Saharan region.

4.6. Ear-and-hearing health care services in South Africa: A rural perspective

4.6.1. Prevalence of hearing loss

In South Africa, an LMIC, hearing loss is the third-highest reported disability after visual impairment and physical disability (StatsSA 2012). The findings of two population-based surveys, one in an urban Western Cape metropolitan area (Cape Town) and one in the rural population in the Limpopo province, differ significantly. In Cape Town, the prevalence rate of disabling hearing loss was estimated to be 4.57% (Ramma & Sebothoma 2016), while in rural Limpopo, the estimated prevalence was 8.94% (Joubert & Botha 2019). The latter is significantly higher than the global prevalence rate of 6.12%, which is influenced by various factors.

4.6.1.1. Associated factors

In both aforementioned communities, two factors - age and hypertension - were associated with hearing loss (Joubert & Botha 2019; Ramma & Sebothoma 2016). The association between disabling hearing loss and advanced age is well-known (Joubert & Botha 2019; WHO 2018; Wilson et al. 2017). The projected global population growth and ageing will significantly increase the number of people affected by hearing loss. It is estimated that between 2015 and 2050, the population will double and triple for those older than 60-80-years-old, respectively (WHO 2018). Hearing loss in these age groups should also be considered beyond its auditory complications because of the association with fall risk (Lubetzky 2020), social isolation, cognitive impairment and depression (Jayakody et al. 2018). Despite the non-preventable nature of age-related hearing loss, early identification and appropriate management are essential to mitigate the impact on the overall well-being, interpersonal communication and QoL of these individuals (Joubert & Botha 2019).

As far as hypertension is concerned, cardiovascular disease, as an associated factor to hearing loss, was confirmed in a systematic review conducted by Rosenhall and Sundh (2006). Low-frequency hearing loss was reported in this population, especially in females. Findings from a South African study supported this association as 5% of individuals between 40-55-years-old diagnosed with cardiovascular disease presented low-frequency hearing loss (Solanki 2012).

In urban areas, a history of head and neck trauma and being male was reported as a significantly associated factor. In some areas of the Cape Town metropolitan area, such as Khayelitsha and Gugulethu, reports indicate a high rate of assault and violent crimes, and many young males are survivors of these crimes. (Nicol et al. 2014). Hearing loss following trauma to head and neck areas has been documented in the literature (Plaks, Khoza-Shangase & Joubert 2014; Ramma & Sebothoma 2016). On the other hand, a rural study showed more females than males with hearing loss, which may be due to the larger female population. In the rural population, the most notable causes of ear disease and hearing loss were impacted cerumen (10%) and OM (Joubert & Botha 2019).

The two population-based studies conducted were the first step in collecting data on ear diseases and hearing loss in South Africa. However, more high-quality population-based data are required to develop evidence-based and contextually relevant strategies and policies on ear-and-hearing health care services in the country (WHO 2017b).

4.6.2. Access to ear-and-hearing health care services

In rural areas, as in the rest of South Africa, the public sector is the main health care service provider. In 2017, 82.21% of the South African population was reportedly dependent on public health care services (StatsSA 2017). The 33.65% of the population who live in rural areas (World Bank 2019) mostly have access to only district hospitals, community health centres and PHC clinics. Poor, vulnerable and marginalised groups, such as individuals in rural communities, often suffer from conditions (such as ear and hearing disorders) that could have been prevented.

The next section discusses the current status of hearing health services and the challenges encountered in accessing hearing health care in the public sector in relation to the availability of services, the accommodative nature of these services, affordability of the services, accessibility of the services and how acceptable the available services are.

4.6.3. Availability of hearing care in the public health care sector

Within the South African context, audiology services are provided by qualified, HPCSA-registered audiologists. Within the public health care sector, the first point of entry for hearing health services are PHC clinics, from where service users are referred to relevant hospitals based on their needs (Khan, Joseph & Adhikari 2018).

Audiology services at community health centres, if available, are limited to basic diagnostic assessment and management. At the district level hospital, audiology services typically comprise screening of patients at risk for hearing loss, as well as diagnostic hearing assessment and management of hearing difficulties. Referrals are made to regional and tertiary hospitals that offer more specialised health care services such as vestibular assessment and management, as well as hearing amplification requiring surgical intervention (e.g. bone-anchored hearing aids and cochlear implants). Comprehensive audiological services are mainly located at tertiary-level (central) and regional hospitals. However, this pathway of care, as described above, is hampered by the limited availability of audiological services, particularly in rural communities (Khan et al. 2018; Pillay et al. 2020).

4.6.3.1. Range of hearing health care services

Despite the WHO recommendations that the primary and secondary prevention of deafness and hearing loss should be integrated at PHC level, audiology services are not typically available where the greatest need is or where the most significant impact can be made.

Regarding the *primary prevention* of hearing loss, there are positive initiatives at the PHC level to prevent deafness and hearing loss. One such initiative is the availability of EPI vaccines at all health care facilities included in the package of free health care services for women and children in

South Africa (Davis 2019). The coverage rate for fully immunised below-1-year-old children was reported at 82.3% in 2016/17, which was slightly lower than the 89.3% reported in 2014/15 (Burnett et al. 2019). This is positive as research has confirmed that immunisation remains the most cost-effective public health intervention (Davis 2019; SANDoH 2014).

Within the South African context, the first step toward the *secondary prevention* of hearing loss was taken in 2007. The HPCSA indicated that the systematic implementation and support of EHDI programmes in infants throughout South Africa should be prioritised (Theunissen & Swanepoel 2008). Disappointingly, the suggestion has not been implemented. A study conducted in the North West and Gauteng provinces of South Africa confirmed that no PHC clinics in these provinces offered formalised infant hearing screening programmes (Khoza-Shangase et al. 2017). In two other provinces, Western Cape and Limpopo, limited infant hearing screening services are available. In the Western Cape province, a systematic infant hearing screening programme was implemented at eight maternal and child health care clinics in the Cape metropolitan area (De Kock, Swanepoel & Hall 2016; Friderichs, Swanepoel & Hall 2012). In the Elias Motsoaledi local municipal area of the Limpopo province, infant hearing screening services are offered at three PHC clinics daily between 07:00–13:00. The services, managed by an audiologist, are offered by appropriately trained and paid community members. The effectiveness of this rural infant hearing screening service was confirmed (Kgare 2018). A retrospective record review indicated an overall coverage rate of 87% and a referral rate of 7%, a reasonably good referral rate for the context. Asmail, Swanepoel and Eikelboom (2016) highlighted that as referral rates increase, larger numbers of follow-up diagnostic assessments are needed. During the record review period, the overall prevalence rate of significant hearing impairment was 0.4/1000 with the prevalence rate of middle ear effusion at 7.8/1000 (Kgare 2018).

At secondary- and tertiary-level hospitals in the North West and Gauteng provinces, targeted infant hearing screening programmes were the predominant approach to early identification of hearing loss (Khoza-Shangase et al. 2017). Although research has been conducted on the feasibility and efficacy of infant hearing screening programmes, this has not led to the implementation of full-fledged programmes in all instances (Kanji 2018). Limited information is available on the current status of infant hearing screening in the other provinces of South Africa.

4.6.3.2. Staffing

Despite the proposed service pathways, audiologists and the required resources for the delivery of audiological health care services are not readily available to potential users at the different levels of care. This situation is not unique, as worldwide (62 countries surveyed) 86% indicated that they did not have enough audiologists to meet community needs (Goulios & Patuzzi 2008). Similar findings were reported for the sub-Saharan African region (Mulwafu et al. 2017). In South Africa, the otorhinolaryngologist-to-population ratio (per 100,000) was 0.46 and the ratio for audiologists was 0.827 in 2015 (Mulwafu et al. 2017). More recent figures indicate a decrease in the ratio for audiologists. The limited number of audiologists in South Africa was confirmed in a recent study by Pillay and colleagues (2020), which indicated an audiologist-to-population ratio (per 10 000) as 0.57. However, as for all health care professionals in South Africa, comprehensive information on the number of practising audiologists is insufficient because of limited information in the HPCSA database. There is evidence that even though health care professionals no longer practise their profession or may have emigrated, many maintain their registration with the HPCSA and may therefore be miscounted as part of the available services (Rispel et al. 2018).

Updated and accurate information regarding the distribution of audiologists between the public and private health care sectors is difficult to obtain. One of the barriers is that sometimes numbers of speech therapists and audiologists are combined in reports, making it difficult to extrapolate the exact number of audiologists practising in different contexts. The total number of speech therapists and audiologists employed in the public health care sector nationally in April 2018 was reported as 712 (Day, Gray & Ndlovu 2018).

There is also no updated information regarding the distribution of health care personnel between urban and rural areas. The distribution of personnel is aggravated by the (1) scarcity of posts for rehabilitation personnel in the public sector (Rispel et al. 2018) and (2) the lack of government funding for hearing health care (Goulios & Patuzzi 2008). The recruitment and retention of health care professionals in rural and underserved areas are global challenges that are well-documented in the literature (Eagar et al. 2013; SANDoH 2011).

To improve access to quality health care and increase the number of health care workers in South Africa, especially in previously underserved areas, the DoH introduced community service for newly qualified health care professionals in 2003 (DoH 2006). Although the one-year community service programme has significantly improved the availability of human resources in the public health sector, significant challenges exist that pose barriers to the delivery of health care services at the PHC level (Ned, Cloete & Mji 2017). Reported challenges include the inequitable distribution of resources (human and material), ineffective management, inaccessibility and lack of transport for professionals to render community-based services (Ned et al. 2017).

The preceding information confirms that with the changing profile and high prevalence of disabling hearing loss in South Africa, it is evident that there is a severe shortage of audiologists to meet the increasing need for hearing health care services.

4.6.3.3. Equipment

Audiologists require specialised equipment to render services. There is a dearth of information on the availability of audiological equipment in the South African public health care sector. A study conducted in 2014 determined the availability of audiological equipment for paediatric assessment and hearing aid fitting in the Gauteng province of South Africa (Teixeira & Joubert 2014). Although a wide range of equipment was available in public sector departments, their availability was not always appropriate for meeting the audiological needs of paediatric patients or was not accessible. In addition, the timely repair of equipment was reported as a significant challenge. This is disconcerting as the lack of functioning and well-maintained audiological equipment may affect the audiologists' ability to provide appropriate, evidence-based audiological services. Moreover, the high staff turnover may result in the under-utilisation of equipment and delivery services that may not be appropriate or meet the patient's audiological needs (Teixeira & Joubert 2014).

4.6.4. Accessibility of hearing health care services

The accessibility of hearing health care services relates to the physical distance or travel time to the service delivery point (e.g. PHC clinic and hospital). Hearing health care services in rural areas in South Africa are currently primarily available at district or regional hospitals that offer outreach services to primary health care clinics on a monthly basis. McIntyre and Ataguba (2017) found that the probability of using a health care service is far lower for individuals who are isolated from health care facilities. These authors report that individuals that live within 30 minutes of a clinic are 10 times more likely to make use of the facility than those having to travel for 90–120 minutes. Similar findings were reported by McLaren, Ardington and Leibbrandt (2014), who found that individuals who live 5 km from the nearest clinic are only half as likely to access treatment when compared with those who live next to the facility.

In a recent South African study, the positive and negative impact of accessibility on the effectiveness of NHS services offered at PHC level was identified (Kgare 2018). Most participants in the study indicated that the PHC clinic where the screening services are offered is easily accessible within walking distance. For participants not within walking distance of the clinic, the limited availability of public transport (buses and minibus taxis) was reported as a challenge. The lack of public transport accessibility in rural areas is well-known (Jennings 2015). This evidence highlights the pressing need for the provision of contextually relevant solutions to the public transport challenges in South Africa. It is suggested that wide-range planning for and implementation of an integrated transport system for individuals located in rural areas will increase accessibility to health care and other services (Mthimkhulu 2017).

4.6.5. Affordability of hearing health care services

Affordability of health care services is one of the main factors that either attracts or deters potential patients (Edusei & Amoah 2014), including hearing health services. Considerations include direct user fees, as well as related and opportunity costs.

Patients accessing public health facilities are classified into three main groups for service fee determination: free services, full-paying patients and subsidised patients. Services at PHC and community health care clinics are free for all users. At the hospital level, services are free for children under six-years-old and the indigent, while being highly subsidised for the rest of the population. Service fees are tiered on a means-tested basis. While public facilities are allowed to charge fees, health care services are mainly provided for free at the point of service. The revenue collected from user fees is less than 1% of total public sector expenditure (Erasmus et al. 2016).

Although user fees are generally affordable, the related costs (such as transport costs and hearing aid batteries) often impact potential users' willingness or ability to access hearing health care services. In South Africa, 55.5% of the chronic poor live in rural and traditional areas (StatsSA 2019). With such a high level of poverty in rural areas, not all individuals presenting ear and hearing-related problems would have the means to pay the related costs.

Research indicates that the utilisation and maintenance of hearing aids fitted within the public sectors were poor (Sooful, Van Dijk & Avenant 2009). The main influencing factor was the cost of accessing health services. The cost of travelling to and from the hospital, as well as paying for repairs and batteries, was reported by participants as significant barriers to the use and maintenance of hearing aids (Sooful et al. 2009).

4.6.6. Accommodative nature of hearing health care services

A variety of factors are related to the accommodative nature of hearing health care services. The focus of this section is on two broad factors: (1) operational aspects (such as hours of operation, appointment systems, waiting times, and waiting lists) and (2) considering the level of health care literacy of patients, as well as their awareness and knowledge of hearing health care services.

4.6.6.1. Operational aspects

The office hours at facilities where hearing health services are available are typically weekdays between 07:30–16:00. As the demand for services far exceeds the supply in relation to available services, there is generally a waiting time for appointments and provision of subsequent hearing aids. If there is a limited budget available for hearing aids, these waiting periods can be significant, e.g. more than 12 months (Sooful et al. 2009). Also, the current referral pathway (from PHC clinics to the various hospital levels) often results in long waiting periods and lists for services.

4.6.6.2. Health literacy levels

Health literacy is defined as the degree to which patients have the capacity to obtain, process and understand the basic health care information and services to make suitable health care decisions (eds. Nielsen-Bohlman, Panzer & Kindig 2004). Literacy is a vital component when accessing medical information (Joubert & Githinji 2014). Research has confirmed the association between low health literacy and poor health outcomes. Individuals with lower health literacy are '1.5–3 times more likely to have poor health outcomes when compared to individuals with higher health literacy' (Protheroe, Nutbeam & Rowlands 2009, p. 721).

A recent study conducted at four PHC clinics in South Africa found that only 17.6% of the participants had adequate health literacy (Marimwe & Dowse 2019). Most patients may experience difficulty of understanding health care instructions and health education materials and may thus be less compliant with treatment. Adequate levels of health literacy would imply that individuals would be able to take responsibility for their own and their family's health (Janse van Rensburg 2020).

Information on hearing health care available to patients is not always appropriate. The quality and readability of pamphlets on hearing and hearing loss in children available at public health care facilities in the Gauteng province were reviewed by Joubert and Githinji (2014). Interestingly, it was found that although most patients were not first-language English-speakers, most pamphlets were only available in English. Additionally, the readability level of these pamphlets was at a sixth-grade level, rather than the recommended fourth-grade reading level (Joubert & Githinji 2014).

4.6.6.3. Awareness and knowledge of hearing health care services

Research conducted in a rural area of South Africa confirmed the general lack of awareness of the audiology profession despite the availability of audiology services at the community and district and regional hospitals (Joubert, Sebothoma & Kgare 2017). The few individuals who were aware of the profession and services confirmed that information was obtained primarily from health care workers at the PHC clinics in the area. According to these findings, health workers conducting health care talks in hospitals and clinics are the primary sources of health-related information (Joubert et al. 2017).

4.6.7. Acceptability of hearing health care services

Acceptability of hearing health care services is influenced by the professional values of service providers and patients' expectations regarding linguistically and culturally appropriate services.

The HPCSA recently released guidelines for speech, language and hearing practice in a culturally and linguistically diverse South Africa (HPCSA 2019). These guidelines highlight the importance of, where possible, providing services in the home language of patients. Patients may feel more competent and empowered when conversing with hearing health care providers in their home language. It has also been found that when they receive health care in their home language and when culture is considered, health interventions are perceived to be more meaningful and effective (HPCSA 2019). Research on the utilisation and maintenance of hearing aids fitted in the public health sector in South Africa confirms this position. Sooful et al. (2009) found that the challenge of language presented complications for clients to fully understand all aspects covered by the audiologist during hearing aid fitting and orientation, especially within the public health care sector. The mismatch between the language utilised by audiologists and the clients they served had a significant impact on treatment adherence (Sooful et al. 2009).

The multilingual nature of South Africa with its 11 official languages complicates the provision of culturally and linguistic appropriate services, as it is nearly impossible for hearing health care providers to communicate with all patients in their preferred language effectively. However, there has been a significant progress towards receiving hearing health care in the language of choice (Moonsamy et al. 2017). The breakdown by population group indicates that in 2018, most of the speech therapists and audiologists employed in the public health care sector were African (41.72%), followed by Whites (31.75%), Indians (18.25%) and Coloureds (8.28%) (Day et al. 2018). Although encouraging, these numbers are not yet reflective of the South African demographic profile and transformation of the profession should remain a priority for training institutions. In order to mitigate these challenges, audiologists should be competent in the languages most frequently spoken in the community where they are employed. If this is not feasible, properly trained hearing screeners (recruited from the community) and trained interpreters should be employed.

4.7. Summary

The most noteworthy challenges regarding access to hearing health services in the rural areas of South Africa are related to:

- **Availability of hearing health services:** The negligible availability of the full range of hearing health services across all levels of care in the public health care sector remains a concern. The main focus of service provision on the tertiary prevention of hearing loss precludes the implementation of comprehensive primary and secondary prevention programmes (such as screening for all age groups) within easy reach of the community. The limited number of audiologists employed in the public sector (specifically in rural areas) hampers the implementation of the full range of services. The implementation of services is further hampered by the reported lack of functioning and well-maintained audiological equipment.
- **Accessibility of hearing health services:** As hearing health services are currently based at district or regional hospitals, the physical location in terms of distance hampers the ability of users to access services easily. This is mainly because of the travel distance, travel time and the limited availability of public transport in rural areas.
- **Affordability of hearing health services:** With the high levels of unemployment and poverty in rural areas of South Africa, most individuals would not have the financial means to pay the related costs (such as transport, hearing aid batteries and repairs) to gain access to hearing health services.
- **Accommodative nature of hearing health services:** The current referral pathway for hearing care services often leads to long waiting times and lists for services, particularly because the demand for services exceeds the supply. When services are offered, low literacy levels of patients on health negatively impact compliance, which thus results in poor hearing health outcomes (such as poor utilisation and maintenance of hearing aids).
- **Acceptability of hearing health services:** Despite the significant improvement in the representativeness of hearing health care professionals in terms of the South African population's demographic profile, more can be done to ensure that patients receive culturally and linguistically relevant hearing health services.

The most significant challenge, however, remains the availability of hearing health services within easily reachable distance for patients. Without these services, the goal of achieving UHC by 2030 will not be realised.

4.8. Solutions and recommendations

The prevention of deafness and hearing loss is non-negotiable even in countries where governments lack the capacity to effectively implement these strategies. In comparison with other countries in sub-Saharan Africa, South Africa has the potential to expand hearing health services to even the most marginalised communities. The NHI bill launched in 2019 recognises that health is a public good, and if hearing health services are implemented according to the WHO's resolution WHA 70.13, all people in South Africa would be able to access quality hearing health services. South Africa, however, faces significant challenges that must be overcome before universal hearing care becomes a reality.

In this section, solutions to the identified challenges to hearing care in rural South Africa are provided, and recommendations for the realisation thereof are outlined.

4.8.1. Community-based service model for the prevention of hearing loss: A South African approach

The establishment of a community-based service model could be important for the successful implementation of a national strategy to prevent and treat hearing loss (Liu et al. 2019). This service model should be aligned with the prevention strategies proposed by Olusanya and colleagues (2014) and the WHO (2018) and be integrated within the framework of the PHC system (WHO 2017a) and NHI. In South Africa, PHC is delivered through the district health system, a relatively self-contained segment of the national health system (WHO 2007). A district typically comprises a well-defined population who live within a delineated administrative and geographical area. All institutions and individuals providing health care in the district (governmental, social security, non-governmental, private or traditional) are included (WHO 2007).

The notion of community-based audiology as a service delivery model in South Africa is not new. In 1997, it was recognised that the use of institution-based models of service delivery has proved to be ineffective in reaching the significant proportion of the South African population who live in rural communities far from clinics and hospitals (Swanepoel 2006; Uys & Hugo 1997). Uys and Hugo (1997, p. 24) highlighted the 'dire need to bring the services to the clients, instead of bringing the clients to the service'.

The most noteworthy benefit of a community-based service is access to hearing health care. In the preceding discussions, the availability, accessibility and affordability of hearing health care were identified as significant challenges to universal hearing care in South Africa. Without adequate numbers of competent hearing health workers to implement comprehensive programmes to prevent deafness and hearing loss, it is time to consider other alternatives. One of the most appropriate approaches would be to shift tasks to other cadres of health workers, such as CHWs. 'Community health worker' is an overarching term for 'laypeople working within their own community in a health promotion, prevention and delivery role' (O'Donovan et al. 2019, p. 2). The WHO (2008) supported task-shifting, made global recommendations and provided guidelines for the rational redistribution of tasks. In order to make more efficient use of the available human resources, specific tasks, where appropriate, are moved from highly qualified health workers to health workers with shorter training and fewer qualifications (WHO 2008). Overall, the evidence suggests that CHWs are key to increasing the availability of and access to basic health services in rural or hard-to-reach areas and, consequently, bridge the health equity gap (Olaniran et al. 2017) and improve health outcomes (Assegaai & Schneider 2019). Chapter 2 in this book also carefully deliberates on task-shifting within the tele-audiology service delivery model to address the capacity versus demand challenge imperative in South Africa.

A systematic review of the role of CHWs in addressing the global burden of ear disease and hearing loss confirmed that this cadre of health workers has the potential to improve access to ear and hearing services for people in remote and underserved areas (O'Donovan et al. 2019). The roles of CHWs in ear disorders and hearing loss included screening, diagnosis and basic treatment of ear diseases. A recent study conducted in South Africa supported this notion, as it confirmed that CHWs can successfully be trained to screen for hearing loss using mHealth technology in vulnerable communities with limited access to hearing health care (Van Wyk, Mahomed-Asmail & Swanepoel 2019). The HPCSA (2018a, 2018b) supported the use of appropriately trained CHWs as screeners in school health and EHDI programmes, with programme planning and management by audiologists.

4.8.2. Proposed community-based service model for the prevention of deafness and hearing loss

The model for community-based audiology services for the prevention of disabling hearing loss is presented in this section. The model outlines the types of prevention activities, location, target population, as well as the proposed resources and staffing requirements for each of the activities (Table 4.1).

As shown in Figure 4.3, an overview of where hearing health services should be situated within each district is provided.

TABLE 4.1: Services, target population, staffing and resources requirements for community-based audiology services.

Services	Location	Target population	Staffing requirements	Resources required
Diagnostic audiology services and management of hearing disorders	Central (district hospital or community health centre)	All ages	• 1 × programme manager • 1 × audiologist for every 3 PHC clinics • 1 × screener or administrator	• Relevant equipment for diagnostic assessments and management of hearing loss (including but not limited to otoscopy, immittance measures, pure-tone audiometry, visual response audiometry, otoacoustic emissions and auditory brainstem response, real-ear measures for verification of hearing aid fittings, cerumen management equipment) • Hearing amplification devices • Transport • Mobile audiology unit for outreach to various sites in the community • Hearing health education material
Infant hearing screening	Primary health care clinic	Infants (0–6 weeks)	1 × dedicated screener per site	• Automated auditory brainstem response (e.g. Maico MB 11) • Hearing health education material
Adult hearing screening	Primary health care clinic	Adults ≥ 18 years (focus on at-risk groups[1])	1 × dedicated screener per site (can be same screener who conducts infant hearing screening)	• Screening equipment (otoscope, immittance measures, screening audiometer) and cerumen management equipment • Hearing health education material
School-based screening	ECD centres and primary schools	Children (3–15 years)	2 × screeners per team (number of teams are dependent on the number of schools in the district)	• Screening equipment (otoscope, immittance measures, screening audiometer) and cerumen management equipment • Transport • Hearing health education material
Community-based screening and health education	Community events[2]	All ages	The team should constitute audiologists and screeners from the various sites	• Screening equipment (otoscope, immittance measures, screening audiometer) and cerumen management equipment • Transport • Hearing health education material
Health education and counselling	All sites and community-based events	Health care workers and public	All staff allocated at different sites (audiologists and screeners)	• Contextually- and linguistically appropriate health education material

Key: ECD, early childhood development; PHC, primary health care.

2. The elderly, individuals on chronic medication (e.g. diabetes, hypertension and HIV), and individuals exposed to occupational and recreational noise.

3. Examples include pension pay points, church events, community meetings and other events.

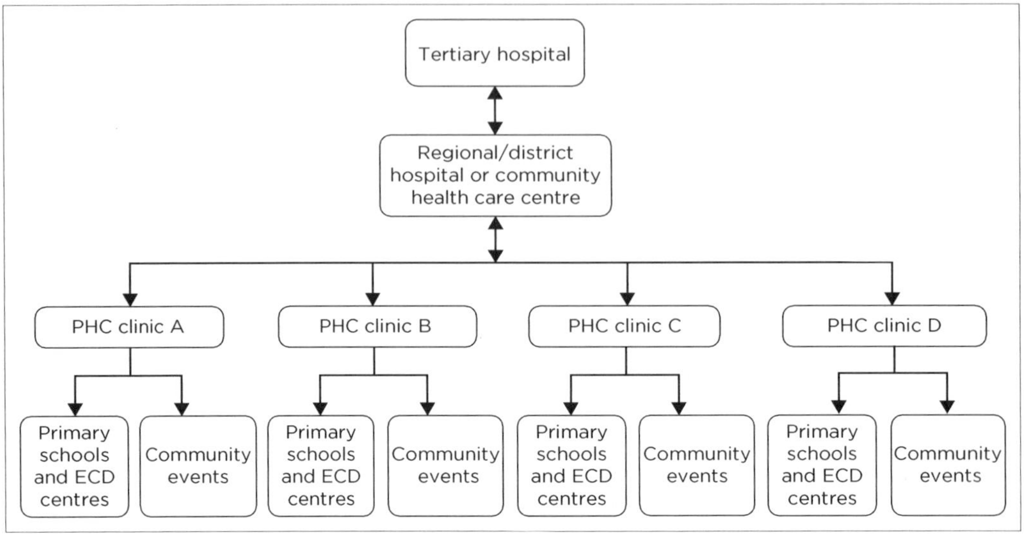

Key: PHC, primary health care; ECD, early childhood development.

FIGURE 4.3: Overview of the location of hearing health care services.

It is proposed that audiologists should be based at either district hospitals or community health centres. The location should be based on the population size within the district to ensure that diagnostic and rehabilitative audiology services are available within an easily reachable distance for the majority of the population. The number of audiologists based here would be dependent on the number of PHC clinics in the districts. Numbers should be adequate so that diagnostic and rehabilitation services at the central site can continue, and community-based services offered by screeners are well supervised and supported by the programme manager and or audiologist.

4.8.3. Roles of different hearing health care staff

The role of the audiologist in this community-based service model is wide-ranging and includes the following:

- To develop, monitor and evaluate all the prevention activities within the community, that is primary, secondary and tertiary prevention.
- To render contextually relevant audiological services, which include the assessment, diagnosis and treatment of hearing disorders.
- To train, monitor, support and supervise the activities of hearing screeners across the different sites (PHC clinics, primary schools and ECD centres, and community events).
- To ensure that all patient information pamphlets are appropriate, of good quality, meet the standards in terms of readability, and are linguistically and culturally appropriate.

The role of the hearing screeners is to implement the screening programmes under the guidance and supervision of an audiologist and educate the community on hearing and the prevention of ear and hearing disorders.

4.8.4. Recommendations

Various strategies can be adopted for the implementation of successful proposed community-based services in rural areas. It is important to:

- Conduct a situation analysis and needs assessment to obtain comprehensive information on the demography, epidemiology, current health status, and potential future health issues and their determinants of the population (WHO 2020c). The analysis should also include an assessment of the hearing health systems' resources (human, physical, financial, informational) and performance, as well as the gaps (resource and performance) in responding to needs and expectations (WHO 2020c). Current, high-quality and contextually specific hearing health data are essential to achieve this (Glenister et al. 2018; WHO 2017a).
- Obtain permission for the services from all the relevant authorities. At the local level, depending on the community, permission must be obtained from the tribal authorities (i.e. village elders and chiefs) or relevant community structures. An important step in obtaining permission is to carefully consider the process of community entry. The success or failure of community-based services will largely depend on the support from important community stakeholders.
- Support for the service, specifically financial support for training, staff and equipment, should also be garnered from the relevant government departments (i.e. Departments of Health and Education) within the district.
- Educate the community and other relevant stakeholders on the importance of ear and hearing health, the risk factors for hearing loss in their community, as well as the identification of potential ear and hearing problems. ear-and-hearing health care education should be multifaceted and can be presented in spoken, written, pictographic and video formats. Regardless of the format, plain language (i.e. no jargon) must be used to present contextually relevant information in language that most community members understand for more guidelines on printed health information material. Examples of activities include health talks (at clinics, schools, pension pay points, and community events), talk shows on local and community radio stations, and distribution of health information material (e.g. pamphlets, posters and videos) at clinics, schools, community halls and local shops, and social media platforms. Refer to guidelines for the development of health information materials developed by Joubert and Githinji (2014), with specific reference to the readability level and structure of printed health information materials.

- Explore public-private partnerships to fund services if government-funded services are not available. There is evidence that such partnerships are successful in existing infant hearing screening services at PHC clinics in the Limpopo province (Kgare 2018). In that programme, equipment and staff were funded by a non-governmental organisation, while the PHC facilities were used as a base for infant and adult hearing screening.
- Train grassroots-level screeners (preferably recruited from the communities where the services are rendered) in the prevention and early identification of common ear diseases and hearing loss across the lifespan. From this cadre, screeners should ideally be dedicated to specific screening programmes (De Kock et al. 2016). *The Primary Ear and Hearing Care Training Resources: Basic and intermediate levels* developed by the WHO (2006) are useful educational resources.
- Integrate services into the school health programme as outlined in the Integrated School Health Policy (Departments of Health and Basic Education 2012). The HPCSA guidelines on hearing screening in school should also be used as a guide for services (HPCSA 2018a).
- Appoint audiologists as the programme managers. The role of the programme manager is to coordinate services, provide ongoing support and training of screeners, and monitor the quality of the services provided.
- Consider the use of a mobile audiology unit or tele-audiology to further increase the availability and accessibility of hearing health services. Diagnostic hearing assessments and hearing aid fittings can thus be successfully conducted in the community. The establishment of tele-audiology hubs, at, for instance, district-level hospitals will provide each community access to a hearing health care provider. This service will minimise barriers to access and increase efficiency (Coco, Champlin & Eikelboom 2006). Examples of successful tele-audiology endeavours are those reported by Coco et al. (2006), Ramkumar et al. (2018), Ratanji-Vanmala, Swanepoel & Laplante-Lévesque (2020) and Van Wyk et al. (2019). The most important consideration for the establishment of community-based audiology services is that it is not a one-size-fits-all approach. The staff structure, services offered and training of screeners should be adapted to suit the needs of each specific community (Coco et al. 2006; O'Donovan et al. 2019; Ramkumar et al. 2018).

4.8.5. Challenges

However, the establishment of community-based audiology services is not without challenges. Although there are limited research studies available on the challenges experienced in setting up and maintaining sustainable community-based services, the following issues were identified:

- **District health structures:** The current district and sub-district health structures in South Africa find it difficult to provide adequate health services (Nxumalo, Goudge & Liz Thomas 2013) but with political will and adequate investment in the capacity building of staff (i.e. training and employment of dedicated hearing screeners from the community) and resource development (i.e. procurement of audiological equipment), it would be possible to establish community-based audiology services.

- **Selection of screeners:** The selection of screeners for a community-based audiology service must be transparent because, in rural communities, the selection of this cadre can be influenced by the power structures within the community (Saprii et al. 2015).
- **Inadequate monetary incentives for screeners:** The monetary incentive that screeners receive for their services shapes their experiences, performance and relationship with the community (Saprii et al. 2015). If this is perceived as inadequate or not market-related (for each specific context), screeners will become demotivated.
- **Staff turnover:** High staff turnover has been reported in the ear-and-hearing health care programmes situated in isolated rural locations, such as services for the Inuit population in Canada (Billard 2014). This not only compromises the capacity to build relationships with all stakeholders in the community but also has implications for the continuity of services and added costs for the training and orientation of staff (Billard 2014).

■ 4.9. Conclusion

In this chapter, the right of people who live in rural communities to access ear-and-hearing health care services was discussed. Health care access was defined, and the five key dimensions that should be considered when determining access were outlined. These dimensions included the availability, accessibility, affordability, accommodative nature and acceptability of services. An overview of the South African health care system and related policies were presented as the background to hearing health care services in South Africa. The importance of the prevention of deafness and hearing loss and the proposed implementation strategies set the scene for the contextualisation of hearing health care services currently available and offered in rural South Africa. Based on the identified challenges, specifically in relation to the availability, accessibility and affordability of services, solutions and recommendations were made for the implementation of a community-based service model for audiology in South Africa.

The community-based service model is designed to prioritise the prevention of ear and hearing disorders. An important component would also be the promotion of hearing health services to increase public awareness, as well as the prevention, treatment and management of ear disease and hearing loss. This can only be achieved by offering services that are (1) person-centred in their approach, (2) responsive to patient needs, (3) able to adapt to the constantly changing hearing health needs, (4) accountable and (5) collaborative in nature.

Chapter 5

Preventing middle ear pathologies in the South African context: A proposed programmatic approach

Ben Sebothoma
Department of Audiology, Faculty of Humanities,
School of Human and Community Development, University of the Witwatersrand,
Johannesburg, South Africa

Katijah Khoza-Shangase
Department of Audiology, Faculty of Humanities,
School of Human and Community Development, University of the Witwatersrand,
Johannesburg, South Africa

5.1. Introduction

Globally, the incidence of middle ear pathologies is persistently high (WHO 2018), with LMICs presenting more cases because of multiple risk factors that exist in these regions. Research studies suggest that middle ear pathology is one of the biggest contributors to acquired hearing loss (Mulwafu et al. 2017a). Within the South African context, early identification of middle ear pathologies can prevent myriad complications and enhance the QoL for the sufferer, consequently reducing the costs associated with treating chronic middle ear pathologies. Traditional audiological service delivery models seem unable

How to cite: Sebothoma, B & Khoza-Shangase, K 2022, 'Preventing middle ear pathologies in the South African context: A proposed programmatic approach', ed. K Khoza-Shangase, *Preventive audiology: An African perspective*, AOSIS Books, Cape Town, pp. 93–109. https://doi.org/10.4102/aosis.2022.BK209.05

to identify signs and symptoms early enough to benefit from preventive health care strategies, regardless of the level of prevention. The key reason why these traditional models of service delivery do not seem to yield significant positive preventive outcomes within the South African context is that these models function in 'silos' within limited resource contexts, outside of contextually conceived health care programmes that are burden-of-disease and priority-list driven (Khoza-Shangase & Riva 2021). Service delivery models that are naïve of context and that ignore contextual realities are bound to yield less positive and unsustainable outcomes.

The SANDoH provides primary health care services by adopting a programmatic approach within the re-engineered primary health care model. Such a programmatic approach includes health care programmes such as:

- a school health care programme
- the prevention of mother-to-child transmission of HIV
- a child immunisation programme
- Integrated Management of Childhood Illness
- Maternal, Child and Women's Health and Nutrition
- HIV awareness
- ward-based primary health care outreach (Fick 2017; Kanji & Khoza-Shangase 2021; Khoza-Shangase & Kanji 2021; King, Mhlanga & De Pinho 2006)
- the First 1000 days programme, TB programmes, MomConnect and other such initiatives (Barron et al. 2016; English et al. 2017; Okeyo, Lehmann & Schneider 2021).

The other South African departments also have similar programmes that are relevant to preventive audiology, such as the Striving for Zero Harm Programme under the Department of Labour (Moroe 2020). The literature indicates that some of these health care programmes use paraprofessionals such as CHWs to promote health care in underserved areas (Schneider et al. 2018). Most of these health care programmes tap into populations with an increased risk of middle ear pathologies, such as young children, people living with HIV and others. Including preventive health care strategies for ear diseases and hearing loss within such programmes, not only is it cost-effective, but it also ensure sustainability as they become part of the government-mandated programmes with budgeting support and political will behind them.

For the South African audiology community to achieve early detection and intervention outcomes within preventive audiology at all levels of prevention, this programmatic approach to service delivery needs careful consideration by policymakers and training institutions in their curricula. This approach may provide an alternative way to prevent middle ear pathologies by enabling wider coverage of cases which would not ordinarily be seen under traditional approaches, including those who are at a greater risk of developing middle ear pathologies across the lifespan. Existing programmes incorporating the current technologies (e.g. asynchronous tele-audiology) and sensitive assessment measures may improve early identification of middle ear pathologies and increase access and coverage. The focus of this chapter is an ear care model that includes task-shifting and telepractice as a human resource strategy, where limited numbers of audiologists and otorhinolaryngologists exist (Mulwafu et al. 2017b).

Middle ear pathologies reportedly affected approximately 700 million people globally in 2018, most of them residing in LMICs (WHO 2018). Evidence from South African studies indicates a high prevalence of middle ear pathologies in both children and adults (Biagio et al. 2013, 2014; Phanguphangu 2017). In a study comprising 140 children aged 2–16 years, Biagio et al. (2014) found a prevalence rate of middle ear pathologies to be 16.5%, with CSOM being the most common type of OM in their sample. In a study conducted in 11 primary schools in the rural Limpopo province, Phanguphangu (2017) found a higher prevalence rate (61%) of middle ear pathologies. Several other studies conducted among adult populations within the same South African context confirmed this high prevalence of middle ear pathologies (Joubert & Botha 2019; Ramma & Sebothoma 2016). It is important to be cautious when interpreting some of these prevalence values as it is possible that where air-bone gap presence in pure-tone audiometry was used to diagnose middle ear pathology in the absence of a complete test battery, the presence of impacted wax and foreign bodies in the ear could have been a confounding variable.

The primary reason for the apparent surge in these pathologies seems to be linked to physiological changes resulting from an incapacitated immune system (Biagio et al. 2014; Khoza-Shangase 2010; Khoza-Shangase & Turnbull 2009; Thobejane & Ntuli-Ngcobo 2014), as well as non-physiological causes, which may be self-induced (Joubert, Sebothoma & Kgare 2017). Among the physiological causes, HIV remains one of the greatest risk factors for middle ear pathologies (Khoza & Ross 2002; Khoza-Shangase & Anastasiou 2020; Sanjar, Queiroz & Miziara 2011; Sebothoma & Khoza-Shangase 2018; Thobejane & Ntuli-Ngcobo 2014; Van der Westhuizen et al. 2013). In a systematic review of middle ear pathologies in adults with HIV, Sebothoma and Khoza-Shangase (2020) found that the prevalence rate of middle ear pathologies can be as high as 50% in this group. In a retrospective record review of 100 paediatric patients living with HIV in South Africa, Khoza-Shangase and Anastasiou (2020) found a prevalence rate of middle ear pathologies to be as high as 30% in their group. Peter et al. (2020) also found conductive hearing loss (CHL) to be the most frequent type of hearing loss among school-aged children living with HIV in another South African study. Overall higher frequency and severity of otorhinolaryngology findings among HIV-positive children when compared with HIV-negative children have been well-documented, with Taipale et al. (2011), for example, finding CSOM (26% vs. 3.8%), dry tympanic membrane perforations (9% vs. 1%) and earlier otorrhea episodes (34% vs. 17%) when exploring otorhinolaryngological manifestations in HIV-positive and HIV-negative children in a developing country.

While the association between HIV and middle ear pathologies is clear in the literature, there is a significant difference between rates of middle ear pathologies in studies. Sebothoma and Khoza-Shangase (2020) suggested that this variation in prevalence rates reported may be because of the different measures used to identify middle ear pathologies (e.g. pure-tone audiometry vs. tympanometry), criteria used to determine normal versus abnormal, as well as the different sample sizes in all the studies. Furthermore, the time period from which the studies were conducted also appears to have an influence on the prevalence rates. For example, studies that were conducted prior to the mandatory treatment of HIV regardless of the CD4 cell number (e.g. Van der Westhuizen et al. 2013) found a higher prevalence of middle ear pathologies than those that were conducted when highly active antiretroviral treatment had become an increasing norm (e.g. Sebothoma & Khoza-Shangase 2018).

As far as middle ear pathologies are concerned, which are caused by non-physiological conditions that are primarily self-induced, studies show local occurrences across the lifespan. Joubert et al. (2017) found that people in rural South Africa use methods such as pouring different oils into their ears or using matchsticks to scratch them when itching or cleaning them. In another South African study conducted in one of the local universities, Khan, Thaver and Govender (2017) found that almost every student interviewed was engaging in self-ear cleaning, with a majority of them (79.6%) using cotton buds. These ear care practices have been shown to cause ear-related injuries (Olajide et al. 2019), which may include tympanic membrane perforations (Khan et al. 2017).

It is unfavourable that the occurrence of middle ear pathologies can be linked to the burden of diseases, such as HIV (Sebothoma & Khoza-Shangase 2020; Thobejane & Ntuli-Ngcobo 2014; Torre III et al. 2016), which is already a significant health challenge in LMICs like South Africa. According to Khoza-Shangase (2020a) and Swanepoel (2006), HIV has also produced an overwhelming burden and an exceptional challenge to ear-and-hearing health care delivery in South Africa. With the current statistics indicating that HIV affects approximately 14% of the population (StatsSA 2019), and with the general lack of knowledge around ear-and-hearing health care that stems from high levels of illiteracy and limited awareness of ear and hearing professionals (Joubert et al. 2017), increased efforts are required to ensure universal access to ear health care. Although measures are in place to limit the spread of HIV (Joint United Nations Programme on HIV/AIDS [UNAIDS] 2019), evidence of new annual infections exists, increasing the burden of the disease further. When examining the progress of South Africa in meeting the 2030 UNAIDS 90-90-90 targets, current data reflecting the status at the end of 2018 indicate that 90% of those living with HIV knew their status, 62% were on treatment (63% in the paediatric population) and only 54% were virally suppressed (UNAIDS 2019). The 2030 targets state that 90% of those living with HIV should know their status, 90% be on treatment, and 90% on treatment be virally suppressed (UNAIDS 2014). Given these factors, there is clearly a need for a model of health care service provision that can allow for increased access to identifying early signs of middle ear pathologies in the general population and not just those self-reporting. This need is particularly high because of the impact associated with these pathologies on the individual affected and on the already pressurised health care system.

Despite the efficacy of current treatments for middle ear pathologies (Vouloumanou et al. 2009), late identification or untreated middle ear pathologies may become chronic (Ibekwe & Nwaorgu 2011), making these conditions challenging and costlier to treat. Further delay in middle ear pathology treatment may cause permanent hearing loss (Kolo et al. 2012), auditory processing difficulties and life-threatening conditions (Sharma et al. 2015). The WHO (2018) also estimated that approximately 50% of individuals with untreated acute otitis media (AOM) will develop CSOM, which places them at a higher risk of permanent hearing loss (Avnstorp et al. 2016). Olusanya, Okolo and Adeosun (2004) found middle ear pathologies to be the greatest risk of hearing loss in school-aged children. The impact of these middle ear pathology complications can have far-reaching consequences and ultimately reduce the QoL of the affected individual (Anderson et al. 2013; Govender et al. 2014; Khoza-Shangase & Riva 2021). Balbani and Montovani (2003) reviewed the literature on children diagnosed with OM and found that these children perceive distorted sound stimuli, which leads to phonetic errors. Haapala et al. (2014) found that children with recurrent OM aged 22–26-months show poor discrimination of small phonetic features.

Sufficient evidence on disease-related factors such as hearing status and the presence of cholesteatoma, history of otological surgery, occurrence of complications, laterality, duration and activity of the disease (Choi et al. 2012) call for careful considerations of health care service delivery models within resource-constrained contexts to achieve positive preventive outcomes.

■ 5.2. Current health care service provision for middle ear pathologies

Health care professionals whose primary responsibilities involve the identification and management of middle ear pathologies include ear and hearing professionals, such as audiologists, general practitioners and otorhinolaryngologists (HPCSA 2011). Although audiologists and general practitioners are often the first point of contact for patients experiencing ear and hearing-related symptoms, depending on the location of patients, these professionals often refer patients who require medical or surgical management to otorhinolaryngologists, particularly where these conditions have progressed to the advanced stage (Kreisman, Smart & John 2015).

Audiologists use different test measures to identify middle ear pathologies in this context. These measures include otoscopy, acoustic immittance measures such as tympanometry conducted in diagnostic audiological clinics and hearing screening programmes (Bezuidenhout et al. 2018; Kanji & Khoza-Shangase 2018; Khoza-Shangase & Harbinson 2015; Mahomed-Asmail, Swanepoel & Eikelboom 2016; Martin & Clark 2019; Petrocchi-Bartal & Khoza-Shangase 2014; Phanguphangu 2017; Ramma & Sebothoma 2016; Sebothoma & Khoza-Shangase 2021). In newborn and infant hearing screening programmes, middle ear function is evaluated through acoustic immittance measures that are mainly only used when there is a *refer finding* during the initial screening (HPCSA 2018; Kanji & Khoza-Shangase 2018).

It is worth noting that measures used to assess middle ear pathologies are not used in isolation but rather are always embedded within the audiological test battery (Martin & Clark 2019). For example, a survey on acoustic immittance practices in South Africa indicated that approximately 70% of audiologists include tympanometry as part of the standard audiological test battery in their practices (Sebothoma & Khoza-Shangase 2021). Similar surveys conducted in the United States have also indicated that acoustic immittance measures are included in the audiological test battery (Emanuel, Henson & Knapp 2012; MacDonald & Green 2001). The utility of tympanometry in screening programmes within the South African context has also been well-documented (Khoza-Shangase & Anastasiou 2020; Khoza-Shangase & Turnbull 2009; Mahomed-Asmail et al. 2016; Ramma & Sebothoma 2016).

While evidence indicates that middle ear assessments form part of the standard audiological test battery in the majority of audiology practices within the South African context, this occurs within a health care service delivery model that the authors of this chapter believe is not efficient nor comprehensive to successfully achieve preventive outcomes for middle ear pathologies within this context. This current model of health care service provision only accommodates patients who are already attending diagnostic clinics and those identified through audiology-specific hearing screening programmes (Mahomed-Asmail et al. 2016), as well as those enrolled in ototoxicity monitoring programmes (Khoza-Shangase & Masondo 2020). Those without hearing or ear-related symptoms are neglected (Ramma & Sebothoma 2017) until they become severe enough to seek health care services once their symptoms become significant. Those not in schools where screenings can occur may not be screened until their middle ear symptoms are severe enough to warrant a consultation, thus unaccounted for in preventive treatment.

The ineffectiveness of the current health care service provision model is also evident in other sectors, such as in occupational settings like mines. Despite the audiological services included in HCPs in mines, middle ear function is also not regularly assessed as part of the hearing assessments

(Sebothoma 2020). Although it is not clear why middle ear assessment is largely ignored in sectors such as mines, except perhaps for cost implications, Moroe and Khoza-Shangase (2018) highlighted that limited involvement of audiologists in HCPs could be one of the key explanations for gaps found in ear-and-hearing health care in this population.

Khoza-Shangase and Moroe (2020) asserted that the availability of resources, in any context, is critical to a profession's ability to fulfil its functions and mandate. Within the South African context, the reason for the significant challenges around resource availability is the lack of human resources in audiological health care services, which is a national crisis. Khoza-Shangase (2019) painted a worse capacity versus demand challenge for the South African public health care sector when compared with the privately funded private health care sector: a sector that must provide services to approximately 80% of the South African population. Because of the limited numbers of audiologists nationally, significant gaps in health care service provision in less popular contexts, such as occupational audiology contexts, exist (Khoza-Shangase & Moroe 2020; Pillay et al. 2020). By February 2019, HPCSA registration records indicated that there were a mere 1589 speech therapists and audiologists, 642 audiologists and 157 hearing aid acousticians to provide health care services to a population of over 55 million, servicing both the public and private health care sectors (Khoza-Shangase & Moroe 2020). These numbers of registered practitioners clearly illustrate the human resources challenge in the provision of ear-and-hearing health care services in South Africa (Pillay et al. 2020), with recognisable implications for the implementation and monitoring of any preventive audiology initiative. This highlights the importance of exploring other health care service delivery models within the South African context.

Surveys conducted in sub-Saharan countries have indicated that there is an extreme shortage of audiologists and otorhinolaryngologists in these regions and that these numbers do not seem to be increasing with the increasing burden of disease (Fagan & Jacobs 2009; Mulwafu et al. 2017b; Pillay et al. 2020). In South Africa, these professionals, where available, are found in health care centres in large cities and private practices. Consequently, a large portion of South Africans are unable to access health care. Indeed they do not reflect the circumstances in SHPs, rural areas, or townships (Fagan & Jacobs 2009). According to a survey conducted in a South African municipality in the Limpopo province, over 80% of the population did not know that health care professionals like audiologists could assist them (Joubert et al. 2017). Consequently, people with middle ear-related symptoms who may want to seek help may be prohibited by the costs of travelling to the clinic where these professionals are located, over and above the health care access costs, as well as the awareness of the existence of the help they require.

5.3. Technology within the current model of ear-and-hearing health care

Technology is currently the topic of scholarly interest and offers promise to address the current challenges facing the provision of health care services to underserved communities (Khoza-Shangase & Moroe 2020; Swanepoel 2015), and this has become amplified by the COVID-19 pandemic. In audiology, research continues to examine whether technological advancements can address the inequality of health care service provision created by the apartheid regime (Mayosi & Benatar 2014). Khoza-Shangase and Moroe (2020) strongly encouraged increased efforts towards the use of tele-audiology within the South African context to mitigate the capacity versus demand challenges and, most recently, to continue the provision of essential ear-and-hearing health care services during the COVID-19 pandemic (Khoza-Shangase, Moroe & Neille 2021a). Because tele-audiology offers promise to increase access to health care in resource-constrained contexts, these authors believe that deliberations around the use of tele-audiology in preventive audiology are timely. As advanced by Krupinski (2015), Khoza-Shangase argued that within the South African context, telecommunication technologies have numerous potential benefits that can enhance health care service delivery, including but not limited to assisting health care practitioners in developing and expanding their practices to locations beyond where they are physically located, expanding reach to patients in remote rural areas, minimising or eliminating travel costs that patients incur when accessing tertiary-level care, strengthening health care services where limited care is available, bolstering access to and enhancing patient satisfaction with specialised care by specialists, and encouraging inter and intra-professional collaboration in rural areas.

The available research findings are promising as they do confirm that technology can be used in underserved areas to increase access and reach, as well as for clinical training and supervision (Khoza-Shangase et al. 2021a). In addition, some of these technological tools can be successfully operated by paraprofessionals, such as CHWs and facilitators, with no previous health background (Biagio et al. 2013), thus facilitating the use of task-shifting. Van Wyk, Mahomed-Asmail and Swanepoel (2019) trained 15 community care workers (CCWs) to conduct hearing screening using the hearTest™ Smartphone application as part of telepractice. Their findings indicated that CCWs can be trained to screen for hearing loss, and with appropriate training ensure that inappropriate referrals, such as false positives, are minimised.

Research has indicated that task-shifting can also be carried out with the use of middle ear measures that have higher sensitivity and specificity in identifying middle ear pathologies. Biagio et al. (2013) found that individuals with no background in health can be trained to successfully capture video otoscopic images or video clips that can be analysed through asynchronous tele-audiology at a later stage by the otorhinolaryngologist. This means that many volunteers can be employed and trained to use video otoscopy in various settings, such as communities, schools and clinics. This would allow for wider coverage of patients in different communities and help with the early identification of middle ear pathologies. Acoustic immittance measures such as tympanometry, which can be operated by paraprofessionals (Erkkola-Anttinen et al. 2014), can also be incorporated into current technology to increase access and ultimately form part of the preventive programmes.

While technological advances are promising to expand health care services to underserved communities (Khoza-Shangase 2021a; Khoza-Shangase & Moroe 2020; Swanepoel 2020), there are also notable challenges with this approach to the delivery of health care services. Currently, technological advances are utilised in isolation, that is, outside established health care programmes. Careful examination of these programmes indicates that they follow the same traditional non-technological model, with the primary focus on schools and clinics (Sandström et al. 2020). Where a programmatic approach is attempted, middle ear assessment is excluded. For example, in Van Wyk et al.'s (2019) study where CCWs were trained to conduct hearing screening using hearScreen™ application, the community health programme that these CCWs were part of excluded middle ear assessment as part of the screening initiative. Patients' middle ear function is measured only when *refer* results are obtained from the hearing screening, which has implications for early identification of middle ear pathologies, as early middle ear pathology may not necessarily cause a hearing loss that will then be identified through hearing screening. Based on the hearing screening that uses hearScreen™, a *pass* result not only translates to a normal hearing threshold (Swanepoel et al. 2014), which does not require further audiological management but also infers normal middle ear function. Given that some middle ear pathologies do not affect sound transduction (Sebothoma et al. 2021), the use of hearScreen™ application alone poses the risk of missing early signs of middle ear pathologies and, consequently, delaying the implementation of timeous intervention – a goal of preventive health care. Similarly, in a majority of the ototoxicity monitoring initiatives forming part of the TB and HIV management programmes, middle ear measures do not form part of the standard monitoring programmes (Govender et al. 2020; Khoza-Shangase 2020b; Khoza-Shangase & Masondo 2020).

■ 5.4. Universal health care coverage and the National Health Insurance within the current model of ear-and-hearing care

Global health and health care are characterised by a renewed emphasis on the goal of achieving universal health access throughout the world (Benatar & Gill 2021; Khoza-Shangase 2021b). Khoza-Shangase (2021b) considered how the

South African hospital sector has distinct divisions between old historical divides (Mayosi & Benatar 2014) and new developments, as well as divisions between public and private health sectors, will benefit from an overhaul that the NHI promises to bring. With the public health sector servicing over 80% of South African citizens who are not privately funded, this author argues that the NHI's proposal of a harmonised approach to health care, where citizens can access health care services in both the public and private sectors at the NHI's cost, irrespective of their socio-economic status, is welcomed. Ranchod et al. (2017) asserted that the NHI is an indication of the South African government's intention to achieve UHC and access to a high quality of care for its citizens. Khoza-Shangase (2021b) cautioned that NHI needs to occur in the context of South Africa trying to attend to the long-term goal of tackling the social determinants of health. This author believes that this approach should also carefully consider the risks and benefits of any initiative adopted to address health challenges within this resource-constrained context, hence the need for preventive audiology programmes, such as the programmatic approach being recommended for the prevention of middle ear pathologies within the NHI plans. Khoza-Shangase (2021b) suggested that such preventive care initiatives would need to be checked for contextual relevance, responsiveness and accountability and that they also need to be systematic and comprehensive, have a strategic plan behind them and involve audiologists at all stages of their development to implementation and monitoring.

Implementation of these initiatives is possible if clear and strategic preventive audiology plans are made within programmes, taking advantage of the NHI bill of 2019, whose goal is that of the WHO's universal health care coverage (Ghebreyesus 2017; WHO 2017), under which universal ear-and-hearing health care coverage falls. However, implementation of the NHI remains challenging as it is a funding model that does not necessarily address the challenges of the human resources challenges, particularly for areas where health care professionals and resources are unavailable (Passchier 2017), as has been illustrated for ear-and-hearing health care professionals within the South African context. Nonetheless, glimpses of the possibilities that the NHI promises to deliver in terms of the universal health care coverage model have been evidenced under the COVID-19 pandemic in South Africa, where a programmatic approach to health care, with a particular emphasis on preventive health care at the primary level, regardless of the financial status of the patient has been clearly demonstrated (Hsieh 2020; Mosam et al. 2020; Reid 2020). COVID-19 has also demonstrated the use of global health teleconsultations and tele-expertise as part of telepractice (Ohannessian, Duong & Odone 2020) within a programmatic approach to health care delivery, which South African ear-and-hearing health care professionals can learn from.

■ 5.5. Programmatic approach: Proposed framework

Khoza-Shangase (2017) argues that health care practitioners must devote attention and resources to programmes to reduce the burdens of disease and programmes funded by the Department of Health. Therefore, they are better resourced and sustainable in achieving preventive outcomes regarding ear health and function. The authors of this chapter hold the same view as far as the prevention of middle ear pathologies is concerned. Owing to the limitation of the current model of health care service delivery, which leads to delayed early identification of middle ear pathologies, the authors believe that a programmatic approach may be a cost-efficient and responsible alternative. A programmatic approach enables several programmes to operate together under the same umbrella (Shapiro & Galowitz 2016). This means that resources allocated to an 'umbrella' programme may be shared or redistributed to improve health care service delivery, which in this case can include auditory pathologies such as early detection of middle ear pathologies.

Because the already existing programmes are budgeted for and have monitoring embedded in them, they already significantly utilise paraprofessionals to play crucial roles (Mottiar & Lodge 2018) such as promoting health in underserved areas (Schneider et al. 2018), conducting screening and home visits (Le Roux et al. 2014), this recommended programmatic approach opens an opportunity for audiology to fit in well within such programmes (O'Donovan et al. 2019). Given that some middle ear pathologies are self-induced (Joubert et al. 2017; Khan et al. 2017), the current scope of paraprofessionals in existing programmes can be expanded to include the promotion of healthy and hygienic practices to reduce the risk of middle ear pathologies. Furthermore, following training in order to adhere to the HPCSA minimum standards, assessments of middle ear pathologies using sensitive measures such as wideband acoustic immittance (WAI) (Hunter & Sanford 2015; Kaf 2011; Shahnaz et al. 2009) are incorporated into current hearing screening, and the utilisation of current technology within a health care service delivery model that uses task-shifting to paraprofessionals can improve the identification and timeous intervention of middle ear pathologies within the South African context.

■ 5.6. Scope of paraprofessionals within the programmatic approach

The available evidence suggests that paraprofessionals can successfully be trained to promote health and conduct certain audiological tests such as smartphone applications (Van Wyk et al. 2019). It is therefore important to carefully plan the scope of paraprofessionals with regard to the prevention of middle ear pathologies. According to the HPCSA, audiologists are responsible for creating training programmes for paraprofessionals, such as volunteers and community workers, and making sure that the minimum standards and regulations are met (HPCSA 2018). The training programme should include community entry to create awareness through communicating with community members. Given that South Africa is a multicultural and multilingual society, audiologists should incorporate the importance of culture and language in health care delivery in their training, as these have a significant impact on health-seeking and health intervention adherence behaviours (Khoza-Shangase & Mophosho 2021). Ensuring linguistic and cultural congruence with the communities served may enhance the understanding and heighten the relevance of the information provided and improve the likelihood of healthy ear-and-hearing health care behaviour.

The training programme should also include training on the use of sensitive middle ear measures such as WAI and video otoscopy to identify middle ear pathologies, especially with more and more WAI normative data in different populations becoming available. As part of the routine procedure, audiology practices are gradually moving towards the inclusion of sensitive middle ear measures to improve early identification and timeous intervention of middle ear pathologies. Video otoscopy (Biagio et al. 2014; Lundberg et al. 2017; Park et al. 2016; Sebothoma & Khoza-Shangase 2018) and WAI (Kaf 2011; Merchant et al. 2021; Myers et al. 2018; Sebothoma et al. 2021; Shahnaz et al. 2009) have demonstrated higher sensitivity in identifying middle ear pathologies. In addition, Keefe et al. (2012) reported that WAI can also be used to predict CHL. Consequently, researchers from various countries have begun to develop normative values for WAI to improve its diagnostic utility (Aithal et al. 2017; Chang et al. 2019; Jaffer 2016; Margolis, Saly & Keefe 1999; Polat et al. 2015; Sebothoma & Khoza-Shangase submitted; Shahnaz, Feeney & Schairer 2013). Over and above their sensitivity, these measures of middle ear pathologies have also been shown to be easy to perform (Biagio et al. 2013; Hunter & Sanford 2015) and, therefore, can easily be incorporated into the tasks transferred during task-shifting to paraprofessionals.

While studies have demonstrated that video otoscopy and WAI are sensitive in identifying middle ear pathologies, their interpretations can only be conducted by qualified professionals. For example, video otoscopic images or video clips require otorhinolaryngologists to analyse and make a diagnosis of middle ear pathology (Sebothoma & Khoza-Shangase 2018). The reduced familiarity with WAI and its technicalities may require audiologists to interpret and make a diagnosis. Because of these restrictions, it is recommended that interpretation of these measures be carried out through tele-audiology or telepractice either via synchronous, asynchronous or hybrid approach, depending on the context and situation where the clinical care is being provided.

Audiologists are, therefore, responsible for thoroughly and carefully training paraprofessionals to take quality video otoscopic images or clips and obtain WAI results, which can be analysed via telepractice by qualified professionals (Khoza-Shangase et al. 2021a; Rushbrooke & Houston 2013; Swanepoel 2015; WHO 2013). The same platform for health care service delivery can then be used for the management and monitoring of middle ear pathologies that are under otorhinolaryngologists' care.

5.7. Task-shifting within a programmatic approach that includes tele-audiology

Ear-and-hearing health care professionals, such as audiologists and otorhinolaryngologists, are the main professionals specifically trained and certified to identify, treat and manage middle ear pathologies and their consequences (Martin & Clark 2019). However, the shortage of these professionals within the South African context (Fagan & Jacobs 2009) has led to their scope of practice prioritising preventive care far less than secondary and tertiary health care services. Consequently, this capacity versus demand challenge may prevent successful and effective implementation for the prevention of middle ear pathologies in the South African context. As a result, some of the tasks required for preventive ear-and-hearing health care may have to be shifted to other individuals who may assist in implementing the preventive programmes - paraprofessionals (WHO 2020).

There is a need for paraprofessionals, such as CHWs, teachers, students, religious leaders, and volunteers, to participate in implementing the ear and hearing preventive programmes. O'Donovan et al. (2019), in their scoping review on the roles played by CHWs, found that these workers can play an important role in addressing ear diseases and hearing loss. In this study, the value of CHWs was located in raising awareness of ear diseases and hearing loss in the community and in promoting community participation in screening programmes.

Students attending the ear-and-hearing health care training programmes can also be involved in health educational activities through initiatives, such as peer education. Peer-led health education has been recognised as a potential strategy for promoting healthy living in school-aged children (Frantz 2015; Mellanby, Rees & Tripp 2000). This strategy encourages students who are thoroughly trained and equipped with the knowledge of a health condition to teach their peers. Ghasemi et al. (2019) conducted a systematic review, which revealed that peer education could have a greater effect on knowledge, attitude, self-efficacy, practice and health behaviour when compared with other methods such as education by teachers, lectures, etc. Several studies have explored the use of peer education in the prevention of HIV, smoking (Dobbie et al. 2019), and obesity and eating disorder (Stock et al. 2007).

However, there is limited evidence of peer-led education in the prevention of auditory pathologies, such as middle ear pathologies. Therefore, the authors of this chapter strongly believe that peer-led education should be explored, particularly in preventing risky behaviours that potentially contribute to the development of middle ear pathologies, such as using matchsticks or pouring unprescribed oil into the ear.

The WHO (2013) recommended the use of telehealth systems to improve health awareness and knowledge of populations in underserved areas. Rushbrooke and Houston (2013) supported that telehealth can also be used to deliver health information and education to communities. Within the South African context, Khoza-Shangase and Moroe (2020) argued that because of the considerable audiological human resources challenges in LMICs and the demand for increasing audiology professionals' management of ear-and-hearing health care in programmes such as HCPs, prudent deliberation around tele-audiology as a platform for health care service delivery in these contexts is necessary. These authors argue strongly that the failure to explore tele-audiology for ear-and-hearing health care in this context signals a squandered opportunity to expand access to preventive audiological health care services to the South African population. They suggest that technological developments, with their recent complementary advances in telehealth, have expanded prospects for alternative and augmentative platforms of health care service delivery that are responsive to context, such as tele-audiology within ear-and-hearing health care preventive programmes. Khoza-Shangase and Moroe (2020) raised caution about the importance of adherence to policies and regulations during implementation, where ethics, human rights and medical law continue to guide the clinical care provided when utilising tele-audiology. These preventive measures also include the use of sensitive middle ear assessment measures that would allow for early detection and intervention before severe or permanent damage has occurred or before more specialised and costly tertiary-level care is required.

Paraprofessionals may also assist in conducting sensitive measures discussed above, such as taking video otoscopic images or video clips (Biagio et al. 2013) and tympanometry (Erkkola-Anttinen et al. 2014). Erkkola-Anttinen et al. (2014) trained parents of 78 children with AOM to obtain daily bilateral tympanograms. The findings of the study revealed that parents were able to obtain 83% of interpretable tympanograms. These results indicate that obtaining acoustic immittance such as tympanometry may not require specialised skills. Given that the procedure for obtaining WAI results and conventional tympanometry is similar (Hunter & Sanford 2015), paraprofessionals may be trained to obtain and record the results electronically within tele-audiology.

Khoza-Shangase, Sebothoma and Moroe (2021b) also argued that primary health care nurses, teacher assistants and trained volunteers can be used to increase access to ear-and-hearing health care. The ability to include paraprofessionals provides an opportunity to cover a wider population within various existing programmes and may ensure continuity of care. This will be particularly efficient and effective when within a tele-audiology programme so that audiologists can continue to provide diagnostic and rehabilitative health care services wherever they are located while remotely managing and monitoring these preventive programmes from across the country.

While task-shifting is a promising health care service delivery model, there are several factors to be considered. The training of paraprofessionals by qualified audiologists or otorhinolaryngologists to meet the minimum standards and regulations as stipulated by HPCSA, and the financing of audiological equipment required to conduct testing such as tympanometry, must be considered and planned for by the relevant stakeholders such as the DoH and HEIs. A lack of consideration of these factors will render this model impossible or unsustainable to achieve. Although health financing continues to be a challenge in South Africa, the authors of this chapter recommend that the audiology community lobby for this forms part of the NHI planning, budgeting and implementation.

5.8. Tele-audiology within the programmatic approach

As tele-audiology has not been widely used in different programmes, careful planning is required. Khoza-Shangase and Moroe (2020) emphasised the need for maintaining and adhering to the HPCSA and Department of Labour regulations, especially within the scope of tele-audiology for paraprofessionals. They further argue that the need for adhering to regulations is important because paraprofessionals will be facilitating tele-audiology such as making recordings, conducting online interactive engagements and real-time videoconferencing in programmes such as HCPs in the absence of an audiologist. This view is also true in other ear and hearing preventive programmes as the currently proposed one for the prevention of middle ear pathologies. The authors of this chapter believe that a similar approach and emphasis should be adopted in all programmes where tele-audiology is going to be utilised. Figure 5.1, adapted from Khoza-Shangase and Moroe (2020), illustrates how tele-audiology can be used in various health care programmes for the prevention of middle ear pathologies within the South African context.

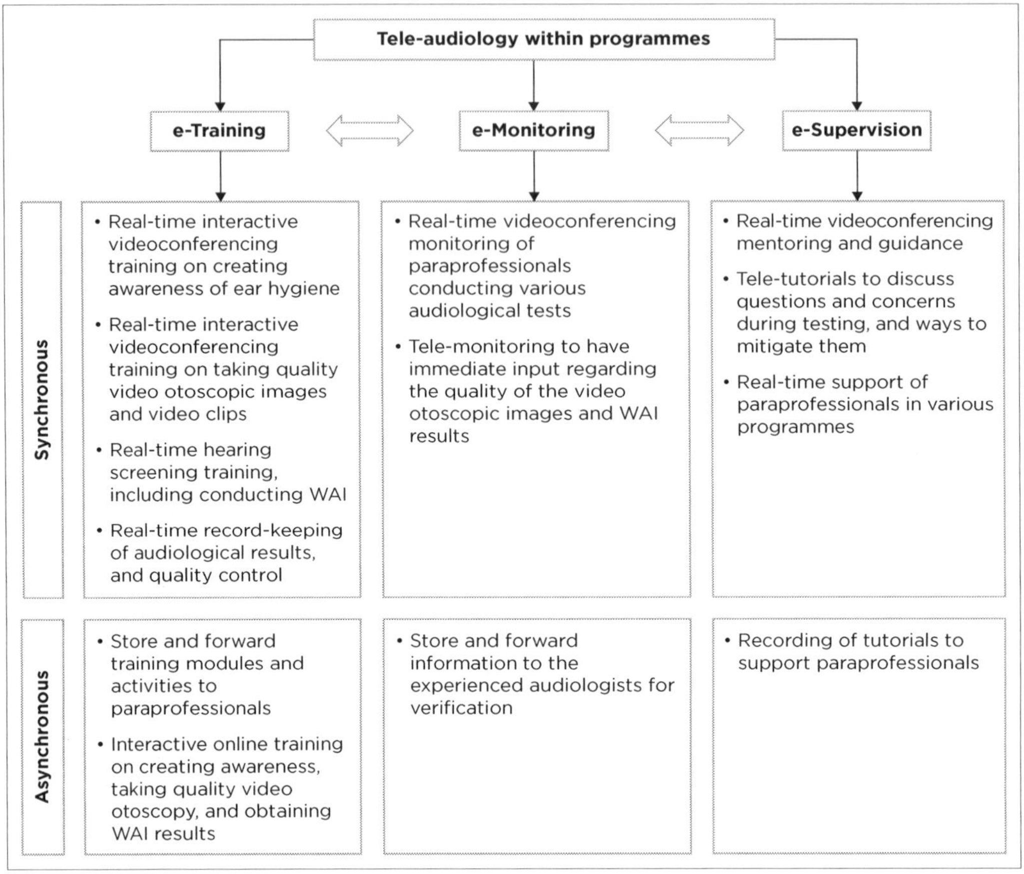

Source: Adapted from Khoza-Shangase and Moroe (2020).
Key: WAI, wideband acoustic immittance.

FIGURE 5.1: How tele-audiology can be used in various health care programmes for the prevention of middle ear pathologies within the South African context.

■ 5.9. Conclusion

Middle ear pathologies are commonly observed, with their high prevalence in LMICs such as South Africa because of various risk factors. While educational activities discussed in this chapter are critical in improving community knowledge and awareness of symptoms of middle ear pathologies and improving knowledge about seeking early hearing health care, these activities may not be sufficient, particularly when middle ear pathologies arise because of a compromised immune system. In these cases, measures with high sensitivity and specificity in identifying middle ear pathologies early become critical at all levels of prevention. As part of a programmatic approach to health care delivery, the authors recommend that middle ear pathologies should not be prevented separately but integrated into other health care and educational programmes. This approach will allow for increased reach, as well as improved monitoring and sustainability of the middle ear pathologies preventive programme.

While access to health care resources in LMIC contexts continues to be a huge challenge for the majority of the citizens, and given the need for UHC, health care professionals and policymakers must begin deliberating on new approaches to health care delivery; approaches that can increase coverage, improve access, and achieve early identification and intervention. While in audiology there is a concerted effort to improve early identification and increase coverage of hearing loss, early identification of middle ear pathologies remains largely ignored. Therefore, the proposed framework suggests a programmatic approach to improve the early identification of middle ear pathologies and increase coverage, especially in people who are already at risk of developing these pathologies. Within already existing programmes in South Africa, the authors propose that audiologists and otorhinolaryngologists do not need to conceive additional programmes but can be incorporated into and collaborate within already existing programmes. Although specific health care programmes are mentioned in the discussion, audiologists and otorhinolaryngologists should not be limited to these programmes but should explore other opportunities to collaborate within health and other non-health programmes, where ear-and-hearing health care is of relevance.

While a programmatic approach may be beneficial, careful planning, implementation and monitoring are required to ensure that current existing programmes are not strained and that health care providers such as paraprofessionals are not overwhelmed with the expansion of their scope of function. Therefore, discussions with relevant stakeholders such as regulators and departmental heads, as well as with political administrators, to map out how such an approach can be accommodated are required, with careful collating of evidence to ensure that future implementation is contextually relevant and responsive, considering barriers and challenges covered in Chapters 2, 3 and 4.

Chapter 6

Ototoxicity vigilance as a preventive audiology imperative within the African context: Pharmaco-audiology explored

Katijah Khoza-Shangase
Department of Audiology, Faculty of Humanities,
School of Human and Community Development, University of the Witwatersrand,
Johannesburg, South Africa

6.1. Introduction

Preventive health care, wherein preventive audiology is located, consists of measures taken for disease prevention at various levels of prevention, as detailed in Chapter 1 of this book. Hearing function can be affected by numerous causes, including drugs or medications used to treat certain conditions, and this is termed ototoxicity. Ototoxicity is a negative response to some pharmaceutical drugs prescribed to treat diseases, where negative effects on the cochlea or auditory nerve signified by cochlear or vestibular dysfunction occur (Ganesan et al. 2018). With the high burden of diseases such as cancer, TB and HIV and AIDS, ototoxicity is one condition that requires

How to cite: Khoza-Shangase, K 2022, 'Ototoxicity vigilance as a preventive audiology imperative within the African context: Pharmaco-audiology explored', ed. K Khoza-Shangase, *Preventive audiology: An African perspective*, AOSIS Books, Cape Town, pp. 111–136. https://doi.org/10.4102/aosis.2022.BK209.06

careful preventive measures as it is preventable, and its degree and effects are significantly minimisable if early detection and intervention protocols are followed. Associations have been proven to exist between medical treatments of these conditions and ototoxicity.

The HPCSA (2018) released national guidelines on the assessment and management of patients on ototoxic medications in South Africa. The HPCSA (2018) guidelines, accessible on the HPCSA website, can only be successfully implemented within LMICs, like South Africa, if contextual challenges such as unavailability of equipment and personnel, limited collaboration among team members, inefficient informational control systems and inefficient health care services are addressed. This implementation should be guided by support from contextualised research evidence.

Recent evidence from the South African context indicates challenges with the implementation of these guidelines because of numerous existing contextual barriers. HPCSA (2018) provided methodical and standardised ototoxicity monitoring guidelines for clinical locations where ototoxic medications are prescribed, with a centrally located clear role of audiologists as part of the treatment team to eliminate or minimise ototoxicity within the South African context. Enough evidence exists to support a pharmaco-audiology vigilance strategy (Khoza-Shangase 2020a) that will permit suitable, precise, well-organised and dependable comparisons of patient data within each patient longitudinally and between patients, as well as between and within different types of treatments and treatment sites. This data comparison can also be performed with other local data or with international data. This chapter argues for pharmaco-vigilance in audiology as one of the key preventive audiology strategies requiring careful consideration within resource-constrained contexts, such as Africa. Risk–benefit deliberations are presented with recommended solutions relevant to the context, including the role of task-shifting and tele-audiology in this scope of audiology practice.

■ 6.2. Context

Evidence indicates that all biologically active substances display several types of harmful and adverse influences on the human body (Guo et al. 2010). While doctors prescribe drugs for disease treatment or prevention, the same drugs can have toxic effects in some patients. This has been seen, particularly where infectious, life-threatening conditions such as HIV and AIDS (Bankaitis & Schountz 1998) and TB (Bardien et al. 2009; Singh 2017) are concerned. A similar concern exists for the treatment of the current novel COVID-19 pandemic (Bogdanov et al. 2021; García et al. 2020; Siemieniuk et al. 2020). In such instances, where sustaining lives is the urgent goal, a newly developed drug may gain approval before the QoL indicators, such as toxic side effects, have been fully established.

The US Food and Drug Administration (FDA) and the European Medicines Agency aligned South African Health Products Authority (SAHPRA) adopts the aforementioned approach too, particularly with the approval of treatments for communicable diseases. If a treatment drug fulfils a clinical need where treatments are not available, such as was the case with HIV or TB therapy and recently COVID-19 pandemic, the SAHPRA adopts an approval accelerating approach, which significantly reduces the time period (a year to a year and a half) ordinarily adhered to drug registration (Rome & Avorn 2020). This has recently played out with COVID-19 where life preservation has been observed to hasten vaccine and drug development processes (Cassidy et al. 2020; Rome & Avorn 2020; Thomson & Nachlis 2020). COVID-19 is an acute infectious respiratory disease that has been reported to be produced by infection with a recently discovered coronavirus that has rapidly spread throughout the world, with various variants emerging in its development course (Duong 2021). Consequently, the WHO director-general, Dr Tedros Adhanom Ghebreyesus, officially proclaimed COVID-19 as a pandemic, which is a public health crisis of global concern (Mustafa 2020). Drug development for such infectious conditions primarily foregrounds sustaining life as a principal goal, with minimal, if any, attention placed on QoL influencing factors such as hearing loss (Burgoyne & Tan 2008; Guastalla & Dieras 2003). This, therefore, highlights the need for post-drug approval pharmaco-vigilance, where drug research focuses on detecting, identifying and categorising side effects of the drug.

The known objective in drug research is, through laboratory investigations, to identify the harmful reactions of recently developed drugs prior to any harm inflicted upon humans (Guo et al. 2010; Tsintis & La Mache 2004). Identifying adverse effects of drugs is what pharmaco-vigilance in the form of ototoxicity monitoring in audiology should be aimed at, with the ultimate goal of minimising or eliminating the toxic effects of the drugs on the auditory and vestibular system. As clear as this goal is, achieving it is not easy and has been met by numerous challenges. Evidence suggests that this failure is because of the lack of South African standardised investigative methods and ototoxicity monitoring practises, as well as an absence of a South African government mandate (Khoza-Shangase 2010a, 2013, 2020a; Khoza-Shangase & Stirk 2016; Stevenson et al. 2021).

As audiological assessment and monitoring are not components of standard initial investigations where adverse drug effects are identified and categorised, preventive audiology measures in the form of ototoxicity monitoring and management become essential not only for clinical practice but also for ethical reasons. Therefore, it is vital for audiologists and audiology researchers to become directly involved in drug development for the early detection of audiology adverse events in the form of vestibulotoxicity and ototoxicity (Bankaitis & Schountz 1998). In resource-constrained contexts such as LMICs, where South Africa is located, efficient identification and prioritisation of which drugs to closely monitor are key, as not all drugs can be monitored. Audiologists should keep an updated log of the major pharmacological agents and health conditions that have been recognised to warrant audiological monitoring to be able to prioritise them in their monitoring programmes. The well-established classes of drugs that have an ototoxic and or vestibulotoxic effect include loop diuretics, platinum-based antineoplastic agents, aminoglycosides, non-steroidal anti-inflammatory agents and, progressively, antiretroviral (ARV) drugs (Bankaitis & Schountz 1998; Bisht & Bist 2011; Khoza-Shangase 2010b, 2013; Khoza-Shangase & Stirk 2016; Rybak & Ramkumar 2007). This recommended prioritisation of health conditions and specific drugs is essential as it would be prohibitive to include ototoxicity monitoring in all clinical drug development trials, especially in environments with a lack of resources, such as is the case in LMICs. This approach has a goal of early identification of ototoxicity and its consequent early intervention, prior to permanent damage, an imperative in primary health care, where prevention is the South African National Health Department's adopted approach.

In his study, Freeman (n.d.) supported the idea of prioritising the issues by asserting that in the South African context, prioritising some health conditions over others because of limited resources available to address all health challenges, including constrained financial and human resources, is necessary. This author argues that it is, therefore, important that the country concentrates its energies and resources on prioritised areas, otherwise minimal progress would be made in attending to health care challenges. Freeman (n.d.) suggested that attempting to address all conditions equally will be less productive than if increased resources are placed into an identified small number of health care conditions as priorities. This prioritisation approach is the position adopted in this chapter where, within the South African context, highly prevalent conditions such as HIV, AIDS, TB and cancer have been spotlighted as strategic diseases in the burden of diseases with an association to ototoxicity (Adams et al. 2012; Khoza-Shangase & Masondo 2021).

■ 6.3. Delving into ototoxicity

In the past decades, post-Apartheid, South Africa continues to be among the LMICs with high mortality rates as well as inadequate health outcomes associated with the distinctive quadruple burden of disease, described as including non-communicable diseases (e.g. cardiovascular diseases and hypertension, diabetes, cancer, mental illnesses and chronic lung diseases), communicable diseases (e.g. HIV, AIDS and TB), injury and trauma, as well as maternal and child mortality (Institute for Health Metrics and Evaluation 2018; Pillay-Van Wyk et al. 2016; Rohde et al. 2008). This quadruple burden of disease's impact has reportedly worsened with the advent of COVID-19, which has disrupted and pressurised the country's economy as well as its health care system (Hofman & Madhi 2020). The treatment for some of these conditions under the quadruple burden of disease banner, which includes over 600 categories of classes of drugs such as platinum-based chemotherapeutic agents, aminoglycosides and loop diuretics, is linked to ototoxicity (Ganesan et al. 2018). Ramma, Schellack and Heinze (2019) highlighted that the increasingly wide range of these drugs, as well as their increased prescription, has increased the incidence of ototoxicity over the years, with Govender et al. (2020) and Paken et al. (2021) locating this also within the South African context.

Despite the established important role that ototoxic medications play in modern medicine, their capacity to cause significant morbidity has also been well-documented (Campbell 2018). The morbidity that is linked to the auditory and vestibular system is largely preventable and its effects minimisable if detected early and preventive measures are implemented timeously. Delayed diagnosis of ototoxicity has been highlighted as one of the main challenges confronted during ototoxicity evaluation and treatment (Ganesan et al. 2018). Ganesan et al. (2018) claimed that diagnosis of ototoxicity often happens after the hearing loss has progressed to a severe degree that already has a significant impact on speech perception, which is a failure in preventive audiology programmes.

Although ototoxicity is argued to be non-life-threatening, evidence indicates that it has a significant impact on QoL as it affects communication, scholastic and occupational outcomes, with documented social consequences for the affected individual across the lifespan (Govender & Paken 2015; Khoza-Shangase 2010b, 2017), and equally significant cost implications for the State. In the paediatric population, the impact on speech and language, as well as social and cognitive development that leads to poor educational and psychosocial functioning outcomes, can be the negative consequences of ototoxicity (HPCSA 2018). Baguley and Prayuenyong (2020) argued for careful monitoring of self-reported QoL impact of the cochlear and vestibular dysfunction because of ototoxicity as part of the surveillance and monitoring programmes as these can cause significant negative psychological and physical outcomes (Manchaiah et al. 2018). The physical outcomes linked to vestibular dysfunction can impact QoL influencers, such as engaging in activities that require good balance like walking, riding, driving and dancing, with consequent psychological effects (Sun et al. 2014).

The WHO (2019) approximated the incidence of disabling hearing loss to be 6.1% of the global population, with causes varying widely to include ototoxicity (ASHA 2015) because of drugs that are usually reserved for treating life-threatening conditions (WHO 2014a). The incidence rates of ototoxicity vary from country to country, depending on prevalent risk factors such as HIV, AIDS, TB and other communicable and non-communicable diseases. For example, in the United States, Landier (2016) approximated the occurrence of ototoxicity to range between 4% and 90%, depending on numerous factors such as the drug under investigation, administrative techniques, age of the patient population and cumulative dose.

It is estimated that, in 2016, the global number of individuals diagnosed with TB was 10.4 million; and of these individuals, 90% were adults, with 74% of them living in African countries (Floyd et al. 2018). Furthermore, the WHO (2014b) estimated that 33 million persons were living with HIV in Eastern and Southern Africa, with an observable constant increase in individuals diagnosed with cancer. The WHO (2020) stated that, globally, TB is the most common presenting illness among people living with HIV, regardless of whether they are on ARV treatment or not, and it is the chief cause of HIV-related mortalities. This organisation reports that sub-Saharan Africa, where South Africa is located, bears the brunt of the dual epidemic, accounting for approximately 84% of all deaths from HIV-associated TB in 2018 (WHO 2020). This dual epidemic has made South Africa the epicentre of HIV and AIDS, with a joint high frequency of TB co-infection. Because of the excessive numbers of individuals on long-term treatment for TB in South Africa, Bardien et al. (2009, p. 440), very early on, claimed that South Africa was '[...] potentially facing the risk of a significant proportion of the population acquiring aminoglycoside-induced permanent hearing loss'. This claim was realised in one of the biggest complaints of negligence against the SANDoH in 2017 for failing to provide proper monitoring, where 123 adults receiving TB treatment in the province of KwaZulu-Natal lost their hearing following TB treatment (Singh 2017). The afore-presented reality raises important implications for preventive audiology, in the form of pharmaco-vigilance, within the African context.

In South Africa, sufficient evidence of links between HIV, AIDS and TB treatments and ototoxicity has been established (Bardien et al. 2009; Govender & Paken 2015; Harris, Peer & Fagan 2012; HPCSA 2018; Hong et al. 2020; Khoza-Shangase 2010a, 2011, 2014; Khoza-Shangase & Jina 2013; Khoza-Shangase, Lecheko & Ntlhakana 2020; Khoza-Shangase & Masondo 2020, 2021; Khoza-Shangase & Stirk 2016; Moodley et al. 2021; Ramma et al. 2019). This evidence calls for careful deliberations by the South African audiology community around preventive ototoxicity strategies. With 7.7 million people living with HIV in South Africa, and 70% of adults on ARV treatment by the year ending 2019 (UNAIDS 2020), with universal coverage being the target, pharmaco-vigilance in the form of ototoxicity monitoring and management must become a critical part of the treatment plan for this population. The current practice, however, shows a lack of uniform, organised and efficient ototoxicity monitoring within the clinical locations where these diseases are assessed and managed, with ad hoc and negligible participation of audiologists as members of the multidisciplinary team (Khoza-Shangase & Masondo 2020, 2021).

The current HIV and AIDS statistics treatment coverage data indicate that there is no universal coverage yet shows evidence of a focused strategy (UNAIDS 2020). Significant progress has been made in the achievement of sustaining the lives of infected individuals as the roll-out of ARV therapy in South African public health care facilities in the first quarter of 2004 (Fairall et al. 2008; Nachega et al. 2006; Nunes et al. 2011). This progress has also been mirrored by advances in medications prescribed, such as fixed-dose combination ARV medication introduced in 2013 (Davies 2013). This new development has been hailed as a significant influence on treatment adherence. Furthermore, the commitment of the South African government to the UNAIDS 90:90:90 strategy by 2030 indicates a clear and directed plan for the efficient management of HIV by this LMIC (UNAIDS 2014).

The aforementioned treatment strategy has a well-defined goal of eliminating or preventing the spread of HIV as well as sustaining the lives of those infected in South Africa. Khoza-Shangase (2020a) strongly argued that in the clinical management strategy of the population with HIV, AIDS and TB, it is imperative that audiologists ceaselessly raise the importance of also foregrounding the *quality* of life that is sustained by ARV roll-out. This author asserts that this additional QoL focus would include otological manifestations (such as auditory and vestibular function) as one of the sensory disabilities found in this population. Consequently, maintenance of at least 90% QoL should form part of the UNAIDS 2030 target of having 90% infected diagnosed, 90% on treatment, and 90% virally suppressed by 2030 (Khoza-Shangase 2020a).

Iatrogenic causes of hearing loss in HIV and AIDS are one of the three main groups of causes of otological manifestations in this population. The other two are primary effects because of the virus itself and secondary causes because of opportunistic infections. Iatrogenic causes comprise the drug-induced auditory and vestibular effects following treatments with medications that are ototoxic in nature (Khoza-Shangase 2018), with these effects constantly changing because of the sustained development in new treatments (Bankaitis & Schountz 1998; Campbell 2018; Kallail, Downs & Scherz 2008). Various extensively used treatments in the treatment of HIV that have documented links with ototoxicity include post-exposure prophylaxis with lamivudine, stavudine and nevirapine, NRTI therapy (nevirapine); zidovudine; and mixtures of zidovudine and didanosine; lamivudine and stavudine; lamivudine, stavudine, didanosine, and hydroxyurea; combinations of lamivudine, nevirapine and stavudine; azidothymidine, lamivudine and efavirenz; antineoplastic medications (e.g. vincristine), antifungal agents (including flucytosine, amphotericin B and ketoconazole), as well as aminoglycoside antibiotics, immune modulators, zalcitabine and didanosine (Bankaitis & Schountz 1998; Kallail et al. 2008; Khoza-Shangase 2010b, 2011, 2014).

Evidence linking these HIV treatments to ototoxicity demonstrates that the ototoxic effects create a burden and a distinctive challenge to the provision of ear-and-hearing health care service delivery in South Africa (HPCSA 2018; Hollander, Joubert & Schellack 2020; Khoza-Shangase 2010a, 2011, 2018, 2020b; Khoza-Shangase & Masondo 2020; Khoza-Shangase & Prodromos 2021; Khoza-Shangase & Van Rie 2017; Swanepoel 2006). The evidence further supports the development and implementation of systematic and standardised ototoxicity monitoring protocols, such as the ototoxicity grading system within a mobile app for resource-limited settings that are recommended by Hollander et al. (2020). These ototoxicity monitoring protocols have pharmaco-audiology vigilance as a primary objective, where elimination of drug-induced hearing loss and determination of the precise compounds causing ototoxicity in this population are done. Nationally, this primary objective can only be attained in a context where locally relevant research, based on reliable data collected using sensitive, valid and reliable assessment measures, is conducted to establish evidence that will facilitate best practice.

In a 2010 South African study by Khoza-Shangase (2010b), where the need for ototoxicity monitoring in patients with HIV and AIDS was examined, findings revealed contextual challenges that seem to have remained the same 20 years later (Khoza-Shangase et al. 2020). These challenges include financial and human resource limitations, lack of required equipment and lack of informational counselling as factors that influence the provision of dedicated, efficient ototoxicity monitoring services. Consequently, a negligible number of individuals on ototoxic treatments undergo monitoring and preventive management (Khoza-Shangase et al. 2020), particularly within the population with TB (Khoza-Shangase & Prodromos 2021).

The importance and value of audiometric testing in the process of early identification of hearing thresholds changes because of drug therapy is widely acknowledged (Hollander et al. 2020; Hong et al. 2020; HPCSA 2018; Ramma et al. 2019). Although it is well recognised and accepted that priority to sustain lives during the treatment of life-threatening conditions such as HIV and AIDS trumps the concerns around the highly ototoxic nature of the agents used, preventive strategies still remain relevant. Sufficient evidence exists that demonstrates that preventive measures, such as prescription of alternative drugs, altered treatment regimens or administration of reduced dosages, are successful options if ototoxicity is identified early in the treatment phase (Khoza-Shangase & Prodromos 2021; Lonsbury-Martin & Martin 2001). Prospective audiological monitoring of high-frequency hearing allows the prescribing doctor to consider and weigh the advantages of alternative treatment and/or amount, mode and frequency of treatment prior to worsening hearing loss to invade the lower range of frequencies that are significant for speech and communication. The value of monitoring hearing thresholds extends beyond medical intervention to rehabilitation, where the audiologist, family and the patient are alerted to hearing challenges early and amplification can be fitted as part of an overall holistic aural rehabilitation programme. Although this is a secondary outcome to an ototoxicity monitoring programme (OMP), with the ideal outcome being complete prevention of hearing loss, early provision of amplification can enhance the patient's QoL and facilitate their adherence to medical treatment. Consequently, in every context, stringent use of and adherence to standardised assessment protocols for early detection of hearing changes become imperative in pharmaco-vigilance preventive programmes.

The implications of pharmaco-vigilance in audiology within the South African context extend to co-existing audiological conditions such as occupational noise-induced hearing loss (ONIHL), where a large number of the mining workforce is affected. Recently, Khoza-Shangase (2020c) found that gold miners with a history of TB treatment present with high-frequency hearing thresholds that are significantly worse than the group without this history. This difference in hearing function in these two groups raises the value of tactical HCPs that incorporate ototoxicity monitoring in those workers with concomitant comorbidities such as TB and HIV or AIDS, with the exploration of prescription of otoprotective or chemo-protective agents in the South African mining population as part of preventive efforts (Khoza-Shangase 2010a, 2010b, 2011, 2017, 2020b).

Stuckler and colleagues (2011, 2013) reported that South Africa appears in the list of countries where the highest incidence of HIV, AIDS and TB is found, with the mining industry being the hardest hit by these conditions. Approximately a third of mineworkers in South African mines were reported to acquire HIV within the first year and a half of working in the mines (Reddy & Swanepoel 2006). AngloGold Ashanti (2012) approximated that 85% of their employees had TB and HIV in the early 2000s. This raises important implications related to the recorded evidence of the compounding influence of synergistic effects of simultaneous exposure to noise while on ototoxic medications for the treatment of HIV, AIDS and TB (Khoza-Shangase 2020c; Valente et al. 2008). The concomitant exposure to these conditions within a chronic hazardous noise exposure environment further accentuates ototoxicity vigilance as a preventive audiology imperative within the South African context.

Research has considered defining ototoxicity and establishing early identification and monitoring guidelines to facilitate deliberations around treatment modifications that would lead to minimal or eliminated ototoxicity (ASHA 1994, 2015; HPCSA 2018). Although numerous guidelines have been developed, their feasibility continues to be uncertain because of various factors, particularly in LMICs. In an LMIC such as South Africa with inadequate resources for basic health care services, there has been a documented lack of standardised practice for ototoxicity detection and monitoring until as recently as 2018, when the HPCSA's SLH Professions Board, for the first time, published national guidelines for ototoxicity assessment and management. This publication is following years of the country's audiologists modifying protocols from HICs, such as the United States of America, to apply within the South African context, with limited success (Govender & Paken 2015). Khoza-Shangase and Masondo (2020), however, argued that for successful application of the HPCSA guidelines to occur within this population, clear scoping of the context with regard to current practices around ototoxicity assessment and management is required, with findings of this exercise affording the audiology community the opportunity to compare the current practice to the endorsed guidelines. In their scoping of the South African context for this very purpose, Khoza-Shangase and Masondo (2020) found considerable lacunae between knowledge and conversion of this knowledge into practice in this area of practice. In their study, these authors report various important findings emanating from this study that bear relevance for the South African context:

1. Although a significant majority of the audiologists sampled (over two-thirds) performed ototoxicity monitoring and management, the protocols utilised were not aligned to either HPCSA guidelines or international standards.
2. Pre-treatment (baseline) assessment was not conducted by a majority of the audiologists, and monitoring was performed irregularly and less frequently than what is recommended in the guidelines, thereby negatively influencing the ototoxicity programmes' ability to detect ototoxicity early for the implementation of early preventive intervention.
3. Non-standard assessment batteries were utilised for assessment and monitoring, raising queries about the reliability and validity of the data that are then used to inform preventive treatment decisions.
4. Collaborative working relationships between audiologists and the rest of the clinical team managing patients on ototoxic medications were inadequate, thus contributing significantly to the less-than-optimal ototoxicity management practices in this context.
5. Specialised treatment institutions, such as TB hospitals, were better equipped and better resourced to be able to adhere to ototoxicity assessment and management guidelines because there was a clinical focus.
6. Within the South African context, where ototoxicity training forms part of the minimum undergraduate curriculum, current findings seemed to indicate that postgraduate qualifications did not influence the audiologists' practices for ototoxicity assessment and management.

Findings from Khoza-Shangase and Masondo's (2020) study offered contextually relevant evidence within the South African context, supporting pharmaco-audiology vigilance as one of the key focus areas for preventive audiology. These researchers resolve that for successful implementation of ototoxicity monitoring and management guidelines within the South African context, a few strategic areas need focus, and these are (1) adherence to guidelines and converting these guidelines, knowledge and policies into practice, (2) clinical assessment and management practices adhered to, (3) suitable allocation of resources for each programme and (4) calculated planning for national ototoxicity assessment and management programmes in context. Such strategic planning should be guided by deliberate benefit versus risk assessments of ototoxicity vigilance within this context, taking South African realities into consideration. Chapter 10 of this book offers interesting cost analysis deliberations that raise important considerations that can influence these benefit versus risk evaluations, although this is done in the area of EHDI in the paediatric population.

■ 6.4. Benefit versus risk of ototoxicity vigilance

Assessments of risk-benefit calculations in pharmacology are well recognised and recorded, where risk-benefit assessments refer to the appraisal of safety indicators in the health care industry, be it medical or surgical signals or both (Guo et al. 2010). Within the South African audiology community and those of other LMICs, careful positioning of pharmaco-audiology within the preventive health care model is needed, where clarity of the role of the audiologist within the team is provided as part of the risk-benefit evaluation of treatment methods. Khoza-Shangase (2017) argued that this repositioning should ensure that audiologists become core and central members of the multidisciplinary and multi-stakeholder team, rather than their current peripheral role, specifically when risk-benefit assessment is made of medications that have been proven to be or have potential to be ototoxic in nature.

In a paper titled *Risk versus Benefit: Who assesses this in the management of patients on ototoxic drugs?*, Khoza-Shangase (2017) highlights important strategic indicators and factors that audiologists must reflect on to engage in more meaningful ways with the process of preventive pharmaco-vigilance. This author highlights the importance of carefully considering the risk-benefit of medications prescribed to treat diseases within LMICs, particularly those that create the biggest burden of disease. With recent South African evidence indicating increasing momentum towards ototoxicity monitoring within the clinical and research communities, although this is non-systematic, non-comprehensive and non-strategic in nature (Khoza-Shangase & Masondo 2020); the value of risk-benefit assessments is highlighted. Alongside risk-benefit evaluations, considerations of challenges impeding efficient OMPs must be addressed. Challenges to be considered include the absence of audiologists in the risk-benefit assessment of treatments during the drug development and monitoring process, lack of appropriate resources such as assessment equipment and alternative treatments, as well as capacity versus demand challenges where limited numbers of audiologists in the country (Pillay et al. 2020) limit their involvement in preventive ear-and-hearing health care. Additionally, the challenge with the restricted collaborative engagement of audiologists with the rest of the members of stakeholders involved in the treatment of patients on ototoxic medications, including paraprofessionals, also needs scrutiny, particularly because this is aimed at safeguarding both quantity and QoL of patients on ototoxic medications.

Within the South African context, where evidence indicates significant health challenges within the public health care sector (Maphumulo & Bhengu 2019), risk-benefit evaluations are paramount. The *challenges within the public health care sector* have been documented to include (1) inadequate and insufficient workforce; (2) inadequate health care professional-to-patient ratios; (3) limited well-functioning public health care facilities; (4) overall scarcity of resources for the population size with consequent demand versus supply incongruence; (5) difficulties with converting knowledge and policies into practice for numerous reasons, including dilemmas with the influences of language and culture in health care; and (6) risk-benefit evaluation quandaries (Coovadia et al. 2009; Khoza-Shangase et al. 2020; Khoza-Shangase & Masondo 2020; Khoza-Shangase & Mophosho 2018, 2021; Maphumulo & Bhengu 2019; Mayosi et al. 2012; Pillay et al. 2020; Scheffler et al. 2009). Maphumulo and Bhengu (2019) argued that although numerous quality improvement programmes have been implemented in South African health care over the years, the desired level of quality service delivery has not been achieved; therefore, these authors stress the importance of the South African government making sure that the application of National Core Standards is done efficiently - and this includes monitoring outcomes of treatments for adverse effects.

Although ototoxicity may not qualify as a 'more severe side effect', it still demands significant focus by the clinical and research community to facilitate ethical clinical care of patients in addition to clinical care (Khoza-Shangase 2010a:575). For a side effect to be regarded as a serious adverse event, literature lists a number of any untoward medical incident, regardless of the dose taken, that can cause patient death, threatens the patient's life, causes hospitalisation or extends hospitalisation and leads to permanent or major incapacity or disability (Moore, Cohen & Furberg 2007; Nebeker, Barach & Samore 2004; Tsintis & La Mache 2004). Although ototoxicity does not quite fall neatly within this definition, Khoza-Shangase (2017) asserted that it does fall under the adverse effects as *it is a permanent or major disability* to the person impacted, regardless of the fact that the person's life is saved by the same ototoxic medication (preventative health care benefits) and hence the importance of risk-benefit evaluation.

6.4.1. Evaluation of benefit versus risk

The procedure that is adopted to guarantee that all medications prescribed to patients are carefully monitored in terms of their effectiveness and examined for their negative side effects is referred to as the evaluation of risk-benefit. In audiology, this denotes ototoxicity monitoring (Bankaitis & Schountz 1998). One component of the risk-benefit evaluation process comprises the evaluation of positive effects or efficacy (comparative evaluation of benefits) and potential harm (risks) of drugs performed early during the drug research and development period, and this is of utmost significance in pharmacology (Juhaeri 2019; Kürzinger et al. 2020). It is well recognised that standard clinical trials must be conducted on all novel experimental drugs, with concessions made for medications explicitly produced for serious diseases and illnesses. In cases such as these, as observed during the COVID-19 pandemic, the United States of America's FDA, and within the South African context, SAHPRA might create an allowance to the standard clinical trial process to speed up the risk-benefit evaluation process of hopeful experimental medications (Blaschke et al. 1995; Cassidy et al. 2020; Rome & Avorn 2020; Thomson & Nachlis 2020).

It is an understandable expectation that the obligation for risk-benefit evaluation rests with the manufacturers whose drug evaluation processes should be continuous (including monitoring during the post-authorisation period). The main objective is to enhance treatment benefits as well as guarantee that adverse events or safety hazards are significantly reduced if complete eradication is impossible (Eichler et al. 2008). However, Khoza-Shangase (2017) argued that long-term negative QoL impacts of drugs might not be effortlessly detected without specialised, precise testing, which is commonly performed by qualified health care professionals, as with audiologists in ototoxicity assessments. These professionals do not normally form part of the initial phases of the drug testing and development process; therefore, it is vital that such risk-benefit assessments are all-inclusive and continuous, with the involvement of all applicable health care professionals. Within a resource-constrained context, like South Africa, where the capacity versus demand challenges exist, the health care professionals might need to be extended to include paraprofessionals. This extension might best be accomplished within a hybrid task-shifting tele-audiology model of health care service delivery, where trained paraprofessionals perform the ototoxicity monitoring under tele-audiology supervision and programme management by audiologists (Khoza-Shangase & Moroe 2020; Khoza-Shangase, Moroe & Neille 2021).

Protocol dictates that risk-benefit evaluation should, at the very least, be performed by a group of stakeholders that includes the patients, relevant health care practitioners advocating for their patients, researchers, pharmacologists, as well as regulatory authorities in charge of drug approval

(Guo et al. 2010; Juhaeri 2019; Khoza-Shangase 2017; Khoza-Shangase & Stirk 2016; Kürzinger et al. 2020; Nebeker et al. 2004; Tsintis & La Mache 2004). Each of the members of this group of stakeholders can be influenced by several factors in their decision-making around risk-benefit evaluation. This is especially true within LMIC contexts where infinite challenges to quality health care exist, where the idea of universal health care coverage is a dream rather than a reality and where significant innovation is required to make it an attainable goal (Benatar & Gill 2021).

6.4.2. Influencing factors to risk-benefit evaluation

Several factors have been branded to influence risk-benefit evaluation, and, as depicted in Figure 6.1, these include (1) nature of the problem, (2) reason for drug use and population requiring treatment, (3) financial factors, (4) stakeholders with interests in the drug and (5) time, data and resources limitations (Council for International Organizations of Medical Sciences [CIOMS] 1998; Tsintis & La Mache 2004).

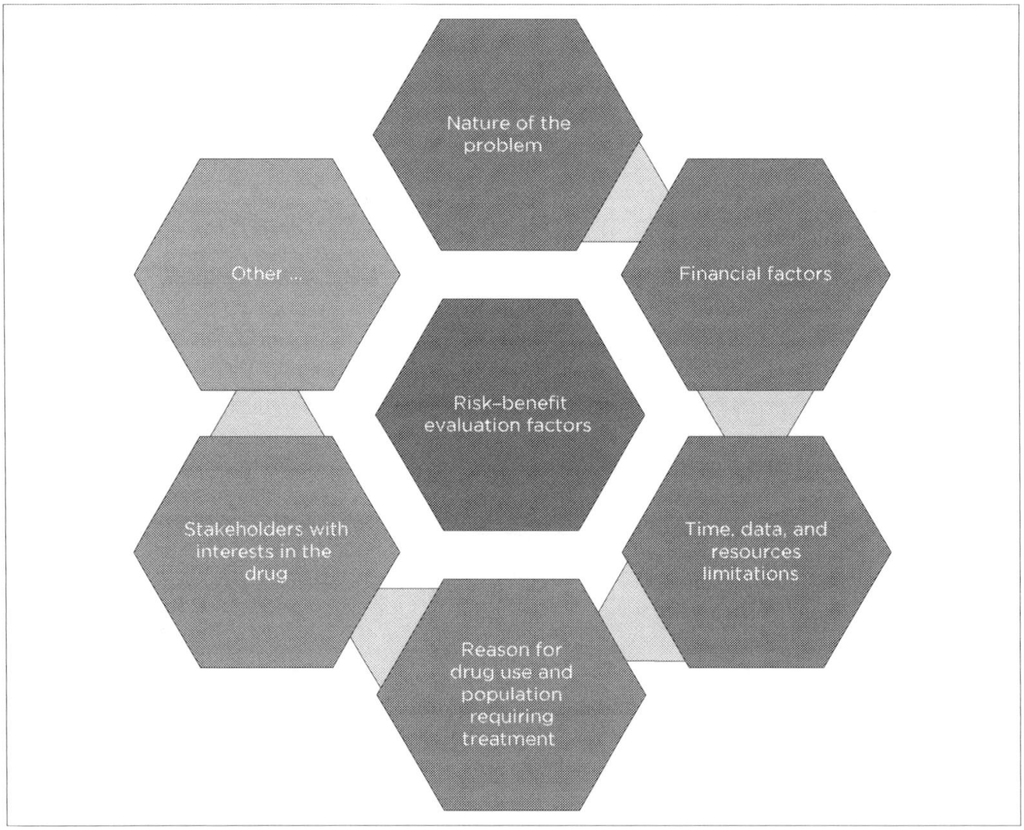

FIGURE 6.1: Factors that influence risk-benefit evaluation.

Khoza-Shangase (2017) carefully reviewed these factors as follows:

1. **Nature of the problem:** This describes the severity of the speculated negative drug reaction as well as its potential hazard to the individual's life. Because QoL adverse reactions such as auditory and vestibular side effects are less prioritised and not ordinarily included under adverse reactions, the nature of the problem can be limiting. Therefore, careful deliberations around the inclusion of QoL indicators, such as hearing and balance function, in the risk-benefit evaluation are required during the drug development and approval processes.
2. **Reason for drug use and population requiring treatment:** Ear-and-hearing health care professionals, such as audiologists, should be knowledgeable about which medications possess elevated acceptable risk and all the circumstances where there are no reasonable therapeutic alternatives. This awareness will guide the planning and development of efficient ototoxicity monitoring and management programmes. Where lifesaving of self-preservation is the goal of the treatment, and no alternative is available, pre-treatment counselling, monitoring and early intervention become essential.
3. **Financial factors:** In financial terms, these factors involve weightings and compromises aimed at economic efficiency. Specifically, differences between costs and benefits are calculated, as part of risk-benefit evaluation, with cost utilised for an individual who reacts similarly to different drugs (CIOMS 1998). These financial factors are particularly significant in risk-benefit assessments, especially in LMICs like South Africa. In LMICs, health departments may possibly approve drugs with less than satisfactory risk-benefit balances because of their lower costs when compared to their alternatives (Coovadia et al. 2009; CIOMS 1998; Mayosi et al. 2009; Tsintis & La Mache 2004). It is for this reason that the role of the audiologists under LMIC contexts as lobbyists should be heightened and centralised. Audiologists' role at this stage would be to ensure that economic factors are not miscalculated because of the exclusion of QoL indicators (e.g. ototoxicity) by pharmaceutical companies during the drug development process. A QoL indicator, such as a permanent hearing loss, can raise substantial economic implications for both the patient and the State if preventive efforts are not successful. For the patient, vocational performance can be negatively affected, which may lead to poor work productivity or loss of employment, and for the State, the country's economy can be directly impacted, and the rehabilitation costs and social/disability grants crippling.
4. **Stakeholders with interests in the drug:** There are numerous groups that have a vested interest in the risk-benefit evaluation, and these include patients, ethics committees, regulatory authorities, doctors, pharmaceutical companies, pharmacologists, other public health care bodies, consumer groups and medical aids (CIOMS 1998). Because all these groups may have

diverse perspectives on the risk-benefit assessment of medications, it is vital to have knowledge of who formed the evaluation team for a certain drug. Khoza-Shangase (2017) argued that the patient's perspective should be at the forefront as objective audiological data collection for ototoxicity and vestibular toxicity is obtained from the patient. In the South African context, sensitivity to contextual factors (including influences of linguistic and cultural diversity) and social determinants of health are important in this process. Evidence indicates that two patients subjected to the same risks and benefits may have diverse perceptions and acceptance of the risk and may also make diverse decisions around the risk (Colopy et al. 2015; Juhaeri 2019; Kürzinger et al. 2020). Moreover, linguistic and cultural diversity within health care delivery in the South African context may compound this level of risk evaluation (Khoza-Shangase & Mophosho 2018). Regardless of these factors, the risk associated with a drug that a patient is taking must be conveyed to the patient so that the patient is able to provide informed consent for treatment and also because appropriate pre-treatment counselling regarding adverse effects has been linked to positive drug adherence (Higashi et al. 2013).

5. **Time, data and resource limitations:** Where the possible major adverse event is urgent, time, data and resources are acutely important. Because ototoxicity may not be viewed as a major adverse event, time may not be argued as an urgency; however, data and resources may be. Adequate data on comparator drugs, alternative treatments or additional treatment modalities must be acquired as soon and as realistically fast as possible. For this to occur, sensitive, valid and reliable standard ototoxicity monitoring practices must be in place nationally, especially in clinical sites where the risk of ototoxicity is high. In such setups, large databases that can facilitate simple reviews of adverse drug reactions can be collated in a standardised manner (Khoza-Shangase & Masondo 2020). The current status of ototoxicity monitoring in South Africa is comprised of limited and non-standard OMPs and would have a significantly negative influence on risk-benefit assessments of any drug, directly impacting successful preventive audiology initiatives within this context. In addition to standardising ototoxicity monitoring protocols, South African audiologists would need to be innovative in addressing the equipment constraints and human resources (capacity versus demand) challenges. This entails adopting innovative health care service delivery approaches such as task-shifting and tele-audiology (Hollander et al. 2020; Khoza-Shangase et al. 2020; Khoza-Shangase & Stirk 2016; Sebothoma et al. 2021).

■ 6.5. Solutions and recommendations

To guarantee that systematic data are gathered for evidence-based practice within the South African context, Khoza-Shangase (2020a) suggested an ototoxicity monitoring protocol. This author suggests that systematic data collation through such a protocol has substantial implications for the South African audiologists' ability to advance their role in drug development and risk–benefit evaluation processes. This expanded role of audiologists is particularly feasible now that South Africa has developed national guidelines on the assessment and management of patients on ototoxic medications (HPCSA 2018).

Over and above pharmaco-vigilance, preventive audiology within ototoxicity rehabilitation within the South African context should include more than early detection, constant monitoring and lessening or averting hearing loss but should also incorporate planning of appropriate early rehabilitative measures (Khoza-Shangase 2020a). Delayed diagnosis of ototoxicity has been reported as the principal challenge in this process because of the highly diverse and unpredictable nature of its presentation (Ganesan et al. 2018; Govender & Paken 2015; HPCSA 2018; Khoza-Shangase & Masondo 2020, 2021). Over and above the diverse and unpredictable nature of ototoxicity, additional factors such as culturally influenced health-seeking behaviours, age, medical conditions and cognitive levels may delay early diagnosis (Ganesan et al. 2018; Harris et al. 2012; Khoza-Shangase 2013; Khoza-Shangase & Mophosho 2018). It is, therefore, imperative that all contextual factors be taken into consideration, together with risk–benefit evaluation outcomes, when planning and implementing a structured programmatic, burden-of-disease-linked OMP.

The HPCSA's guidelines (2018) suggested that an ototoxicity programme should always commence with informational counselling where patients' awareness around ototoxicity symptoms is raised. This process involves educating campaigns where patients are taught what symptoms to look out for to report to the attending health care professionals, such as audiologists, pharmacists, nurses, doctors and paraprofessionals involved in their clinical care. These guidelines further highlight that, although symptom awareness training is important, the fact that ototoxicity can go unnoticed until it has caused significant damage stresses the importance of objective clinical assessments that afford health care practitioners with audiometric data to enable comparison of function before, during and after the drug administration.

The current status of ototoxicity monitoring in South Africa is sub-optimum and requires urgent attention for preventive programmes to be successful. This reality is despite the availability of the HPCSA (2018) national guidelines. Besides ensuring comprehensive and standardised implementation of national guidelines, the South African audiology community needs to attend to the pressing challenges that are deemed responsible for the limited availability of programmes and lack of adherence to national guidelines – capacity versus demand and equipment limitations (Khoza-Shangase & Masondo 2020; Khoza-Shangase & Stirk 2016; Pillay et al. 2020). As far as the capacity versus demand challenge is concerned, the use of trained non-audiological screeners (paraprofessionals) to implement OMPs adhering to recommended guidelines should be seriously considered. In a recent retrospective record review study by Stevenson et al. (2021), an OMP conducted by CHWs was found to be limited as it fell short of meeting recommended guidelines such as performance of baseline measures, conducting repeated measures at recommended intervals and timeframes, inclusion of ultra high-frequency (UHF) measures, and other important recommendations, including efficient record-keeping that is crucial in an OMP. The author believes that this could have been because of the lack of training of CHWs and the lack of audiologists' involvement in the running and management of the programme that has been raised about this particular programme. Although one strategy of addressing the human resources challenge is the utilisation of paraprofessionals, it is important that this is done within a tele-audiology health care service delivery model with audiologists as programme managers responsible for training, supervision and monitoring programmes from remote locations. Chapters 2, 3 and 5 deliberate on this approach for preventive audiology in other areas within the scope of audiology.

Within the large audiologists neglected HCPs in the South African context, Khoza-Shangase (2020a) asserted that if ototoxicity monitoring does not become incorporated into the treatment programmes of workers with HIV, AIDS or TB, workers' hearing is placed at a higher risk, with ONIHL outcomes being far worse (Khoza-Shangase 2020c). These negative consequences would be because the workers have not benefitted from various treatment options, including the prescription of alternative TB drugs such as bedaquiline (Khoza-Shangase & Prodromos 2021), as well as reduced dosages or altered treatment regimens (Lonsbury-Martin & Martin 2001) – all aimed at addressing both quantity and QoL of the infected individual. Other immediate preventive measures, such as redeployment of an employee to a less noisy environment while they are under ototoxic treatment, cannot be applied, thus failing to reduce the risk by circumventing the synergistic effect of noise exposure and ototoxic drugs on the ear (Boettcher et al. 1987; Li & Steyger 2009; Morata 2007). Hearing conservation programmes, therefore, need to be cognisant of the complexity of ONIHL as an occupational health condition and the significance of paying attention to the influence of the burden of disease and the treatments involved on preventive audiology outcomes. Hearing conservation programmes that are naïve to the influence of the burden of disease fail to guarantee stricter monitoring of workers, customised administrative controls for target workers and consideration of alternative protective measures for workers at increased risk, such as prescription of otoprotective agents. All this evidence raises policy and practice review implications in the conceptualisation and implementation of HCPs within this context (Khoza-Shangase 2020a).

As guided by the HPCSA (2018) guidelines, which are comparable with international ototoxicity monitoring guidelines from HICs, for example, ASHA and the American Academy of Audiology, ototoxicity monitoring protocols must be implemented in a manner that allows for simple analysis and comparison of the data collated, so that findings can facilitate evidence-based decision-making that guarantees that preventive targets are achieved. Included in such protocols should be reliable and sensitive measures such as extended UHF audiometry and diagnostic otoacoustic emissions, performed in clinical environments with efficient record-keeping systems in place for longitudinal data analysis. Such protocols will ensure early detection of subclinical changes in hearing function, facilitating medical interventions such as drug and or dosage alterations, as well as potential utilisation of otoprotective agents and so on, to slow down and or eliminate ototoxicity (Khoza-Shangase 2020a).

The HPCSA (2018) guidelines advocate that patients should undergo pre-treatment baseline measures to record current hearing thresholds. Baseline measures are important for use when tracking hearing thresholds during and after treatment. The guidelines recommend that repeated measures should be conducted bi-weekly, with a plan in place to conduct a comprehensive assessment within 24 h or before the next scheduled treatment on the patient should their thresholds worsen when compared to baseline data. Grading criteria for significant ototoxic changes in the patient's hearing thresholds should be predetermined, and this allows for the severity of the hearing threshold shift to then be graded in accordance with the adverse event scale specific to hearing, as recommended in the guidelines (HPCSA 2018). To ensure that the patient is not lost to follow-up and late-onset ototoxicity is not missed, for patients where a shift was detected, the HPCSA guidelines recommend that follow-up assessments be repeated once monthly until stabilisation in hearing function is achieved, and no additional change is measured. For continuity of care, as far as medical management and aural rehabilitation of the patient with ototoxicity is concerned, the HPCSA guidelines advocate for a multidisciplinary team approach where the main goal is to adopt a comprehensive management plan for the patient (HPCSA 2018).

Khoza-Shangase (2020a) suggested an ototoxicity monitoring protocol for the South African context. This tabulated protocol specifies equipment and resources, functions of each, as well as pass and referral criteria that can be used as a checklist for the establishment of OMPs. Although this protocol is specific to the HIV and AIDS population, it is generalisable to most populations at risk for ototoxicity within this context. This protocol considered the validity and reliability of the assessment measures, accessibility, as well as feasibility of implementation within the South African context and is guided by contemporary evidence on the presentation of ototoxicity in this population. Firstly, this protocol presupposes adherence to national as well as international audiological and health and safety norms and standards. Next, the protocol recommends measures that consider resource constraints such as time, human resources, and specialised equipment availability, over and above conventional audiometry. Finally, the protocol has considered the impact of linguistic diversity by excluding speech audiometry. The current lack of appropriate speech audiometry tools and incongruence between languages spoken by audiologists versus patients' was an important consideration in this protocol – in the interim, until these challenges have been addressed.

Accuracy and validity of results in an OMP also rely on appropriate equipment calibration over and above control for patient variables such as confounding variables such as the burden of disease, noise exposure, age and genetic risk factors, to name a few. During all audiological evaluations, standard precautions are similar to those recommended by Hall (2000) and Bess and Humes (1990). These precautionary processes comprise efficient equipment care and calibration, optimise testing environments that entail testing in a soundproof booth or sound-treated space where noise levels are monitored and correct transducer placement including proper DPOAE probe placement and considerations of the transducer type for UHF test-retest reliability (Khoza-Shangase 2020a). For enhanced validity and reliability, it is also advantageous to control for the influence of fatigue on behavioural audiometry testing by testing all patients in the mornings (Khoza-Shangase 2011; Schellack et al. 2015), especially because most of the patients on ototoxic medications are frequently clinically unwell during these monitoring sessions.

Once the OMP is in place, it is vital to have clear guidelines regarding medical intervention in the programme (ASHA 1994; Campbell 2004; HPCSA 2018; WHO 2017). If ototoxicity is detected early with consequent prompt medical intervention, the additional decline of hearing thresholds to the extent of affecting lower frequencies that are crucial for speech understanding may be reduced (Campbell 2004; Duggal & Sarkar 2007). Specific to multidrug-resistant tuberculosis (MDR-TB) burden of disease, the WHO (2014a) emphasised the significance of active surveillance for established adverse side effects of MDR-TB treatment through close monitoring programmes. Audiologists involved in OMPs should have appropriate guidelines for specific burdens of disease, for example, cancer and HIV and or AIDS, in place. Should adverse effects be detected early in MDR-TB, the WHO (2014a) suggested intervention approaches. These approaches, as far as ototoxicity intervention is involved, include the following:

1. Record hearing thresholds and compare them to the pre-treatment audiogram.
2. Where early signs of ototoxicity are recorded:
    - Raise the dosing interval from, for example, every day to three times a week.
    - Replace an aminoglycoside with capreomycin if it was the initial injectable in the regimen.

3. If hearing thresholds continue to worsen regardless of the said modifications, stop the injectable drug and add other agents to enhance the regimen of the drug.

In the amended MDR-TB treatment protocol, drugs that have shown to be minimally ototoxic such as linezolid and bedaquiline have been spotlighted as first-option drugs. Bedaquiline is a significant breakthrough in TB treatment as the first drug in the new classes of TB treatments since 1971 developed specifically for MDR-TB (Danckers et al. 2014). The amended MDR-TB treatment protocol has not been nationally implemented in numerous countries because it is expensive, although it has been approved by the WHO (Bistline 2018; WHO 2019). The limited national roll-out of bedaquiline is said to be because of multiple barriers to programmatic introduction such as '[...] technical expertise and guidance, confusion about pharmaco-vigilance requirements, challenges with registration and import and difficulties obtaining the other medications needed for successful treatment outcomes' (Guglielmetti et al. 2017, p. 167). Nonetheless, South Africa is ahead of the pack as the first country worldwide to have adopted the amended MDR-TB treatment protocol in its national TB treatment policy (Bistline 2018; Guglielmetti et al. 2017; McKenna 2018; WHO 2019), and this protocol adoption has positive implications for patients with MDR-TB and the role of audiologists in their management, particularly because bedaquiline is prescribed only when changes in hearing function are noted; not as a first-line drug yet.

In Khoza-Shangase et al.'s (2020) study investigating the impact of medical interventions for reducing ototoxicity during treatment for MDR-TB in South Africa, results provided evidence encouraging vigilant and consistent utilisation of preventive medical intervention procedures to preserve hearing function during treatment with ototoxic drugs. In this study, frequently implemented medical intervention strategies proved to be considerably useful as preventive measures. These strategies included dosage reduction and discontinuing the ototoxic drug, substituting it with a less toxic drug (bedaquiline). Such contextually relevant findings have the potential to positively sway political will through the delivery of evidence that clearly promotes early ototoxicity detection and monitoring. In another South African study, where the aim was to describe the audiological function in adult patients with MDR-TB on bedaquiline treatment, the less ototoxic nature of bedaquiline was established (Khoza-Shangase & Prodromos 2021). Such evidence has implications for risk-benefit evaluations within a resource-constrained context like South Africa.

For risk-benefit evaluation, it is important that the audiology research and clinical communities perform context scoping exercises, risk-benefit and options evaluations, as well as make a determination on appropriate options available for the context, as depicted in Figure 6.2.

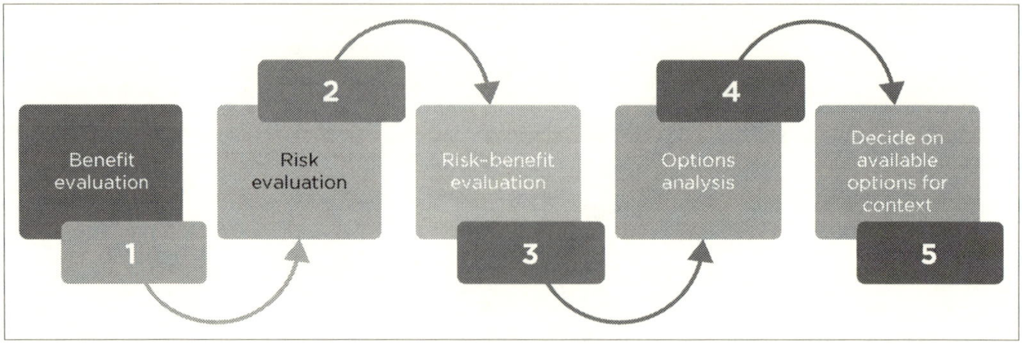

FIGURE 6.2: Stages of risk-benefit evaluation in ototoxicity assessment and management within the South African context.

As far as scoping the context is involved, specifications and descriptions of the medicines and where these are sold or prescribed within the South African context should be determined (Juhaeri 2019; Kürzinger et al. 2020). As new medicines continuously get introduced into the market, continuous updating of this data must occur, with a careful recording of indications for the prescription that is founded on influences such as the burden of disease and the various levels of care within the South African context. Once indications for prescription have been determined, one or more less ototoxic substitute drugs or treatment modalities (including surgical intervention) must be identified. Finally, scoping the context also involves determining and categorising features of ototoxicity and vestibular toxicity, such as the time of onset and development, as well as the severity of hearing loss, vertigo, tinnitus or any grouping of these symptoms.

As far as benefit evaluation in risk-benefit assessment is concerned, Khoza-Shangase (2017) maintained that, although it does not commonly concern audiologists, it remains an essential consideration for audiologists working in ototoxicity. Benefit evaluation entails research into the incidence or prevalence, as well as the development course of the target illness or disease. This process also involves determining the function of the drug (prophylaxis, cure, etc.) and how this affects toxicity tolerance (Colopy et al. 2015; CIOMS 1998; Juhaeri 2019; Kürzinger et al. 2020). Moreover, the benefit evaluation includes a process of contrasting efficacy data and universal toleration data to alternative treatments, where alternative treatments include interventions such as surgery or other interventions and the choice of no treatment (CIOMS 1998; Tsintis & La Mache 2004).

As far as risk evaluation, the audiologists' role must be repositioned to be more meaningfully and more centrally located in the risk-benefit evaluation process. This aspect of the process becomes the locus of the establishment of the weight of evidence for the suspected risk (in this case, ototoxicity) as far as prevalence or incidence are concerned. Here, 'risk profiles' and their frequent reactions for the specific ototoxic drugs as well as parallel profiles for substitute treatments are documented, and comparisons are made between these drugs (CIOMS 1998; Tsintis & La Mache 2004). Proper and accurate comparisons rely on efficient record-keeping, as alluded to earlier. These records would include longitudinal data of audiograms and distortion product grams, with careful cognisance of confounding variables such as concomitant treatments, noise exposure and ageing, in the interpretation, hence the importance of efficient record-keeping systems (Khoza-Shangase 2020a; Khoza-Shangase et al. 2020; Ntlhakana, Khoza-Shangase & Nelson 2020; Perez 2015). The ability to prevent, forecast and reverse ototoxicity is another aspect of risk evaluation that must be considered, with approaches such as the utilisation of oto-protectors, dose modification, frequency and methods of administration changes being important strategies that can be adopted (Le Prell et al. 2014; Perez 2015). Moreover, at this point, considerations around alternative therapies, including the option of no treatment, are engaged with. Within the South African context, as earlier presented, bedaquiline is one such alternative therapy (Conradie et al. 2014; Khoza-Shangase & Prodromos 2021).

The above-listed considerations facilitate systematic and comprehensive risk–benefit evaluation that leads to effortless summarisation of the treatment goal, treatment efficacy and treatment benefits. Furthermore, the risks' prevalence, duration, incidence, and severity are outlined. A risk–benefit summary is also calculated with all considerations listed, considering alternative therapies and no treatment options.

Once the risk–benefit relationship has been determined, option analysis becomes the last step in the risk–benefit evaluation that audiologists must participate in. At this stage, an options list is compiled, and this list must entail all suitable options for action, a portrayal of advantages and disadvantages and possible outcomes of each option being considered (impact analysis), as well as recommendations on consequence monitoring or assessment methods (CIOMS 1998). This options analysis process meets significant barriers for audiologists in LMICs because of the influence of limited financial resources on unrestrained priorities number. Regardless of this reality, existing options incorporate (1) no change where evidence of ototoxicity concern is absent; (2) 'watching and waiting' where tracking of future ototoxicity presentation is done to collate additional evidence; (3) rigorous extra data collection/new studies conducted through the use of standardised protocols; (4) alterations to the medicine or its utilisation or modifications to the drug information; (5) limitation of drug accessibility, pausing of drug licence or experimental-status permission, voluntary or forced removal of the medicine from the market; as well as (6) announcement of new or bolstered information to the relevant stakeholders such as health care professionals or the general public about the outcomes of risk–benefit evaluation of a specific drug (Colopy et al. 2015; CIOMS 1998; Khoza-Shangase 2017; Kürzinger et al. 2020; Tsintis & La Mache 2004).

It is recommended that principles such as equity, accountability and objectivity should direct all decisions made during the process of risk–benefit evaluation, where collaborative decision-making is done by relevant multidisciplinary teams and several stakeholders (Coplan et al. 2011; Juhaeri 2019; Khoza-Shangase 2017; Kürzinger et al. 2020; Tsintis & La Mache 2004). These principles should guide audiologists during the mandatory pre-treatment counselling where ototoxic drugs are prescribed to safeguard that informed consent is obtained from the patient. Although limited minimally ototoxic alternative treatment options are accessible, particularly in LMICs, it is still an ethical duty that patients are counselled pre-treatment on possible negative side effects of the drugs on auditory and vestibular function. This raised awareness of anticipated ototoxicity symptoms will expediate early detection and diagnosis of ototoxicity as the patient may be knowledgeable and, thus, more likely to adhere to attending ototoxicity monitoring appointments. Khoza-Shangase and Jina (2013) also claimed that pre-treatment counselling also encourages treatment adherence as the probability of defaulting on treatment because an experience of uncomfortable, unexplained, unanticipated and unknown negative effects is significantly lessened.

In preventive audiology care during treatment with ototoxic medication, early detection of the damage remains crucial even though the drug-induced damage to the cochlear is unrecoverable. As part of primary prevention, early detection allows for the provision of intervention options such as altering the drug to a potentially less ototoxic regimen (as in the case of bedaquiline in MDR-TB treatment), preparation of audiological intervention and where significant hearing impairment has occurred, provision of amplification devices may be the only intervention choice and so on. Konrad-Martin et al. (2014) supported this position when they asserted that an efficient OMP is one that also makes audiological rehabilitation post-treatment easier, particularly because a good rapport between the audiologist and the patient would have been established already during the repeated assessment sessions.

As far as medical intervention is concerned, efforts towards the development of therapeutic agents that are not toxic to the ear should be increased by research, clinical as well as pharmaceutical communities, with systematic research trials in place to enhance the range and level of evidence collated for accurate risk–benefit assessments within the South African context (Khoza-Shangase 2017). Additionally, these increased efforts should extend to the development of and investigations into otoprotective agents that are crucial in the toxicity-related prevention of hearing loss, including compounds such as d-methionine (sulphur-containing compound), ACE magnesium and

N-acetylcysteine (HPCSA 2018; Kros & Steyger 2019; Le Prell et al. 2014; Sheth et al. 2017). Moreover, these investigations should include research into restorative care, which comprises hair cell regeneration through neurotrophins (Wissink et al. 2006; Zheng & Gao 1996). These protective and restorative intervention approaches are particularly of significant relevance in LMIC contexts for tactical cost saving for the State through the elimination of expenditures linked to lawsuits, procurement of assistive devices, rehabilitation and social grants in the long term.

■ 6.6. Conclusion

Hearing function can be affected by drugs or medications used to treat certain conditions, and pharmaco-vigilance in the form of ototoxicity monitoring becomes imperative in resource-constrained contexts such as LMICs, where the burden of disease is high and health care priorities compete with many other priorities in resource allocation. With the high burden of diseases such as TB, cancer, HIV and AIDS in South Africa, ototoxicity is one morbidity requiring careful preventive measures as it is preventable, and/or its degree and effects are significantly minimisable if early detection and intervention protocols are followed. The associations that have been established between treatments of the listed conditions and ototoxicity call for carefully constructed, implemented and monitored OMPs that take cognisance of contextual realities as described in this chapter. Considerations of contextual realities will ensure contextual relevance and responsiveness of protocols and programmes adopted towards preventive audiology goals.

Although the HPCSA released guidelines on the assessment and management of patients on ototoxic medications (HPCSA 2018), contemporary evidence from the South African context indicates significant challenges with the feasibility of implementation because of various factors. However, sufficient evidence exists to support the establishment and adoption of a clear national pharmaco-audiology vigilance strategy, where audiologists are centrally located. The current chapter has proffered careful deliberations around pharmaco-vigilance as one of the key preventive audiology strategies within the South African context. Considerations around risk-benefit evaluations of ototoxicity monitoring have been advanced, with thoughts around the role of task-shifting and tele-audiology in the implementation of ototoxicity monitoring and management in preventive health care initiatives shared. The chapter has proposed solutions to challenges raised, with a recommendation of an ototoxicity monitoring protocol that can be applied within this context to guarantee systematic data collection that can be utilised for evidence-based development. Such an evidence base will facilitate best practice and contribute towards early identification and intervention of ototoxic hearing loss within this population.

Audiologists should play a significant and strategic role in this process by establishing efficient OMPs with efficient data management systems that allow for contextually relevant evidence to be developed. The contextual relevance should take cognisance of the burden of disease influence on ototoxicity, over and above relevant resources required for appropriate data collection that can be used in risk-benefit evaluations. The role of audiologists in risk-benefit evaluation needs lobbying and advocating, similarly to their expanded involvement in drug development, approval and monitoring processes for both new and marketed drugs. This expanded role of audiologists will facilitate their engagement in Advisory Panels on benefit, risk and cost analysis and management of potentially ototoxic therapeutic, with them offering advice on public education and awareness programmes on ototoxicity. All these recommendations raise important implications for the audiology training curricula at both undergraduate and postgraduate levels, as well as implications for continued professional development initiatives in South Africa.

Chapter 7

The earlier the better: Framing EHDI within preventive audiology

Amisha Kanji
Department of Audiology, Faculty of Humanities,
School of Human and Community Development,
University of the Witwatersrand,
Johannesburg, South Africa

7.1. Introduction

There are 466 million individuals with hearing impairment globally, which equates to approximately 6.1% of the world's population. Of these individuals, 7% are children (WHO 2020a, 2020b). The main regions affected by disabling hearing impairment (> 40 dB in adults and > 30 dB in children) are South Asia, Asia Pacific and sub-Saharan Africa, with prevalence rates that are almost four times that of higher income regions (WHO 2018a). Unless appropriate public action is taken to address hearing impairment, these figures could increase. Projections by the WHO suggest that the number of individuals with hearing impairment could increase to 630 million by the year 2030 and to 2.5 billion by the year 2050 (WHO 2020a, 2020b, 2021).

The World Health Organization estimates that 60% of diagnosed hearing impairment is because of preventable causes, such as vaccine-preventable

How to cite: Kanji, A 2022, 'The earlier the better: Framing EHDI within preventive audiology', ed. K Khoza-Shangase, *Preventive audiology: An African perspective*, AOSIS Books, Cape Town, pp. 137–155. https://doi.org/10.4102/aosis.2022.BK209.07

diseases, ear infections, birth-related causes and ototoxic medication (WHO 2016, 2021). More specifically, 30% of childhood hearing impairment results from infections and 17% from complications at birth. The remaining 13% of hearing impairment is related to ototoxicity, congenital non-genetic malformations and other maternal prenatal causes (WHO 2016). Prenatal and postnatal infections that account for 30% of childhood hearing impairment include rubella, cytomegalovirus, mumps, meningitis, measles and chronic ear infections, with meningitis and rubella collectively being associated with over 19% of childhood hearing impairment (WHO 2016). Chronic ear infections are reported to occur mostly in countries in the South-East Asia, Western Pacific and African regions, where the prevalence may be as high as 46% (WHO 2013). This high prevalence may be because of poor identification in primary care practice, poor or limited access to appropriate preventive interventions and comorbid factors such as malnutrition, HIV and exposure to contaminated water that increase the risk of developing these infections (Monasta et al. 2012; Taipale et al. 2011). Complications at birth include lack of oxygen, low birthweight, prematurity and neonatal jaundice, which can be addressed and prevented through appropriate maternal and child health care practices (WHO 2020a). These causes of hearing impairment may not be the same across countries, possibly contributing to the unequal distribution of prevalence rates of hearing impairment across the world (WHO 2013).

The proportion of hearing impairment associated with preventable causes is much higher in LMICs (75%) as opposed to HICs (49%) (WHO 2020a). This difference may be because of the overall higher occurrence of infections (e.g. rubella, mumps, measles, cytomegalovirus, etc.) in LMICs such as those within the sub-Saharan African region, and more effective maternal and child health care in HICs (WHO 2016). Furthermore, coverage and access to health health care services have been variable across Africa, especially among the lowest-income countries in this region. However, between 1990 and 2013, some countries have significantly increased health care coverage and made progress towards addressing barriers to health such as financial challenges (Dovlo 2020). These financial challenges have been addressed through an increase in the average government budget devoted to health. Increased health coverage is linked to SDGs.

The United Nations' (UN) SDGs are the plans to achieve a better and more sustainable future for all and are aimed at addressing various global challenges, which are outlined by the 17 goals. These 17 goals include, but are not limited to, *poverty, hunger, health and well-being, gender equality, inequalities, climate change, education,* and *peace and justice* (United Nations 2018). Health is centrally placed in the SDGs, more specifically SDG 3, which comprises 13 targets. These 13 targets cover all major health priorities, namely those not achieved as part of the UN millennium development goals (MDGs), new health priorities including non-communicable diseases and environmental challenges and implementation-related targets pertaining to health systems and UHC (WHO 2017). The drive towards SDGs and UHC has created opportunities for the strengthening of primary health care services and its workforce. However, regular monitoring of both SDGs and UHC will facilitate the identification of bottlenecks to implementation and subsequent amendments to related policies and plans (WHO 2017), which is vital when considering changing health priorities as a result of the burden of disease, as well as the role of social factors and inequalities on disease patterns (Bradshaw et al. 2019).

South Africa's burden of the disease consists of communicable and non-communicable diseases. Communicable diseases include HIV, AIDS and TB, maternal and child mortality and non-communicable diseases include hypertension and cardiovascular diseases, diabetes, cancer, mental illnesses and chronic lung diseases, as well as injury and trauma from violence (WHO 2018b). WHO outlined four strategic priorities to be targeted in cooperation with South Africa between 2016 and 2020. These comprise (1) strengthening national efforts towards achieving UHC; (2) reduction in the prevention of communicable diseases (specifically HIV, TB, hepatitis and vaccine-preventable diseases); (3) support of the prevention of non-communicable diseases; and (4) supporting South Africa to meet its global health obligations and contribute to international health and development (WHO 2018b). While these strategic priorities (particularly the second and third) link to preventive health care associated with the burden of disease, it is important to consider the association between such diseases, their prevention and hearing impairment. Meningitis, measles and rubella are some of the infectious diseases that are still reported as significant determinants of hearing impairment in children in LMICs (Swanepoel, Koekemoer & Clark 2010). Addressing preventable causes of infant hearing impairment such as infectious diseases, environmental causes and poor prenatal and perinatal health care services are important in reducing the burden of hearing impairment, especially in LMICs (Olusanya 2009). Preventive strategies related to infectious diseases, including immunisations and vaccinations that are reported to have the potential to assist in reducing infectious diseases contributing to hearing loss, with a consequent decrease in the rates of hearing impairment (Butler 2010). Hence, the significant burden of disease and the status of health care services within South Africa warrant consideration of preventive strategies for hearing impairment within the broader focus of preventive audiology with the aim of reducing the burden of hearing impairment.

Early detection of and intervention for hearing impairment should therefore be viewed within the broader primary, secondary and tertiary health care initiatives. This chapter will begin by describing the South African health care context. Thereafter, the various levels of prevention will be discussed, with a specific focus on their relation to EHDI. Preventive strategies (where applicable) will be discussed in reference to specific frameworks, the national health strategy as well as the re-engineering of primary health care (PHC) within the South African context. Risk factors for hearing impairment will be discussed. Where relevant, these factors will be evaluated in terms of how they may be addressed within the broader health care context's primary preventive strategies to minimise risks being realised as causes of hearing impairment. A secondary prevention strategy will be discussed for audiological screening and assessment. Alternatively, tertiary prevention strategies will be addressed to reduce difficulties associated with hearing impairment through early intervention (EI) health care services.

■ 7.2. Health care in South Africa

Health care in South Africa is managed and steered by the DoH, which is responsible for health policy and derives its mandate from the constitution and the *National Health Act* (NHA) *61 of 2003* (Maphumulo & Bhengu 2019; Schellack et al. 2011). The NHA states the right for all to have access to health care services, which is an important consideration in preventive health care. More specifically, the NHA specifies *patient rights within the health care system*, namely:

1. the right to emergency medical treatment at the nearest health facility (whether private or public)
2. the right to full user knowledge related to one's health status, the availability of procedures and their associated risks, costs and benefits, and the right to refuse treatment
3. the right to informed consent
4. the right to participation in decision-making regarding one's treatment
5. the right to information about health care services for all across all provinces, districts, and municipalities
6. the right to confidentiality
7. the right to lay a formal complaint about treatment at a health facility.

Apart from these rights, the NHA outlines the structure of the health care system, specifying the power and responsibility at national, provincial and district levels, and considers both public and private components of the health care system (Stevenson 2019).

The South African health care system comprises nine provincial health departments that are mandated to provide health care services (South African Government 2020b) and are responsible for the daily management and functioning of health care facilities (hospitals and clinics) and programmes (Stevenson 2019). The vision of the National Development Plan (NDP) is to ensure a long and healthy life for all South Africans. In line with this plan, the DoH focuses on sustainably expanding the prevention and treatment of HIV, AIDS and TB, renewing public health care facilities and ensuring the provision of specialised tertiary hospital services (South African Government 2020b).

Aligned to the five health-related NDP goals is the DoH Strategic Plan 2015–2020, which outlines strategic goals. These strategic goals include promotion of health and prevention of disease (with the reduction of the burden of disease), progress towards UHC through the NHI Scheme and improvement of health care facilities for NHI implementation, re-engineering of primary health care, improving health facility planning through implementation of norms and standards, improving financial management, development of an efficient health management information system, improving quality of care and improving human resources for health (DoH 2015). Within the time frame of the DoH Strategic Plan, the programmes recently funded and implemented by the DoH in 2018/2019 can be argued to have contributed toward primary and secondary prevention as a result of a focus on HIV, AIDS, TB and maternal and child health care. Other programmes were related to administration, NHI, primary health care services, hospitals, tertiary health care services and human resource development, and health regulation and compliance management. Despite programmes varying at the provincial level, programmes related to the DoH funding in 2018/19 included administration, district health care services, emergency medical services, provincial hospital services, central hospital services, health sciences and training, health care support services and health facilities management (Stevenson 2019). These general findings highlight the differences between national and provincial health plans and apportionment of funds as well as a possible lack of coherence in terms of prioritisation of health care needs. These findings are further supported by a study conducted in the Free State province, whereby stakeholders attributed poor disease and management outcomes to fragmented system operations and poor policy coordination in the public health care sector (Malakoane et al. 2020).

The health care system comprises public and private sectors, with an emphasis on primary health care (Schellack et al. 2011). The public health care sector serves or is accessed by the majority (84%) of the population; while the private health care sector serves only 16% of the population (Naidoo 2012). However, the number of health care professionals in both these sectors is disproportionate to the population being served, with approximately 30% of health care workers working in the public sector. This not only contributes to a considerably higher ratio of patients to health care professionals in the public sector (DoH 2011; Van Rensburg 2014) but also highlights the reality of a lack of and inequitable access to health care services by the large majority of South Africans.

The current South African two-tiered health system with public and private health care sectors has been critiqued for being unsustainable, with a paucity of financial and human resources. Despite increased access to public health care, the quality of services has been associated with dissatisfaction (DoH 2011; Naidoo 2012; South African Government 2018). The South African government has promulgated a NHI bill (RSA) that will be gradually phased in, with the objective of improving access to quality health care service through UHC and strengthening and improving the under-resourced public sector (DoH 2011; Matsoso & Fryatt 2013). The NHI bill 2019 recommends the re-engineering of PHC that aligns with preventive care (RSA 2019). The re-engineered PHC services will predominantly be focused on community and home-based services which will be aimed at promotion, prevention and quality curative and rehabilitative health care services (DoH 2011). These health care service are proposed to be delivered through four streams, namely:

- **District clinical specialist teams:** The district clinical specialist teams will aid the delivery of priority health care programmes at a district level as well as address the high maternal and child mortality rates (DoH 2011; Feucht 2013; Naidoo 2012).
- **Integrated school health programmes:** Integrated school health care programmes will be implemented through mobile clinics for school-aged children and will focus on a range of promotive, preventive and curative health care service inclusive of screening for health-related barriers such as visual, hearing, cognitive and developmental impairment (DoH 2011, 2015; Naidoo 2012). It will also include oral immunisation against missed EPI vaccines. Private oral, eye and audiology practitioners will be contracted based on the need for these health care service to provide corrective interventions to deal with the issues that have been identified (DoH 2017).
- **Municipal ward-based primary health care outreach teams:** These teams will facilitate community involvement in the detection of health-related issues placing individuals at risk for disease and in need of preventive, curative and rehabilitative health care services; as well as provision of health promotion education (DoH 2011, 2015; Naidoo 2012). This stream will include CHWs who will have the responsibility of conducting health assessments within households and making necessary and suitable referrals to a PHC facility. Early childhood development interventions can be targeted and propelled forward through these PHC teams. PHC re-engineering may be used to promote the care and development of young children. The use of CHW within the PHC teams may facilitate links between services within the health sector and external partners and may also assist in the scaling up of community and home-based programmes. This scaling-up process will, in turn, address key health care service delivery gaps such as the need to strengthen health care services for pregnant women and children their the first 1000 days of life; strengthen early identification and referral systems for children at risk, specifically those with disabilities; and improve health care for three- to five-year-old children, specifically those not attending Early Childhood Development (ECD) centres (Albino & Berry 2013).

- **Contracting of private health care practitioners at a non-specialist level:** Private health care practitioners will comprise the fourth stream so as to assist in decreasing the burden of disease and enhancing access to health care. Speech therapy, audiology and other allied health care services are said to be prioritised with the goal of addressing ECD and physical barriers to learning (DoH 2015).

Despite efforts over the years to restructure the health care system and the commendable goals that have been set by the government to improve the quality of health care for all South Africans, key challenges persist. These challenges need to be carefully considered and addressed within the greater health care context in order to facilitate the successful achievement of the set goals. A systematic review of literature from 1996–2018 aimed at identifying challenges in practice that compromise quality in the health care sector and strategies employed by the government to improve the quality of health delivery revealed that millions of individuals residing in South Africa suffer from preventable harm daily (Maphumulo & Bhengu 2019). Reasons for this include, but are not limited to, challenges related to unequal distribution of resources, management and leadership (Nabhan et al. 2012):

> Preventable harm refers to (1) harm with an incidence that can be reduced through detection, intervention or prevention of cause, (2) detection of the cause before harm takes place, (3) the use of efficacious, evidence-based intervention that can reduce or eliminate the harm resulting from a causal event. (n.p.)

Crisis-increased disease burden and slow progress in restructuring the health care system (Maphumulo & Bhengu 2019). In addition to these challenges, Young (2016) reported public health care facilities as being inadequate because of long waiting times, poor health care service delivery in terms of care, poorly maintained infrastructure and poor hygiene and infection control resulting in poor disease control in prevention practices. These inadequacies, in turn, contribute to increasing morbidity and mortality rates. Approximately one in seven patients attending public sector hospitals in South Africa is at risk of getting a health care-associated infection because of poor infection control and prevention measures, more specifically as a result of poor hand hygiene compliance (Patel et al. 2016). The hands of health care professionals are responsible for 50%–70% of all health care-associated infections and are the primary route for spreading diseases (Peters et al. 2018). Audiologists have a great degree of contact (direct and indirect) with patients during screening, diagnostic assessment and management. While healthy patients may have a general resistance to infections, neonates and infants in neonatal intensive care have lower resistance and remain more susceptible to infection (Khan et al. 2019). Hence, hand hygiene through handwashing and the use of hand sanitisers, the use of personal protective equipment (PPE), and sterilising and disinfecting of equipment are crucial for minimising the spread of infectious diseases in audiology-specific clinical practice (Ehlert & Naudé 2014;

Khan et al. 2019; SASLHA 2011). The risk of health care associate infections may be further exacerbated by overcrowding in hospitals, high patient-to-professional ratios, old infrastructure, poor cleaning and transfer of patients with drug-resistant infections between hospitals (Dramowski & Whitelaw 2017).

In addition to these infections, South Africa currently faces a multiple burden of disease, which consists of HIV and AIDS, TB, maternal and child mortality, high levels of violence and injuries and increasing non-communicable diseases such as cardiovascular diseases, diabetes, chronic respiratory conditions and cancer (Mayosi et al. 2012a; Pillay-Van Wyk et al. 2016). Health priorities in South Africa have been focused on addressing aspects related to the burden of disease, some of which link to MDGs 4–6 and as well as SDG 3. The MDGs 4–6 were focused on reducing the mortality of children under five-years-old, improving maternal health and combatting HIV, AIDS, malaria and other diseases (Chopra et al. 2009; Mayosi et al. 2012b). Similarly, the current SDG 3 comprises several health targets including, but not limited to, reducing maternal mortality, ending preventable deaths of newborns and children under five-years-old, ending epidemics related to communicable diseases and reducing premature mortality associated with non-communicable diseases (WHO 2020c).

The vision of the NDP 2030 is to ensure a long and healthy life for all South Africans. Hence, the current health priorities include the upliftment of public health care facilities, access to specialised tertiary hospital services and the sustainable expansion of treatment and prevention of HIV, AIDS and TB (South African Government 2020b).

■ 7.3. Levels of prevention

Preventive strategies have proven to be an important aspect of health care and consist of stages related to primordial, primary, secondary, tertiary and quaternary prevention. Together, these strategies are aimed at preventing the onset of a disease or condition by reducing risk and also aim to minimise the complications related to a manifested condition or disease (Kisling & Das 2019).

Primordial prevention is the earliest prevention strategy and is aimed at reducing risk towards an entire population through environmental and social changes. It is typically expressed in laws and national policies, such as improving access to health care to decrease the risk of late or no identification of a condition or disease (Kisling & Das 2019). The 2013–2017 strategic plan for the prevention and control of non-communicable diseases in South Africa indicates population-wide and community-based interventions to promote healthy lifestyles as a means of addressing primordial prevention (DoH 2015). However, this needs to be considered in light of the high levels of poverty and unemployment in South Africa, which contribute to the growth of non-communicable diseases and require additional interventions related to poverty alleviation, job creation, improved public transportation and more equitable health care services (Bradshaw et al. 2019; DoH 2015). While national policies and strategic plans exist in South Africa, this alone will not translate into the control of non-communicable diseases as policies must be translated into action at various levels of society, including community level, and is further dependent on the readiness of the South African health system to implement and monitor proposed strategies successfully (Puoanei et al. 2017).

Primary prevention, on the other hand, focuses on the population or individuals susceptible to having the condition or disease and is aimed at preventing the disease from occurring in healthy individuals through limiting risk exposure. Examples of primary prevention include immunisations against vaccine-preventable diseases such as measles, diphtheria, TB, poliomyelitis and tetanus (Kisling & Das 2019). In South Africa, vaccinations are provided through the EPI schedule (which should form part of the free health care services for women and children in the public health care sector) as well as the Integrated School Health Programme as an outreach to schools (Davis 2019). Ensuring the highest possible coverage of childhood immunisation against the target diseases of the EPI as well as against mumps, rubella and meningococcal meningitis is a vital contributor to the primary prevention of related hearing impairment (Olusanya, Neumann & Saunders 2014).

Secondary prevention is aimed at early detection of the disease or condition and is often executed through screening for early disease or disorders. In audiology, this refers to hearing screening that is either universal (for everyone) or for high-risk groups. In the paediatric population, this typically involves newborn and infant hearing screening as well as routine hearing screening at school entry (Olusanya, Neumann & Saunders 2014).

Tertiary prevention aims to reduce the effects of the disease or condition once already present in the individual through rehabilitation or other forms of intervention. Within the context of preventive audiology, tertiary prevention may include the timely provision of assistive technology followed by effective aural rehabilitation. This may, however, prove to be challenging in some LMICs that are poorly resourced and where hearing aids or cochlear implants, as well as inclusive educational support, are costly or not readily available (Olusanya, Neumann & Saunders 2014).

While tertiary prevention is focused on intervention, quaternary prevention is aimed at protecting individuals from interventions that are likely to cause more harm than good. In the context of medical practice, quaternary prevention is the action of identifying a population or patient that is at risk for over-medicalisation, protecting patients against invasive medical interventions and offering ethically acceptable interventions or procedures. It further highlights the need for critical engagement by health care professionals in terms of their own practice and ethical limitations with the aim of constructing good practice (Jamoulle 2015; Tesser 2017). Although not specifically defined in terms of audiology, the author believes that this can be viewed in light of evidence-based best practice, ethical practice and contextually relevant and responsive practice within the profession. To ensure effective action in addressign hearing impairment, it is vital that these stages of prevention be viewed in relation to the early detection and intervention for hearing impairment (Kisling & Das 2019).

7.4. Prevention in the context of early hearing detection and intervention

Early hearing detection and intervention refers to the prompt identification, diagnosis and provision of intervention for newborns and infants with hearing impairment in order to afford them the opportunity to develop to their maximum potential (HPCSA 2007). The term encompasses aspects related to secondary and tertiary prevention. Early hearing detection and intervention principles outlined by the Joint Committee on Infant Hearing (JCIH) and the HPCSA may also be considered within primary, secondary and tertiary prevention (HPCSA 2007, 2018; JCIH 2007; JCIH et al. 2013).

Primary prevention in EHDI may be considered in the broader context of maternal and child health by addressing the environmental and or medical risk factors that may predispose an unborn child to develop a hearing impairment (Alvarez 2008). With regard to secondary prevention, EHDI may be viewed in terms of early identification initiatives that, if followed by prompt intervention, will reduce the developmental difficulties associated with hearing impairment. Tertiary prevention, on the other hand, may relate to efficient, effective and contextually relevant and inclusive intervention for children with hearing impairment and their families (Alvarez 2008).

While primary, secondary and tertiary stages can be viewed in terms of EHDI, primordial prevention can be viewed as absent. Primordial prevention may be argued more broadly in terms of the future implementation of the NHI policy in South Africa. However, it cannot be currently justified, specifically in relation to EHDI, because of a lack of government mandate for UNHS. Nevertheless, it is vital to consider the role of audiologists within the various stages of prevention. Olusanya, Neumann & Saunders (2014) asserted that as the costs of rehabilitative health care service are enormous in LMICs, primary prevention plays a critical role in reducing the burden of hearing impairment.

7.4.1. Primary prevention

Primary prevention requires an understanding of the risks and causes of hearing impairment within a context, given region or population (Olusanya,

Neumann & Saunders 2014). The HPCSA's (2018) EHDI guidelines outline risk factors for hearing impairment for LMICs such as South Africa, with the acknowledgement that these risk factors may differ among contexts and may be influenced by social determinants of health as well as maternal and child health (Colella-Santos et al. 2014; Kanji & Khoza-Shangase 2018). Kanji and Khoza-Shangase (2019) argued that to identify risk factors within a particular context it is important to note the differences between cause and risk. Risk increases the chance of acquiring a condition, while cause guarantees the occurrence of the condition (Rifkin & Bouwer 2007).

There are a number of preventable causes that have been demonstrated to contribute to the prevalence of hearing impairment in sub-Saharan Africa, with the most significant being perinatal conditions, middle ear disorders, infectious diseases and ototoxic medication (WHO 2016).

A review of literature pertaining to the prevalence of hearing loss in sub-Saharan African countries revealed that, of perinatal problems, birth asphyxia and neonatal jaundice alone or as complications of difficult delivery resulting from poorly skilled birth attendants increased the risk of hearing impairment in infants (Abdalla & Omar 2011). These findings highlight the need for a greater focus on maternal and child health care. Ninety-six per cent (96%) of births in South Africa take place at a health facility; thus, the quality of care provided at these facilities is of utmost importance (SADHS 2016). The 2008 Saving Mothers Report highlighted poor management of emergency deliveries with the recommendation to address the gaps in health care workers' knowledge and skills (National Committee for Confidential Enquiries into Maternal Deaths 2008). The NDoH subsequently developed and tested a training programme related to Essential Steps in Managing Obstetric Emergencies, which resulted in the improvement of quality health care (Bhardwaj et al. 2018).

Ear infections, in addition to infectious diseases such as mumps, rubella, measles and meningitis make up 31% of the 60% of preventable causes of hearing impairment (WHO 2016). Otitis media, more specifically, has been reported to be more common in LMICs due to risk factors such as poor hygiene, nutrition and housing (Abdalla & Omar 2011). These risk factors relate to social determinants of health. Through education of expectant mothers regarding hygiene measures and timely medical and surgical treatment when appropriate, infections such as OM can be reduced (WHO 2016).

Infectious diseases associated with hearing impairment in sub-Saharan Africa comprise measles, mumps and meningitis, the incidence of which can be reduced through immunisations. Of these infectious diseases, rubella and bacterial meningitis are listed as risk factors for hearing impairment within the HPCSA's (2018) EHDI guidelines. Vaccination remains the most cost-effective public health intervention that protects children from vaccine-preventable diseases (Davis 2019). The World Health Organization (1995) recommended ensuring the highest possible coverage of childhood immunisation against the diseases of the EPI as well as against mumps, rubella and meningococcal meningitis (WHO 1995). In South Africa, immunisations are available and provided free-of-charge at public health care sector clinics, with the first vaccines given at birth (South African Government 2020a). Scientific literature has highlighted the effectiveness of the EPI in South Africa with a reduction in childhood mortality and protection against illness and disability (Dlamini & Maja 2016). South Africa has made significant strides with regard to EPI and has been at the forefront of introducing new vaccines (Dlamini & Maja 2016).

While the above-mentioned primary prevention strategies are not directly linked to the scope of practice of the audiologist, Abdalla and Omar (2011) asserted that many of the identified conditions contribute to the disease burden of hearing impairment as a result of a lack of awareness of their complications. This emphasises the need for public education campaigns. Audiologists may thus have a role in organising collaborative workshops with primary health care professionals and mothers at antenatal clinics, community health care clinics and primary health care clinics. The focus of these workshops would be the audiological and subsequent developmental complications associated with these prevalent conditions if unaddressed, as depicted in Figure 7.1. WHO's training manuals on primary ear-and-hearing health care may serve as useful resources for the establishment of training programmes for primary-level health care providers (WHO 2006).

Although there is no clear framework guiding disease prevention and control as part of primary prevention, the factors contributing to the preventable causes of hearing impairment are suggestive of primary health care as a strategic framework. Primary health care is related to the social model of health, which is based on the argument that when basic health needs are met first, better health gains are obtained (Keleher 2001). It encourages an integrated approach to health care and prevention and emphasises community participation in health with regard to health promotion (Dookie & Singh 2012). It can be argued that the PHC approach further aligns with the future plans of primary health care re-engineering in South Africa as it (1) suggests the prioritisation of primary care by the government with a focus on equity and (2) recognises the interrelated relationship or link between risk factors and their resultant condition.

While addressing these risk factors as part of primary prevention may be valuable in decreasing the prevalence and incidence of hearing impairment in newborns and infants, it is acknowledged that not all causes of hearing impairment can be eliminated using this prevention strategy. This highlights the need for comprehensive and effective secondary and tertiary prevention strategies for early identification and intervention of hearing impairment.

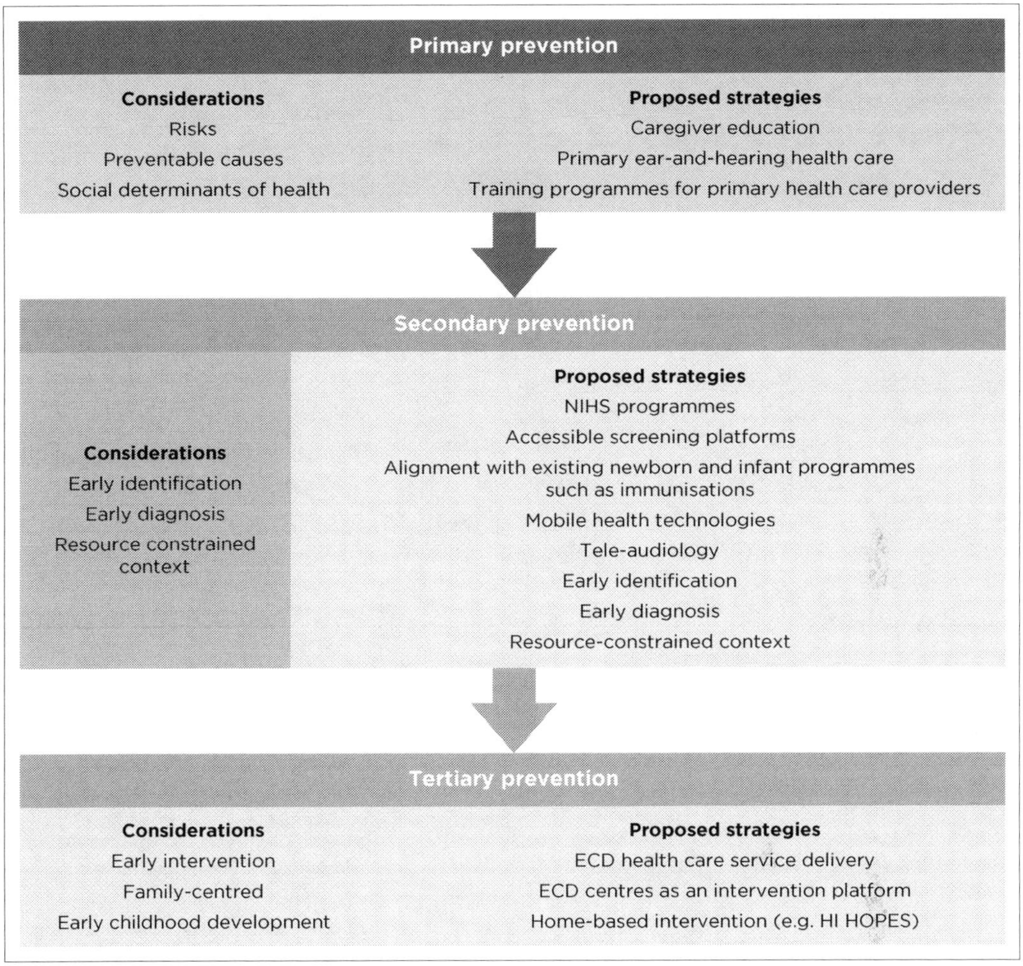

Key: ECD, early childhood development; NIHS, newborn infant hearing screening.

FIGURE 7.1: Prevention in the context of early hearing detection and intervention: Considerations and proposed strategies.

7.4.2. Secondary prevention

Secondary prevention emphasises the early detection or identification of hearing impairment. Although early hearing detection is conducted through screening programmes, these programmes may differ based on the onset of hearing impairment being screened for. Newborn and infant hearing screening (NIHS) programmes, for example, are targeted toward the early identification of permanent, congenital hearing impairment, whereas school-based hearing screening programmes are focused on the identification of acquired hearing impairment. Therefore, the aim of school-based screening is the identification of permanent hearing impairment that may have been missed as a result of NIHS programmes in some contexts.

Secondary prevention may be best achieved through NIHS programmes. This is evidenced by a number of justifications. Firstly, NIHS programmes promote the early identification of permanent hearing impairment and have demonstrated positive outcomes if followed by prompt diagnosis and EI. Secondly, permanent hearing impairment may be non-preventable through primary prevention, such as those resulting from genetic causes. Thirdly, progressive or acquired hearing impairment may occur post-lingually. It may also be transient in nature and not have the same degree of impact on development, particularly if it is because of infections such as OM which can be addressed within primary prevention and managed medically (Qureishi et al. 2014; Upadhya & Datar 2014). Finally, the implementation of NHS programmes as a secondary prevention strategy will reduce the risk of undetected or late identified permanent hearing impairment in school-going aged children. This would be best achieved through UNHS, as not all newborns and infants with hearing impairment may present with risk factors (Kanji 2016a; Kanji & Khoza-Shangase 2019). However, UNHS may not be feasible in LMICs where primary prevention initiatives (as an initial step to prevention) are focused on other health care priorities such as those relating to the burden of disease. Hence, risk-based hearing screening may be an interim approach (Kanji 2016b). Irrespective of the screening approach, international guidelines recommend a 1-3-6 principle, whereby screening is conducted by the infant's first month of age, diagnosis is confirmed by or at three-month-old and intervention is initiated at six-month-old (JCIH 2007). The updated JCIH (2019) position statement has encouraged states who have achieved the 1-3-6 principle to strive towards a 1-2-3 month timeline. Contextual differences have been noted in South Africa, where HPCSA (2018) guidelines recommend initial hearing screening by the infant's first month and no later than six weeks if programmes are linked to immunisation visits. Diagnosis of hearing impairment should be confirmed by no later than at four-month-old and intervention should commence by no later than eight-month-of-age.

There are a number of platforms proposed for NIHS, with the most common being hospitals. Screening in hospitals is advantageous for two reasons. Firstly, it reduces the number of times that parents or caregivers have to return for appointments. Secondly, it assists health care professionals with coverage rate in that babies have been screened before discharge (Olusanya 2006). However, studies conducted in Nigeria, and more recently in South Africa, have proposed primary health care clinics and midwife obstetric units (MOUs) as screening platforms. As part of this, we will be able to ensure a more comprehensive level of coverage, take into account home births, and deal with capacity demand and baby discharges on weekends, thus emphasising the advantages of decentralising health care services (explicitly hearing screenings) to PHC facilities aligned with the re-engineering of PHC in South Africa. Findings from South African-based studies revealed that despite missed cases because of discharge outside of the audiologist's working hours, the MOU three-day assessment was feasible. Immunisation clinics have also been reported to be feasible provided that appropriate equipment is used, the programme is overseen by an audiologist and the non-audiologist personnel conducting the screening are adequately trained (De Kock, Swaepoel & Hall III 2016; Khoza-Shangase & Harbinson 2015 Khoza-Shangase et al. 2017). Hence, linking NIHS services as secondary prevention to existing EPI programmes within primary prevention may be a beneficial approach toward achieving improved coverage rates within EHDI programmes.

The appropriate use of technology for screening and sufficient human resources are important within all contexts when such screening programmes are implemented. With regard to technology, objective, physiological, measures such as otoacoustic emissions (OAEs) and automated auditory brainstem response (AABR) have been reported as valid and feasible, even in LMICs (Neumann et al. 2019). There are, however, differences between the two measures in terms of sensitivity and specificity. Literature indicates 80%–100% sensitivity for AABR and 81%–100% for transient evoked OAEs and 96%–100% specificity for AABR and 97%–99% for transient evoked OAEs (Institute of Health Economics 2012; Pasupathy & Kumar 2018; Shetty, Koohnoor & Rajalakshmi 2016). Literature related to distortion product OAEs has indicated a high sensitivity but lower specificity (Pasupathy & Kumar 2018). The choice of measure has varied globally, with transient evoked OAEs and AABR being more commonly adopted in comparison to distortion product OAEs (Kanji Khoza-Shangase & Moroe 2018). Despite these valid and feasible measures, human resource challenges have been reported to be a challenge within sub-Saharan Africa. This shortage requires creative solutions with regard to preventive audiology (WHO 2007). One such solution may be the use of task sharing.

Task-sharing refers to the redistribution or reallocation of specific clinical tasks, where appropriate, to less specialised health workers. This allows for more efficient use of human resources within resource-constrained contexts (WHO 2007, 2021). It is argued that training a new community health worker can take between a week and a year, depending on the competencies needed. This is as opposed to the years it would take for new health care professionals to obtain a qualification. Hence, task-sharing would reduce delays in increasing the workforce within health care systems that have adequate checks and balances and would protect both health workers and patients (WHO 2007). The use of non-specialists as screeners at primary health care facilities has been found to be cost-effective (Engelman 2014). Olusanya et al. (2007) argued that the use of highly skilled personnel like audiologists may not necessarily result in the rapid spread of NHS because of the lack of human resources. This lack of human resources may in turn limit health care service delivery and is one of the challenges faced in South Africa. The HPCSA's (2018) EHDI guidelines provided a useful curriculum training guide for non-professional screeners, and the inclusion of CHWs within municipal ward-based PHC teams may serve as a useful means of identifying newborns and infants who have not been screened. It would also help address loss to follow-up audiological services that would be imperative to ensuring preventive audiology within an already resource-constrained context. Although audiologists may be involved in the initial training of CHWs, a 'train-the-trainer' approach could be explored with oversight from an audiologist. The costs for training and equipment purchases and maintenance need to be carefully considered through stakeholder engagement, particularly as a lack of adequate financial resources and inadequate training have been reported in literature exploring the implementation of municipal ward-based PHC teams (Nelson & Madiba 2020; Sodo & Bosman 2017).

Digital health (the use of ICTs for health) has been given due consideration as a means of addressing health care challenges globally and can be utilised in various areas of medicine and public health, including the management of electronic health records, provision of remote health care services through telehealth, distant learning for health care workers through e-learning and health information and health care service provision through mobile telephone technology (mHealth) (Olu et al. 2019). Programmatically, digital health has been successfully applied to the prevention of non-communicable diseases in sub-Saharan Africa, such as maternal and child health (Pillay & Motsoaledi 2018), immunisation (Crowley, Fink & Karlan 2014) and HIV and AIDS management (Peter, Barron & Pillay 2015).

The use of mobile health (mHealth) technologies has been recognised as an integral, programmatic approach to the delivery of health care services in South Africa. mHealth will assist in addressing needs related to information communication, health education and data management (DoH n.d.). Data management has been a challenge within EHDI programmes in South Africa. The lack of a data management system has led to challenges in tracking newborns and infants along the EHDI pathway or identifying those who have been lost to follow-up (Moodley & Störbeck 2017). A systematic review of 40 studies was used to evaluate the effect of mHealth interventions on health outcomes in South Africa. Findings indicated that while mHealth interventions using mobile phones and text messages were targeted at improving treatment adherence, there was insufficient evidence of the effect of mHealth interventions on health-related outcomes (Ojo 2018). The use of mHealth in audiology, more specifically, has been reported to provide accurate, low-cost hearing screening in community-based contexts, with CHWs being able to conduct hearing screening after one four-hour training session (Swanepoel 2017). However, this mobile hearing application has been focused on screening using pure-tone audiometry and is currently not applicable to NIHS programmes that require the use of objective, physiological measures. Telepractice may therefore be another consideration for LMICs like South Africa (Figure 7.1).

Telepractice in audiology allows the delivery of distance assessment and intervention health care services by linking clinicians and patients (ASHA 2020). Results from a scoping review aimed at describing the use of tele-audiology health care services to aid in audiological management for children in both rural and urban settings, as well as determining strengths, challenges and clinical implications of such health care service, revealed that tele-audiology improved access and coverage in rural areas (Govender & Mars 2016). However, findings also highlighted a dearth of diagnostic studies, insufficient staff training and the need to ensure consistency among protocols and procedures (Govender & Mars 2016). Synchronous or 'live' tele-audiology assessment may prove to be challenging because of connectivity issues in rural and remote areas or because of limited clinician time (Swanepoel, Koekemoer & Clark 2010). In these instances, an asynchronous approach can be used as an alternative health care service delivery method through remote interpretation of audiological findings (Swanepoel, Koekemoer & Clark 2010). This approach could facilitate much wider coverage of audiological health care services and may be beneficial for diagnostic audiological assessment of infants such as tele-ABR. While tele-ABR has been explored within a number of studies, its practical implementation is low as a result of significant challenges. This includes additional training required for telehealth facilitators to be competent and confident to place electrodes on newborn babies as well as the cost of ABR equipment required for these assessments (Brennan-Jones, Eikelboom & Swanepoel n.d.). In HICs, the use of telepractice in audiology as a means of performing diagnostic ABRs was the second most common service implemented after tele-intervention (Houston, Behl & Mottershead 2018) and would be classified under tertiary prevention.

7.4.3. Tertiary prevention

Early intervention for children with hearing impairment is a vital tertiary prevention strategy following diagnosis. Early intervention includes fitting of amplification and family-centred intervention. Early intervention falls within the broader ECD framework, which is aimed at providing equitable access to ECD programmes, health care service and resources for children, families and communities. The ECD framework ensures that these programmes and health care service are inclusive and culturally relevant (DoH Culture and Employment n.d.).

Early Childhood Development is one of the priorities of the South African government and is guided by the National Integrated Policy for Early Childhood in 2015 and the inclusion of ECD within the 2030 NDP. The policy refers to the provision of ECD services and defines this period as being from conception until the year before children enter formal schooling. For children with a disability, this is modified to the year in which they turn seven-years-old (RSA 2015). The NDP is aimed at transforming ECD service delivery in South Africa to ensure universally available and equitable access to these services (RSA 2015). While South Africa has made good progress from a policy perspective, many of the services defined in the policy have made little or no progress over the past few years, particularly with regard to nutrition, early learning and caregiver support. Reasons for this lack of progress may be because of severe fiscal constraints and inadequate institutional resources and planning required to coordinate, manage and monitor ECD service delivery. Therefore, there is a need for a central hub and plan for the coordination and mobilisation of services, capacity development for delivery of quality health care service and effective, routine monitoring service to measure the progress of childhood outcomes (KiDS 2019).

An ECD centre is a partial care facility that provides early learning and development to children from birth until the year before they begin formal school (ages four to five). In the Foundation Phase of Grade R, with the help of ECD programmes, children are taught early learning and development *(DoE National Curriculum Framework [NCF] for Children From Birth to Four Years Old of 2015; DoE Curriculum and Assessment Policy Statement [CAPS] of 2012)*. ECD centre-based programmes can potentially serve as platforms for EI with the inclusivity of children with hearing impairment if staff working at these facilities are adequately trained. These centre-based programmes will not only increase the access to EI for this population but also result in upskilling of ECD practitioners. South Africa has very few schools catering to hearing-impaired children, with little curriculum support available in special education or disability (SEND) schools, inadequate learning and teaching materials, and a limited number of multidisciplinary professionals supporting hearing-impaired children.

In South Africa, there are various types of ECD centres that include standard nursery and preschool facilities for children aged three-years-old or older. Some of these schools may also offer childcare services for younger children. Crèches and daycare centres are also ECD facilities that cater mostly for young children from infants to six-years-old (StatsSA 2016). However, statistics have indicated that 47% of children between nought- to six-years-old did not attend an educational institution. Significant differences were noted between provinces that were suggestive of the rural-urban access gap, as well as a lack of affordability by families residing in specific provinces. More specifically, approximately 49% of three-years-old children did not attend any ECD learning programme, close to 29% of children aged four-years-old did not participate in ECD learning and at least 13% of those five- or six-years-old did not attend any ECD facility. Government investment in ECD programmes is of utmost strategic importance because of its ethical rationale around social justice (StatsSA 2016). Early Childhood Development programmes should consider children's rights, factors related to social inclusion and exclusion and the provision of preschool services for young children as a means to promote social justice (Aubrey 2017).

In order for tertiary prevention to be effective for EHDI, EI needs to commence soon after diagnosis. Home-based EI programmes may be a suitable option when considering the lack of universal access to services (Figure 7.1). The HIHOPES programme is one such programme in South Africa and has been implemented within five of the nine provinces. These programmes are family-centred as per the EHDI guidelines. They focus on language development, amplification options, schooling options, as well as facilitate decision-making for parents or caregivers of children with hearing impairment regarding communication modality (HIHOPES 2019; Störbeck & Young 2016). There is evidence to suggest the positive contribution of home-based EI toward auditory and speech development within a two-year period (Yang et al. 2015). Findings from a systematic review of the literature including studies on home-based interventions indicate better language outcomes in children receiving intervention before six-months-old (Meinzen-Derr, Wiley & Choo 2011; Shekari et al. 2017; Yoshinaga-Itano & Mah-Rya 1998).

■ 7.5. Conclusion

Prevention has been argued to have cost-effective and risk-reducing benefits. Sufficient evidence exists that justifies increased and focused efforts on preventive approaches to health care delivery. All three levels of prevention are vital for EHDI, particularly as each level addresses an aspect within the continuum of care for all newborns and infants. Secondary and tertiary prevention entails more involvement from the audiologist. The plans by the South African government regarding re-engineering of PHC and UHC may form a good platform for the integration of preventive audiology, more specifically, secondary prevention. Because human resources are a challenge, creative solutions need to be sought to address this in order to ensure widespread implementation of NHS programmes, which is the initial first step to any EHDI programme. Solutions in this resource-constrained context include task sharing, tele-audiology and considerations for mHealth technology as a means of data management and tracking. Tele-audiology may also extend into tertiary prevention through the provision of tele-intervention for newborns and infants diagnosed with hearing impairment. Home-based EI programmes are equally important as precursors to schooling to ensure effective tertiary intervention for children with hearing impairment.

Chapter 8

Early hearing detection and intervention: Considering the role of caregivers as key co-drivers within the African context

Katijah Khoza-Shangase
Department of Audiology, Faculty of Humanities,
School of Human and Community Development, University of the Witwatersrand,
Johannesburg, South Africa

■ 8.1. Introduction

Early detection of hearing impairment in children with a consequent timely and effective intervention programme is necessary to minimise the negative effects on the development of the child. Such EI programmes need to be multidisciplinary, technically and technologically sound and, most importantly, should consider the specific family, community and country context in which the child functions. The aim of this chapter is to explore evidence on the role of caregivers within families in EHDI programmes while arguing for caregiver-centred or FCEI approaches to all EHDI processes within the African context.

How to cite: Khoza-Shangase, K 2022, 'Early hearing detection and intervention: Considering the role of caregivers as key co-drivers within the African context', ed. K Khoza-Shangase, *Preventive audiology: An African perspective*, AOSIS Books, Cape Town, pp. 157–177. https://doi.org/10.4102/aosis.2022.BK209.08

Globally, there is a paradigm shift towards the inclusion of caregivers in care and decision-making. This is also consistent with the National Health System in South Africa requiring caregivers to become active partners in the EI process for their children with hearing impairment. As children develop and acquire skills such as language within the context of a family, the family's cultural beliefs and practices, values, expectations, experiences and child-rearing influences must be considered when planning and providing intervention. This chapter includes research-anchored, evidence-based perspectives and information that can be referred to for the development of programmes. It is contextualised within the African context while being cognisant of international trends and standards. The chapter deliberately adopts an approach that explores challenges with systems and resources, which can be argued to be a problem-based perspective rather than an asset-based perspective to sharpen the focus on areas that need careful scrutiny and consideration in planning and implementing contextually responsive FCEI for the hearing-impaired child.

Early intervention is used broadly to denote intervention methods with children from birth to the age of three (Guralnick 2005). More specifically, this intervention targets aspects that provide health care services for hearing-impaired children and their families for the purpose of lessening the deleterious effects of the hearing impairment (Bowe 2004; Guralnick 2005). As part of preventive audiology measures detailed in Chapter 1, early audiological intervention involves ensuring that all hearing-impaired infants and toddlers are identified early and, where necessary, enrolled into timely and appropriate audiological, educational and medical intervention (Kanji & Khoza-Shangase 2021; Moeller 2000). According to international guidelines, EHDI programmes aim to identify hearing impairment within one month of birth, diagnose it by three months and provide intervention to children with hearing impairment by six-months-old (the 1-3-6 target timelines). This programme is implemented to ensure that they develop and achieve milestones that are in line with their hearing peers (JCIH 2007). The HPCSA adjusted these 1-3-6 target timelines for the South African context to be as follows: completion of hearing screening by six-weeks-old, diagnosis by four-months-old and commencement of intervention by eight-months-old (HPCSA 2018). Kanji and Khoza-Shangase (2021) considered that these adjustments are appropriate, accounting for the various South African screening platforms and other contextual factors such as home births, discharge timeframes and scheduled immunisation visits at the primary health care (PHC) level. However, the author believes that further deliberations on these targets would need to be held by the HPCSA, audiology community and the NDoH when the implementation of the NHI, under the re-engineered PHC, becomes realised.

Because of the high prevalence of babies born daily with permanent sensorineural hearing impairment in South Africa, there have been increased efforts toward the implementation of EHDI programmes (Kanji 2021a; Khoza-Shangase 2019). The prevalence rate of hearing impairment in children is four to six per 1000 live births in a LMIC like South Africa (Olusanya & Newton 2007); a figure that is higher than the usually reported 1–3 per 1000 births for HICs (Swanepoel, Störbeck & Friedland 2009). Therefore, a preventive approach to ear-and-hearing health care, and developmental impairments, is prudent for LMIC contexts, like South Africa, where the burden of numerous diseases, economic and socio-political challenges compete for the same resources (Kanji & Khoza-Shangase 2021).

Early hearing detection and intervention programmes have three key components, which include NHS, diagnosis of hearing impairment and the implementation of intervention services. A review of published evidence in these three components globally suggests that some advancement has occurred in the growth of EHDI programmes in the past three decades (Alvarez 2008; Bezuidenhout et al. 2018; De Kock, Swanepoel & Hall III 2016; HPCSA 2018; Kanji 2021b; Kanji & Khoza-Shangase 2018a; Kanji & Krabbenhoft 2018; Khoza-Shangase & Harbinson 2015). This progress has been limited in LMICs, with evidence of positive outcomes where it has been successfully implemented (Erbasi et al. 2018; Guralnick 1998; HPCSA 2007; Khoza-Shangase 2019; Khoza-Shangase & Michal 2014; Khoza-Shangase, Kanji & Ismail 2021a; Maluleke Khoza-Shangase & Kanji 2018; Maluleke, Khoza-Shangase & Kanji 2019; Moodley & Störbeck 2017; Olusanya 2006; Olusanya, Neumann & Saunders 2014; Olusanya et al. 2007; Störbeck & Young 2016).

Early hearing detection and intervention's documented positive effects include those on social and communicative functioning, achievement of developmental milestones, including motor, cognitive, speech, language and hearing development, as well as academic performance and consequent vocational outcomes (Graydon et al. 2019; Guralnick 2005; Khoza-Shangase 2021b; Wroblewska-Seniuk et al. 2017). There is extensive evidence that undetected hearing impairment has profound effects on the language abilities and skills of the infants, which may result in language delays of at least 2–4 years (Khoza-Shangase 2019; Lang-Roth 2014; Maluleke et al. 2018, 2019; Moodley & Störbeck 2017). Consequently, long-term financial benefits are derived from EHDI for the hearing-impaired child, family and the State (Khoza-Shangase 2021b; Moeller 2000; Yoshinaga-Itano 2004). Furthermore, parent-child interactions are strengthened; a supportive family environment is provided and an overall improvement in the QoL is achieved (Kanji & Khoza-Shangase 2021; Moeller 2000; Olusanya 2005; Olusanya & Newton 2007; Rossetti 2004; Yoshinaga-Itano 2004). These effects make it justifiable for considerable attention to be directed towards earlier identification and intervention for hearing-impaired children.

In South Africa, unfortunately, there is a substantial lag between the age at identification and that at the initiation of EI services (HPCSA 2018; Kanji 2021b;

Khoza-Shangase, Barratt & Jonosky 2010; Khoza-Shangase & Harbinson 2015; Khoza-Shangase & Michal 2014; Petrocchi-Bartal, Khoza-Shangase & Kanji 2021; Pillay, Moonsamy & Khoza-Shangase 2010). Previously, researchers have reported delays in identification, diagnosis and intervention in specific settings and geographic areas, such as healthy and high-risk infants, HIV, neurological conditions, etc. (Harrison & Roush 1996; Khoza-Shangase & Rifkind 2010; Khoza-Shangase & Anastasiou 2020; Noorbhai 2002; Thompson 1991). These delays in EI services as well as the failure to implement EHDI as a standard of care in South Africa have been linked to various reasons. Financial constraints and capacity versus demand challenges have been reported as the main factors (Khoza-Shangase 2021a). However, White (2003) strongly argued that EHDI benefits far outweigh the costs.

White (2003) advanced three pieces of evidence that justify the expenditure involved in the implementation of national EHDI programmes. Firstly, hearing impairment is the most frequently occurring condition of all congenital disabilities; secondly, undiagnosed hearing impairment has severe effects on the developing infant; and lastly, there is sufficient evidence proving the positive outcomes associated with the early identification of hearing impairment (Maluleke et al. 2019; Olusanya & Newton 2007; Rossetti 2004; White 2003). Petrocchi-Bartal and Khoza-Shangase (2016) asserted that with almost 20 infants born with hearing impairment on a daily basis in South Africa, EHDI has become an intervention imperative for the South African audiology community. This goal has recently been endorsed by the publication of the HPCSA's (2018) *Early Hearing Detection and Intervention Guidelines* aimed at advocating for EHDI within the South African context while facilitating standardisation in practice that is both internationally comparable and contextually relevant and responsive.

This goal is far from being achieved in the South African context, given the many challenges making EHDI implementation significantly different from that in the United States (Khoza-Shangase 2021a; Petrocchi-Bartal & Khoza-Shangase 2014, 2016). Khoza-Shangase (2019) offered three challenges that hinder EHDI programme implementation in South Africa: (1) lack of prevalence and incidence data as well as evidence on use and efficacy of different interventions, (2) the non-systematic, non-integrated, non-comprehensive and decentralised nature of EHDI in this context and (3) urgency to develop, implement and monitor well-resourced EI that is holistic and multidisciplinary and takes into consideration the hearing-impaired child's caregiver and the uniqueness of the South African context.

■ 8.2. Background

Globally, attention to caregivers' opinions, views, perceptions, as well as their role and value in the EHDI process, as important co-drivers of any intervention programme, remains limited in both the clinical and research community (Khoza-Shangase 2019). Khoza-Shangase (2019) argued that:

> [*T*]his reality is more pronounced within the South African context where linguistic and cultural diversity incongruence between the majority Black South Africans and the mainly White English/Afrikaans speaking clinicians exist. (p. 74)

This incongruence negatively influences the ability of the intervention practitioners to (1) critique their contextual relevance and responsiveness to the needs of families, (2) modify and or develop more effective evaluation and treatment strategies and (3) enable Afro-evidence-based clinical health care service provision (HPCSA 2019).

To ensure effective EHDI, a receptive, cohesive and integrated system that centres caregivers and families of children with hearing impairment and sees the caregivers as key co-drivers of EHDI success must be in place. Primary preventive programmes such as prenatal education classes about risk factors and development stimulation, suitable screening, referral channels, evaluations, constant monitoring and rigorous planning are several aspects requiring consideration for an effective EHDI programme (Khoza-Shangase 2019). These programmes must be guided by the audiology principles for EI (Khoza-Shangase et al. 2010; Maluleke et al. 2018; Prendergast, Lartz & Fiedler 2002; Spivak et al. 2009).

While there is mounting unanimity that the goal of practising evidence-based health care which involves caregivers and the context where the patient is coming from is sound, caregiver involvement can be challenging when health care delivery continues predominantly within the medical model (Khoza-Shangase 2019). The beliefs and experiences of caregivers or families impact the quality of adequate EI practices, particularly in LMIC contexts (Russ et al. 2004). This needs to be acknowledged if proper reflections on planning, implementation and monitoring of caregiver-centred interventions are to occur.

At the inception of EI as a model of care, EI programmes were child-focused and their outcomes were measured against the performance only of the child (Guralnick 1998; Iversen et al. 2003). With the realisation and recognition of the role that caregivers and families play in all aspects of the intervention process, increasing focus is now being placed on child-centred to family-centred intervention approaches (Iversen et al. 2003; Maluleke, Khoza-Shangase & Kanji 2021a). Family-centred care is promoted as an essential feature of best practice for hearing-impaired children, from identification to intervention (Gravel & McCaughey 2004; Maluleke, Chiwutsi & Khoza-Shangase 2021b; Moeller et al. 2013). Schlebusch, Samuels and Dada (2016) raised the important issue of family routines as a basis for family-centred interventions and their influence on family QoL and appraisal of disability, thereby highlighting the importance of partnering with and supporting families.

Sass-Lehrer (2004) propositioned that an intervention approach for hearing-impaired children that prizes collaboration with families while enabling and developing self-efficacy in parents may produce more positive outcomes and facilitate more active engagement and adherence in the intervention programme. Sufficient evidence has since been garnered that proves that caregivers are core to the success of EI programmes (Khoza-Shangase 2019; Majid et al. 2017; Maluleke et al. 2021a; Ravi et al. 2016). In a systematic review exploring current evidence reflecting trends in caregiver or FCEI for children with hearing impairment, Maluleke et al. (2021a) identified four major themes of relevance in the data: (1) caregiver involvement, (2) caregiver coaching/ information sharing, (3) caregiver satisfaction and (4) challenges with FCEI. Generally, their findings reveal the following:

1. Ample evidence exists for FCEI, with caregivers demonstrating a compelling need for their comprehensive participation in the intervention.
2. Cultural and linguistic diversity needs to be considered in methods of caregiver intervention involving coaching and information sharing, with considerations around time and manner of delivery.
3. Challenges identified in caregiver-centred interventions were identified and comprised logistical challenges, professional-related challenges and caregiver-related challenges.

As far as the challenges were concerned, Maluleke et al. (2021a) found evidence of logistical challenges related to the delivery of FCEI. In LMIC contexts such as India, Nigeria and South Africa, the lack of available and accessible free public sector health care services negatively influenced caregivers' involvement in FCEI (Adedeji et al. 2015; Bezuidenhout et al. 2018; Merugamala et al. 2017; Samuels, Slemming & Balton 2012). The lack of availability of public sector EHDI in such LMIC contexts highlights implications for systematic and integrative development and execution of international level gold standard EHDI programmes at the different levels of health care in these contexts.

Additional logistical challenges were reported by Elpers et al. (2016), Larsen et al. (2012) and Khoza-Shangase (2019), where caregivers raised concerns about difficulties with numerous appointments that their hearing-impaired child had to attend. Most of these appointments were reported to be in two or three locations and often after having been placed on a long waiting list. Additionally, time and financial costs are linked to caregivers having to travel far to access health care, where often they have to travel with extended family members, especially when there is no consistent mode of transport, and a language barrier exists between the caregiver and the health care provider (Elpers et al. 2016; Khoza-Shangase 2019; Merugumala, Pothula & Cooper 2017). Maluleke et al. (2021a) strongly argued for the decentralisation of hearing health care services, with the exploration of alternative models of service delivery within the South African context to overcome these challenges.

One of the potential models of health care service delivery that Swanepoel and Hall (2010) recommend in health care provider-constrained contexts, like South Africa, is tele-audiology. Khoza-Shangase (2021a) proposed that tele-audiology combined with task-shifting as defined by the WHO guidelines (WHO 2008) be adopted as one of the health care service delivery models that can help caregivers and FCEI. The value of tele-audiology has been strengthened by the COVID-19 pandemic, with telepractice, in general, having been demonstrated to be an increasingly immediate need for clinical health care service provision.

Blaiser et al. (2013) suggested that the use of tele-intervention could facilitate caregiver involvement and lead to optimal outcomes for hearing-impaired children. Similar to Blaiser, Khoze-Shangase and Sebothoma in Chapter 2, argue that tele-intervention, as part of tele-audiology, has the potential to meet the caregiver preventive audiology goals in a cost-effective manner. In their study, Blaiser et al. (2013) found that children in the tele-intervention group-involving caregivers performed significantly better on the expressive language test than the in-person group. An assessment of home visit quality revealed that the tele-intervention group achieved better as well. Khoza-Shangase and Sebothoma deliberate on advantages and disadvantages, as well as considerations around tele-audiology within the South African context, to make sure that all variables are considered before implementation within this context.

Behl and Kahn (2015) took the health care service delivery model of utilising telepractice for FCEI further in their survey on provider perspectives on telepractice for serving families of hearing-impaired children. Their findings revealed large differences in hardware and software, with various providers presenting trepidations relating to data security, Internet connectivity and skills required to deliver telepractice health care services. Khoza-Shangase, Moroe and Neille (2021b) also highlighted the training challenge where gaps in telepractice were identified in training curricula globally. Behl and Kahn's (2015) findings highlighted important aspects that need resolving and strategising around if telepractice will form part of FCEI, particularly in LMIC contexts where the use of ICT in ear-and-hearing health care remains significantly behind (Khoza-Shangase & Moroe 2020).

In the review by Maluleke et al. (2021a), three challenges relating to professionals were identified, and these included caregivers reporting that (1) health care providers did not prioritise their child's hearing health and disregarded concerns raised until a late stage, and these providers were being poorly informed about EI programmes resulted in delayed intervention (Elpers et al. 2016), (2) they had been referred from a general children's clinic for a hearing evaluation but were not directed exactly to the right people and place (Merugamala et al. 2017) and (3) the professionals lacked knowledge or understanding on what their child's challenge was (Khoza-Shangase 2019).

Challenges relating to caregivers included limited knowledge of treatment options for hearing impairment (Elpers et al. 2016), lack of understanding of children's development and family activities (Balton, Uys & Alant 2019) and cultural power dynamics that often undermine the mother's concerns and earlier suspicions of the hearing impairment (Merugumala et al. 2017). Maluleke et al. (2018) asserted that maternal awareness of infant and childhood hearing impairment may trigger earlier suspicion and subsequent EI, particularly where delayed-onset hearing impairment that cannot be detected via universal newborn hearing screening programmes (UNHS) is concerned, as it is within the South African context. This elevated maternal awareness can be attained through expanding the health education offered to mothers as part of antenatal and postnatal care at immunisation clinics to include risk factors for hearing impairment, knowledge of developmental norms, childhood hearing loss and its effect on speech and language development (Fitzgibbons, Beswick & Driscoll 2021; Kanji & Khoza-Shangase 2019; Maluleke et al. 2018), as well as issues around health-seeking behaviours (Conroy et al. 2016).

The challenge around family power dynamics and their influence on health-seeking behaviours and caregiver involvement in EI identified in Maluleke et al.'s (2021a) study requires significant attention within the African context. Conroy et al. (2016) reported that there are three social structures that serve as influencing factors to health care access in South Africa. These factors include gender dynamics that see the male partner controlling decisions around health and health-seeking along with its associated patriarchy, as well as the existing economic inequalities. These authors maintain that these social structures bestow females very restricted power to source health information, decide on what is best for their health and take measures to improve health. Mophosho (2018) argued that the same influences are at play in Speech-Language therapy consultation practices within the South African context. Furthermore, Ganle et al. (2015) reported that, in other sub-Saharan countries, health care decisions are commonly taken by the women's partners or a family elder. These power dynamics have serious implications for EHDI that is naïve to family and community involvement (Maluleke et al. 2021b). Therefore, EI within the African context needs to move away from child-centred and mother-centred approaches to models of care that involve the family.

Early intervention practitioners within the African context must become conscious of the intricacies involved in contextual decision-making dynamics and investigate means of navigating them in the provision of EHDI within an FCEI philosophy. Maluleke et al. (2021a) argued that acknowledging that family-child interactions are central in any intervention represents a major shift in paradigm, where the caregiver is no longer viewed as a peripheral player in child-focused interventions. In this paradigm, the health care service delivery model drives health care providers to focus on strengthening family interactions, an approach advocated by Woods et al. (2011), with

Kuo et al. (2012) contending that this approach primarily defies the unilateral responsibility for decision-making by the health care provider paradigm.

The HPCSA (2018) also advocated that after diagnosis of hearing impairment, EHDI services must be family-centred, be conducted within a community-based model of care and must consider the influence of culture. Maluleke et al. (2021a) argued that, within the South African context, establishing FCEI programmes for children with hearing impairment can contribute to alleviating the injustices and inequities related to health care access (Khoza-Shangase & Mophosho 2018; Nkonki et al. 2011). This is particularly relevant in South Africa, where health care access is considerably influenced by an over-burdened health care system, as well as linguistic and cultural incongruence between health care providers and the majority of the patients accessing health care (Pillay et al. 2020). Predictably, these challenges generally affect the already vulnerable sections of the population, notably in rural and poor black communities (Khoza-Shangase & Mophosho 2018, 2021; Nkoki et al. 2011; Störbeck & Young 2016).

Consideration of internationally recommended best practices in FCEI is important; however, this should be done without contextual blindness. Moeller et al. (2013, pp. 430–443) offered 10 important principles that guide FCEI with auditory-impaired children. These *10 foundational principles* which should be considered within the South African context include (Moeller et al. 2013, pp. 430–443):

1. early, timely and equitable access to health care services
2. family/provider partnerships
3. informed choice and decision-making
4. family social and emotional support
5. family infant interaction
6. use of assistive technologies and supporting means of communication
7. qualified providers
8. collaborative teamwork
9. progress monitoring
10. programme monitoring.

8.3. Exploring evidence on the role of caregivers in early intervention with solutions for the African context

8.3.1. Identification/detection and caregivers

Regardless of the significant expansion in early hearing detection since the year 2000 globally, including the increased efforts within the African context that includes deliberations on the feasibility and the benefits of early

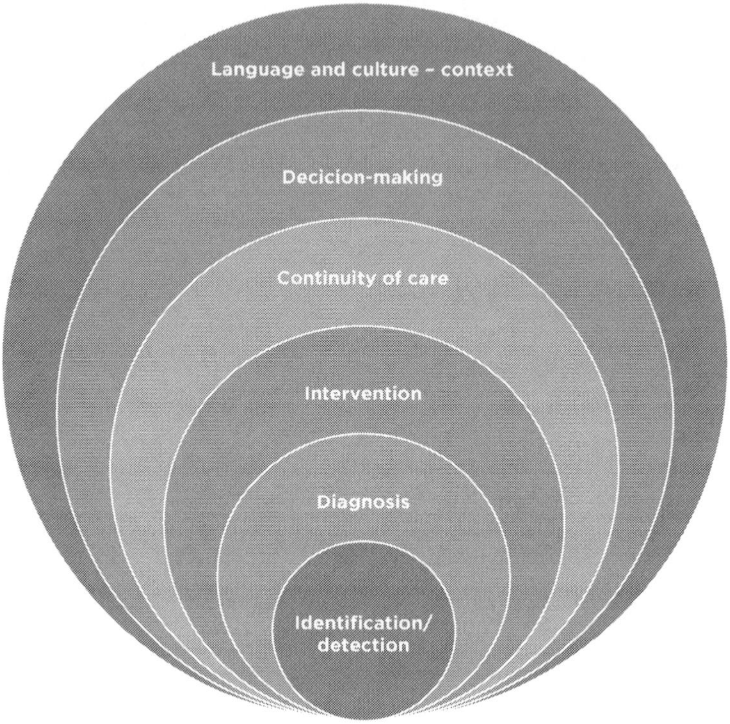

FIGURE 8.1: Overview of areas where the role of caregivers is explored.

identification and intervention, substantial challenges still exist. Key to these challenges within the African context, the author believes, is the involvement, informed and empowered involvement, of caregivers at the identification/ detection phase, as depicted in Figure 8.1. Caregiver involvement is important for the future development of EHDI programmes in all aspects including:

1. **Screening protocols:** Stipulate location(s) (where) and time (when) to implement screening protocols.
2. **Follow-up, return rate for diagnostic audiology evaluation and all future rehabilitation sessions:** Empower caregivers to see the benefit and value of the health care services that audiologists provide from identification of the hearing impairment to aural rehabilitation.
3. **Risk factors:** Raise caregivers' awareness of risk factors for congenital and acquired hearing loss to facilitate preventive ear-and-hearing health care benefits.
4. **Early intervention progress monitoring:** Empower caregivers to know what to expect of their hearing-impaired child in their auditory, speech, as well as language development. Caregivers should be an integral part of the

regular surveillance that is conducted on developmental milestones, communication development, auditory skills, academic development and so on.

5. **Quality control:** Empower caregivers in a health care system where patients migrate within the country to different health facilities (Vearey, Modisenyane & Hunter-Adams 2017), so that caregivers can form part of an efficient data management system, wherein they exercise their right to access information (where they keep updated records of their child's records) as part of an integrated system. This is important to monitor and improve the quality of EDHI services.

In an Australian study, Russ et al. (2004) found evidence that highlighted a need for parents to be provided with greater emotional support and counselling during the hearing screening and diagnosis period. Because of strong emotions such as shock and denial in their study, at the point of receiving the diagnosis of a hearing impairment, as well as exasperation because of communication challenges with health care providers causing delays in diagnosis, these authors recommend that additional training be provided to health care providers on effective communication with caregivers, with a strong focus on periods when parents are most vulnerable to strong emotions. Within the South African context, this communication training should consider the influences of language and culture (HPCSA 2019; Khoza-Shangase & Mophosho 2018).

Russ et al.'s (2004) study also found that parents experienced challenges with testing for children with additional medical and developmental challenges, confusion about certain surgical procedures that their children underwent, such as tympanostomy tube insertion, as well as difficulties with wearing hearing aids. Consequently, these authors recommend the provision of more and varied strategies for parents to facilitate and support hearing aid use in very young children, with specialised approaches to testing for children with comorbidities. Such flexibility in addressing contextually relevant needs is key to ensuring buy-in and adherence to intervention by caregivers and families. Ravi et al. (2016) asserted that parents and caregivers of a newborn have a fundamental role to play during the hearing screening and intervention process. These authors believe that decisions taken by caregivers on the EHDI process rely significantly on their views, attitudes and knowledge.

Within the South African context, Swanepoel et al. (2009) bemoaned the fact that although EHDI programmes are becoming the benchmark for positive outcomes for the hearing-impaired child as well as their families and communities where they come from; these programmes are scarce and awareness around them reduced. These authors believe that despite sub-Saharan Africa's relatively mature economic and fairly developed health care infrastructure, limited evidence and data on infant hearing impairment and limited availability and access to EHDI programmes exist, and this has an impact on caregiver-centred care. This impact was found in a caregiver-focused South African study exploring factors compromising EI health care service delivery to their hearing-impaired children (Khoza-Shangase 2019). In this study, caregivers reported a number of challenges including a lack of community awareness about hearing impairment, extending to inadequate skills and knowledge of health care professionals and teachers about hearing impairment and its impact on the child; variable and contradictory health care professional views about the child's diagnosis and treatment; insufficient numbers of schools and health care facilities for their hearing-impaired children, with those that are available located long distances away from where they reside; as well as high costs associated with the health care services required by their hearing-impaired children, such as health care expenses and special boarding school costs. Khoza-Shangase (2019) concluded that these findings have a place in clinical, training, policy and advocacy planning for the South African context, for both access and success of FCEI.

In another South African study, Scheepers, Swanepoel and Le Roux (2014) investigated why parents decline NHS and default on follow-up rescreening in two private health care facilities. Their findings revealed follow-up return rates that were lower than set benchmarks, with the most commonly named reasons for screen refusal being cost, caregiver knowledge of NHS and health care professional knowledge and teamwork. In this study, 96% of caregivers suggested that if costs had been incorporated in the birthing package or been paid for by the medical aid, they would have consented to NHS. These findings, although not on a sample and health care sector that is accessed by the majority of the South African population, the public health care sector, where over 80% of the population who are not privately funded access health care (Ranchod et al. 2017), still reveal valuable lessons. The public health care sector in South Africa has well-documented resource constraints (Khoza-Shangase 2021a); however, current findings from the privately funded private health care sector still indicate the need for such primary preventive health care services to be free of charge with health care awareness and education around health conditions screening and EI forming part of prenatal classes within the South African context. Scheepers et al. (2014) concluded from their study that within the South African private health care context, incorporating NHS as a mandated birthing service is chief to increased coverage and pre-emptive notices and better communication with caregivers critical to reducing loss to follow-up.

Kanji and Khoza-Shangase (2018b) found different results from their South African study, which was, however, conducted in the public health care sector. These authors found that explanations for poor follow-up return rates varied, with the most shared reason being moving place of residence. In this study, maternal age seemed to have an influence on the return rate as older mothers tended to return more with their newborns for diagnostic assessment than younger ones. Kanji and Khoza-Shangase (2018b) concluded that, within the

South African public health care sector, follow-up default can be significantly improved by efficient appointment scheduling where follow-up appointments are made on the same day as other medical follow-up services – despite the documented contextual challenges. Some of the contextual challenges found in Kanji and Khoza-Shangase's (2018b) study included failure to reach patients telephonically for appointment reminders, families moving their place of residence away from the province or city where the health care facility is, caregiver work commitments, as well as economic challenges such as lack of money for transport to the hospital. It is the hope of the author that the proposed NHI, which has the goal of UHC and access to a high quality of health care (Ranchod et al. 2017), regardless of financial standing and distance from health care facilities (DoH 2017), will achieve this primary preventive ear-and-hearing health care service. This approach will succeed if caregivers are incorporated as key co-drivers of EHDI, in line with what Popich, Louw and Eloff (2007) raised over 10 years ago when they highlighted the importance of caregiver education and involvement in prevention strategies for communication disorders within the high disease burdened South African context, where risk factors to hearing impairment are high.

In another South African study on influencing factors to follow-up return rate in a risk-based hearing screening programme, Kanji and Krabbenhoft (2018) found that friendly audiologists, good and clear communication between caregiver and audiologist as well as appointment reminders as factors most frequently reported as positive contributors to caregivers' attendance at follow-up appointments. A key challenge found in this study was residing a long distance from the health care facility. These results corroborate earlier findings of demographic, socio-economic and interpersonal factors influencing follow-up return rate, with sufficient evidence suggesting the necessity for efficient scheduling in all-inclusive appointment days (Babalola & Fatusi 2009; Say & Raineb 2007; Tsawe et al. 2015).

Majid et al. (2017), in a study investigating the effects of perceived attitude and anxiety on awareness of UNHS among caregivers in Malaysia, found results contrary to previous commonly reported findings. Caregivers' perceived attitudes were found to be more influential to their awareness of UNHS than their anxiety. These authors posit parents' lack of belief in early detection of hearing impairment in children because they believe their children are not old enough to undergo audiological assessment influences their uptake of UNHS. Moreover, these authors postulate that the socio-economic position of the caregivers may have influenced their inability to keep UNHS screening appointments because some of them may have to work to earn an income while some may view it as a futile exercise to honour such appointments. These authors also argue that the poor relationship they found between caregivers' awareness of UNHS, and anxiety may be because of caregivers' religious beliefs in their context. In a Brazilian study, Cavalcanti and Guerra

(2012) found that mothers who were less educated, earned a low income, attended less prenatal care visits and had more than one child were more likely to non-adhere to the UNHS programme. Because of their conclusion that socio-economic factors may negatively influence the effectiveness of hearing screening programmes in poorer regions, these authors advocate for advancements in health care politics, tracking systems and public awareness if efficacious and sustainable programmes are to be implemented.

Without taking into careful cognisance evidence around caregivers and the process of early detection and identification of hearing impairment, implementation of early hearing detection in LMICs will remain intangible. Fragile health care systems that are insufficiently funded lead to inadequate UNHS programmes. This challenge needs to be addressed as it has implications for human resources, equipment availability and so forth. Despite caregivers observing the need for health care services, there is no access to them due to a lack of resources. There is a high incidence of loss to follow-up at different stages of the programme in these countries, creating a barrier to the attainment of the positive effect of early hearing screening programmes. Strategies must be established to develop and enhance family involvement and commitment from this early stage of the EHDI programmes.

8.3.2. Diagnosis and intervention

Scarinci et al. (2018a) explored the views of caregivers about the information and support they obtained after their child's diagnosis of hearing impairment. Their findings revealed general caregiver satisfaction with the information received from sources that included information counselling with audiologists and medical professionals as well as written information. For the small minority of caregivers (11%) who indicated a break in information transfer about their hearing-impaired child, a nuanced analysis revealed two themes that described the diagnostic period as a difficult and emotional experience for caregivers. These are (1) questions around what should be prioritised between the provision of support or information during diagnosis and (2) traversing through the maze of accessing EI services following a diagnosis of hearing impairment. These findings demonstrate the heavy and total reliance of caregivers on audiologists at this very crucial part of the EHDI process. These findings also raise serious implications for audiologists involved in this diagnostic period to be as comprehensive, transparent and supportive as possible, as this is the gateway to a lifelong EHDI journey for the hearing-impaired child and their family.

Swanepoel and Almec (2008, p. s44) argued that parental knowledge and attitudes about infant hearing impairment are key to the effective implementation of EHDI programmes, especially in LMICs where 'concerns have been raised of cultural-based ignorance and resistance towards childhood disabilities'. While it is believed that without caregiver knowledge and buy-in, EHDI programmes will not succeed within the African context. The author is strongly opposed to the inference that diverse views and beliefs about disability can be labelled as ignorance or resistance. This is especially significant within the African context, where cultural beliefs and practices significantly vary from the Western norms that generally guide health interventions such as EHDI. Clinicians adopting such positions within this context go against evidence from global health (Flood & Rohloff 2018). Khoza-Shangase (2021a) highlighted that cultural beliefs and practices within the African context have significant implications for health-seeking behaviours, as well as health intervention adherence behaviours. These views are buoyed by evidence on global health care that shows that populations from non-dominant cultures in any context have worse health outcomes compared with the dominant cultures (Flood & Rohloff 2018). Flood and Rohloff (2018) emphasised the importance of indigenous languages and cultures in the conception and implementation of health care programmes, and argued that conceptualisation and delivery of health care programmes that do not utilise the patients' language will most likely lead to less efficacious interventions and, therefore, less positive outcomes. Consequently, EHDI initiatives within the African context must take into consideration cultural and linguistic influences if they are to be successful and be collaborative with family and caregivers in nature (Khoza-Shangase & Mophosho 2021).

Kyarkanaye, Dada and Samuels (2017) further emphasised this collaboration between practitioners and caregivers of children receiving EI within the South African context by arguing that this partnership is a pivotal precept of early childhood intervention (ECI). In their study exploring caregiver perceptions of collaboration in ECI teams in South Africa, these authors found that caregivers understand collaboration in ECI services; however, in relation to family-centred practices, caregivers seemed to undervalue this collaboration. This undervaluing was illustrated by how caregivers viewed professionals' opinions as more worthy for successful caregiver professional collaboration, more important than their own involvement in teams. These authors postulated that these caregivers' undervaluing of their own important role may reflect the nature and character of the medical model approach under which EHDI falls. Khoza-Shangase and Mophosho (2018) argued that power dynamics at play in health care interactions within the South African context, driven by linguistic and cultural incongruence between the majority black African patients and the majority white health care practitioners influence the views held and expressed in these interactions. The majority of interactions within such a medical and Westernised model of care are influenced by power dynamics that regard professionals as the experts who are knowledgeable about what is best for the hearing-impaired child and their family. Watermeyer, Kanji and Cohen (2012) claimed that in post-apartheid South Africa, the challenge of cultural non-congruence between patients and health care providers reproduces historical power dynamics that leaves patients feeling isolated and marginalised and unable to probe or request clarification when communication breaks occur. This result produces a systematic barrier where the patient and family are excluded from accessing effective care (Mophosho 2018). Maluleke et al. (2021a) argued that through FCEI programmes, this cycle of exclusion is eradicated as family involvement and its role is empowered, facilitating opportunities for caregivers to advocate, make decisions and become equal partners with EI professionals in their child's care, as advanced by Sass-Lehrer (2015) and Swanepoel and Almec (2008).

In their study on maternal views on infant hearing impairment and EI in a South African community, Swanepoel and Almec (2008) found that over half of their sample were knowledgeable about at least three common causes of infant hearing impairment (ear discharge, medication, congenital) and that over half (57%) held a culturally based view of the cause. Regardless of the cultural beliefs held about the cause of hearing impairment in this study, maternal attitudes toward hearing screening and intervention were positive, as 99% of the mothers in this study indicated that they would have their baby's hearing screened in the neonatal period and that they would agree to have their hearing-impaired child be fitted with hearing aids as part of intervention. In Changsha, Hunan province, China, Wang et al. (2017) found that caregivers indicated knowledge of more risk factors for infant hearing impairment than in the South African study by Swanepoel and Almec (2008). Similar to the findings in the South African study, regardless of the knowledge of risk factors, 99% of the mothers conveyed a willingness to enrol their baby in hearing screening immediately after birth. Wang et al. (2017) also raised the need for caregiver awareness programmes about ear-and-hearing health care, prevention of hearing impairment because of preventable causes, as well as timely early identification, early diagnosis and intervention of hearing impairment.

Over 10 years ago, Van der Spuy and Pottas (2008) lamented South Africa's deficiency in data reporting the mean age of identification, diagnosis and intervention for hearing impairment because of inadequate systematic or routine screening programmes. This situation, unfortunately, remains so currently (Khoza-Shangase 2021a). Khoza-Shangase (2021a) believed that the perpetuation of the status quo is because of the lack of a government mandate on EHDI. Van der Spuy and Pottas (2008, s. 30) also found that successful EHDI significantly depends on the 'ongoing support, guidance, and commitment that parents obtain from the paediatric audiologist'. This ongoing support is reinforced by Störbeck and Pittman (2008), who argued for moving beyond hearing screening within the South African context. Störbeck and Pittman (2008) examined data on hearing-impaired infants and their families registered with a family-centred, home-based intervention programme (HI HOPES) over a period of 1 year to monitor the efficacy of this FCEI within the

South African context. Their findings showed substantial improvement in language abilities where identification had occurred before the 7-months-old, with a high level of approval from families who were part of the programme, highlighting the value of caregiver support and involvement in EHDI programme success.

Parent support and empowerment in programmes such as the HI HOPES programme can be extended to include parent-to-parent support for families of hearing-impaired children. Mehta et al. (2020) reported the value of this strategy where caregivers joined a multidisciplinary team of speech therapists, audiologists, and educators to assist the hard of hearing. These authors found high levels of satisfaction in families where peer support was introduced, with a parent possessing a shared experience being viewed as the person best positioned to provide assistance and counsel soon after the diagnosis of childhood deafness, while counselling and advice of the teacher or therapist as most useful in the preschool period after this initial period. An overwhelming majority (97%) of the participants stated that they would endorse peer-support as being valuable.

Kiling et al. (2019) reported that young children with disabilities in LMICs confront a variety of environmental risks that have an influence on their development, with interventions that do not include caregiver support within communities being one such risk factor. These authors suggest that barriers such as stigma and discrimination that children with disabilities face within these contexts can be alleviated by the provision of interventions that are community-based and inclusive of basic health care services as well, with ongoing caregiver support and collaboration being key. Within the South African context, dealing with stigma, discrimination and inclusion within communities, for example, through community-based rehabilitation programmes, with involvement of different sectors, is recommended. Moreover, because hearing impairment is a lifelong disability, a life cycle approach to caregiver support should be adopted where intervention does not end in the early years but extends to support areas such as access to schooling, access to social grants and career guidance. This support should not be confined to the child with hearing impairment but to the empowerment of the mother or caregiver as well.

Yoshinaga-Itano et al. (2017) found that maternal education level had an impact on vocabulary outcomes of hearing-impaired children who were screened at one-month-old, diagnosed at three-months-old and received medical intervention at six-months-old. Because children who had mothers with higher levels of education had higher vocabulary quotients, these authors conclude that as part of EHDI, intervention strategies to assist mothers with lower levels of education are important. In this study, the importance of appropriate support for parents who are hearing-impaired or hard of hearing is highlighted, with specific recommendations made for fully integrating adults who are hearing-impaired or hard of hearing in the intervention process. Incorporation of hearing-impaired or hard of hearing parents in the intervention programme also facilitates positive entry into the Deaf community for the child, an important consideration should that be an identity the child and family want to adopt (Yoshinaga-Itano 2014). In another Longitudinal Outcomes of Children with Hearing Impairment (LOCHI) study from Australia by Ching et al. (2018a), higher maternal education level was found to be related to superior speech-language outcomes, better functional performance, enhanced psychosocial development and higher cognitive abilities, thereby highlighting the importance of caregiver support as part of FCEI.

8.3.3. Decision-making throughout the EHDI process

Where caregivers are not supported and incorporated into EHDI programmes, even with evidence showing that this enhances language outcomes (Yoshinaga-Itano et al. 2017), the child-family needs, contextual relevance and contextual responsiveness of the intervention become questionable (Khoza-Shangase & Mophosho 2018). Crowe et al. (2014) asserted that for caregivers to make appropriate decisions regarding the choice of communication mode or language that their hearing-impaired child adopts, it is critical that interventions empower them to make informed decisions.

These authors put forward four themes they identified as the most important factors that influence caregiver decision-making. These themes, which have relevance for the South African context, were (1) sources of information, (2) practicalities of communication, (3) impact of children as individuals and (4) caregivers' decisions impacted by their children's future lives. As far as the theme 'sources of information' was concerned, diverse sources of information were described and this included information that caregivers obtained through personal research as well as lived experiences and preferences, information from professionals and, lastly, the views and opinions of family and friends.

As far as 'practicalities of communication' was concerned, access to and use of communication within the family and the community was an important influence on caregiver decision-making, over and above solid acquisition of one language or communication mode prior to the introduction of another. Theme three described the effect that each child's traits, such as their own communication mode preference and communication skills, including their ability to perceive speech through their residual hearing, as well as the presence of other comorbidities, have on caregivers' decision-making. And lastly, theme four related to caregivers being influenced by their aspirations for their children's future lives when making decisions for their hearing-impaired children.

Important considerations included explicitly nurturing a sense of belonging, developing future prospects and accomplishments and offering children the chance to select their own mode of communication.

Crowe et al.'s (2014) findings are consistent with recent results from the LOCHI study by Ching et al. (2018b), where findings reinforce the importance of comprehensive parental support and sharing of unbiased information that allows parents to make informed choices, support and information that facilitates decision-making that has considered all options in order to get the needs of their hearing-impaired children met. In Ching et al.'s (2018b) study, findings also highlighted the importance of continuity of care where caregiver support is provided continually for implementation of their choices as they adjust to their children's changing communication needs, as well as their developmental demands. Khoza-Shangase (2021b), for example, argued that there is an urgent need for continuity of care at school for the hearing-impaired child as part of EHDI goals, to make sure that the benefits of EHDI are not lost. It is in this context that Ching et al. (2018b, p. 154) concluded that 'parent decisions around communication mode are rarely made in isolation but occur within a larger decision-making matrix that includes device choices, EI agency choices, and "future-proofing" the child's ongoing communication needs'.

Continual family involvement and support are further illustrated in Scarinci et al.'s (2018b) Australian study where the authors justify the significance of this continued support by emphasising that the communication journey of a hearing-impaired child is frequently an intricate, multifarious process in which the child's utilisation of language or method of communication may frequently vary. Their study raised five key themes that shaped caregiver decisions. These themes are consistent with other reviewed studies and hold relevance for the South African context. They include '(1) family characteristics, (2) family access to information, (3) family strengths, (4) family beliefs and (5) family-centred practice' (Scarinci et al. 2018b:123).

■ 8.4. Conclusion

Findings from the afore-reviewed studies lead to several conclusions:

- Firstly, they strongly affirm the importance of caregiver collaboration and involvement in all EHDI processes, including ensuring that they are provided with unbiased information about available options. This information should include all accessible possibilities and technologies provided in a balanced manner that presents the risks versus benefits of each option for informed choices (Ching et al. 2018b). It should be acknowledged, though, that caregiver information sharing does not come without challenges on the professionals' side. Laugen (2013) highlighted that as important as the provision of comprehensive information at an early stage of the EHDI process is, this can also be overwhelming to many families. Caregivers struggle with making decisions when ambiguous information has been shared with them.

- Secondly, these studies highlight that no intervention can occur without knowing what the caregivers' communication, developmental and life goals are for their hearing-impaired child. These goals shift and adjust depending on the changing needs of the child and the child's immediate environment (Ching et al. 2018b; Crowe et al. 2014; Guralnick 2005). Hence, Maluleke et al.'s (2021a) argument for family-centred EHDI approaches within the African context where there is a strong acknowledgement of the importance of continually supporting caregivers and families as central in their hearing-impaired children's communication development journey becomes relevant.
- Thirdly, as part of the importance of family-centred care, these studies show that parents make 'sacrifices' (Ching et al. 2018b), which require that they obtain community support in the implementation of EHDI. The role of family-centred care in offering families increased understanding of EHDI, and the influence of their decision-making at each step of the process is essential. Such an approach will facilitate the transfer and carry-over of intervention goals to the context, thereby facilitating positive EHDI outcomes for the hearing-impaired child in all spheres of their life in their daily life and context. This is particularly important as Erbasi et al. (2018) reported that the role and nature of parental involvement in their hearing-impaired child's intervention are complex and multi-layered in nature combining a wide range of behaviours and practices, which have critical consequences for FCEI. Erbasi et al. (2018, p. s15) identified five important themes defining the nature of parental involvement to consider in FCEI plans, and these included (1) parents work behind the scenes, (2) parents act as 'case managers', (3) parents always have their child's language development in mind, (4) parents' role extends to advocacy for all children with hearing loss and (5) parents serve a number of roles, but at the end of the day, they are parents.

These findings clearly illustrate the 'sacrifices' (Ching et al. 2018b) that parents make, which justify the importance of extensive and continual support, as well as empowerment within family and community-centred models of intervention delivery.

It is important that, even within this FCEI, efficient team models are explored that ensure that care is coordinated and not fragmented when working with other team members to minimise stress for the already stressed parents.

Family-centred early intervention is key to positive outcomes for children with hearing impairment, and this is particularly true for the South African context with all the presented contextual challenges of a LMIC's culturally, linguistically and socio-politically diversity. Family-centred early intervention, as a philosophy from which early interventionists base the development and empowerment of families for positive outcomes of the child with disabilities (Dalmau et al. 2017; Epley, Summers & Turnbull 2010), should drive all clinical care initiatives. This approach is particularly appropriate for the South African context as it is based on principles that embrace the Afrocentric ethos of *ubuntu* as asserted by Khoza-Shangase (2019, p. 77).

Caregivers' involvement in the entire EHDI process throughout their child's development journey is influenced by a number of factors, including but not restricted to the features, assets and values of each family, their access to information, delivery of family-centred services (Scarinci et al. 2018a), maternal factors including mother's age, educational level, trust in the health care system, as well as the intervention programme itself (who is involved - the experts and how they share the expertise, how it is run - including tele-intervention and where it is provided). Although there is no single factor that parents name as the reason behind their lack of or suboptimal involvement in the EHDI process, but rather an interaction of numerous influences over time, one predominant theme is evident from the evidence reviewed. At the core of EHDI success are caregiver involvement and family-community-centred approaches. The evidence reviewed raises implications for research, teaching and clinical health care service provision that put caregivers at the centre of all EHDI initiatives, including all preventive efforts from prenatal care to intervention where negative sequelae of hearing impairment are minimised or eliminated.

While FCEI is being proposed in this chapter, it should be acknowledged that having nuclear families is not always the norm in South Africa. The structure, form, role and function of South African families differ significantly from Western notions of family imposed by colonialism and apartheid, its social and economic factors, and burdens of disease such as TB, HIV and AIDS. These factors, which have a huge impact on FCEI, disrupted family structures, leading to child-headed households, orphans, children cared for by grandparents, single parenting, unmarried women having children, teenage pregnancies and so on. So, while these may not fit the scope of this chapter, they must be acknowledged and raised as matters to consider to ensure that despite all of these challenges, efficient strategies are explored for the provision of FCEI service that is relevant within this complex environment.

Chapter 9

Preventive audiology in the context of deafblindness

Nomfundo F. Moroe
Department of Audiology, Faculty of Humanities,
School of Human and Community Development,
University of the Witwatersrand,
Johannesburg, South Africa

Khetsiwe P. Masuku
Department of Speech Pathology, Faculty of Humanities,
School of Human and Community Development,
University of the Witwatersrand,
Johannesburg, South Africa

9.1. Introduction

Although children with disabilities can live complete and satisfying lives, evidence suggests that for most of them, disability can restrict these lives significantly. These restrictions can limit their development and negatively impact their social participation and educational outcomes, impacting their employment possibilities and their consequent QoL. This is particularly true for deaf-blind children. As such, there is a need to advance these children's well-being and QoL. This can be achieved by focusing on health promotion, prevention and the minimisation of the impact of disability-related sequelae on a deaf-blind child. Therefore, in this chapter, the primary, secondary and tertiary prevention interventions for deaf-blind children are explored, with

How to cite: Moroe, NF & Masuku, KP 2022, 'Preventive audiology in the context of deafblindness', ed. K Khoza-Shangase, *Preventive audiology: An African perspective*, AOSIS Books, Cape Town, pp. 179–197. https://doi.org/10.4102/aosis.2022.BK209.09

careful consideration of the African context. Furthermore, recommendations on enhancing the QoL of deaf-blind children are provided.

The first five years of life is a period of rapid growth in which the developing brain is most pliable and responsive to stimulation and learning. This serves as a cornerstone for imminent educational and skills training and learning (Global Research on Developmental Disabilities Collaborators [GRDDC] 2018). The United Nations' 2030 SDGs seek to improve the health status of all children, including those with disability, going beyond survival (GRDDC 2018).

Approximately 15% of the world's population lives with a disability severe enough to alter their daily lives (Groce 2018). Eighty per cent of persons living with a disability live in LMICs (Vesper 2019). Based on these statistics, it can be argued that HICs are better resourced than LMICs, hence the significantly reduced incidence of disability in these countries. Of this population, it is not clear how many are children and present developmental disabilities, although evidence suggests that globally, disability among this population continues to be a notable public health concern (Groce 2018; Krahn, Walker & Correa-De-Araujo 2015; WHO 2018).

'Developmental disabilities are a group of conditions resulting from impairments affecting a child's physical, learning or behavioural function' (GRDDC 2018, p. 1100). Although children with developmental disabilities might have a good QoL, for some disability impacts their development, social engagement, access to education, health and ultimately employment outcomes (Blackburn, Read & Spencer 2012; GRDDC 2018). This is even more relevant for children who present a multisensory disability such as deafblindness.

■ 9.2. Deafblindness

Deafblindness is a distinctive multisensory disability characterised by varying degrees of hearing and visual impairment. Various authors have offered definitions for deafblindness (Anthony 2016; Dammeyer 2014; Ehn et al. 2019; Jaiswal et al. 2018). For the purpose of the chapter, deafblindness is defined as a (Wolford 2016):

> [*C*]ombined vision and hearing loss causing such severe communication and other developmental and educational needs that the student cannot be accommodated in special education programmes solely for students with deafness or students with blindness or in special education programmes solely for students with multiple disabilities. (p. 1)

Contrary to other definitions of deafblindness, Wolford (2016) explicitly highlighted the need for reasonable accommodation deaf-blind children, as these children must be provided with health care services responsive to their unique needs.

Deafblindness is a lifelong and progressive condition (Dammeyer 2014) that can be congenital or acquired in nature, has multiple causes and can be categorised into four distinct categories (Moroe 2021):

- **Category 1:** Congenital/prelingual deafblindness - from birth or early onset before the child develops language.
- **Category 2:** Acquired/post-lingual deafblindness - those who simultaneously develop both visual and hearing impairments during their lives.
- **Category 3:** Congenital single sensory impairment (vision or hearing) and then subsequently acquire another (vision or hearing) impairment.
- **Category 4:** Age-related dual-sensory impairment of vision and hearing loss in varying degrees and order and time of onset.

Deafblindness is a unique and complex impairment because of its defining feature; 'the notion of synergy - the sum (deafblindness) is greater than the parts (hearing and vision impairment)' (Simcock 2017, p. 814). Globally, the prevalence of deafblindness (Wolford 2016; Zwanenburg & Tesni 2019) with Blackburn, Read and Spencer (2012) placing the prevalence at 0.01 in 2012.

Similarly to global trends, the incidence of deafblindness is reportedly low in South Africa (Maguvhe 2014). However, Maguvhe (2014) argued that despite the low incidence of deafblindness locally, our communities seem to have neglected deaf-blind individuals form part of our communities. This author attributes this sentiment to the fact that even within the population of persons with disabilities, deaf-blind individuals are still a minority with their rights and needs are not adequately considered and addressed (Maguvhe 2014).

Unfortunately, not much is known about South African deaf-blind children. Presumably, South African deaf-blind children have similar experiences to their counterparts in other parts of the world. However, South Africa is an LMIC with limited resources regarding the availability of special educational needs or disability schools for learners with deafblindness. Additionally, deaf-blind children lack access to adequate health care professionals. According to Moroe (2021), the experiences of deaf-blind children are more pronounced in this context than those of their peers in HICs because of the stigma associated with disability.

The contribution of deafblindness on the developing child is multiplicative in that it is a combination of two vital senses - vision and hearing - which are foundations for communication, socialisation, orientation and mobility, access to information and daily living (Jaiswal et al. 2018). Vision and hearing are distance senses as they connect the individual to the world that extends beyond their personal body space and reach (DB-LINK 2017). Furthermore, these senses facilitate accidental learning of language and other important concepts without early planned instruction (Marschark & Hauser 2012).

Consequently, the impact of deafblindness extends far beyond early development, such as communication and learning, as experiences are restricted to the here and now (Moroe 2021). Therefore, if the contribution of deafblindness in developing children is not mitigated, their well-being and QoL may be affected, ultimately hindering the achievement of the SDGs. There is thus a need to focus on health promotion by preventing or minimising progression and the related sequelae of the disability on the developing child.

Health promotion is concerned with empowering people to be self-determined and improve their health (Olukemi 2019). Prevention, on the other hand, is concerned with 'measures not only to prevent the occurrence of disease, such as risk factor reduction but also to arrest its progress and reduce its consequences once established' (Duplaga et al. 2016, p. 478). Interestingly, health promotion is rarely promoted among people with disabilities despite disability being associated with poor health promotion practices (WHO 2010). The reality is that, when compared to people without disabilities, people with disability have a greater need for health promotion as they are at risk of the same health conditions in addition to the disability that potentially makes them more susceptible to health conditions. However, people with disabilities and their families have limited access to information and resources that promote and maintain good health (WHO 2010). Therefore, there is a need to promote health through primary prevention and secondary prevention where a condition already exists so that the impact of the health condition does not become progressive (tertiary prevention) (WHO 2010).

■ 9.3. Preventive health

Contextualising health prevention, specifically to deafblindness in children, entails three aspects: (1) stopping the disability from occurring in the first place (primary prevention), (2) early identification and intervention to halt the progress of the symptoms and sequelae of the disability (secondary prevention) and (3) rehabilitation to mitigate the adverse effects of an already existing health condition (tertiary prevention) (WHO 2010). The authors of this chapter acknowledge that the above-mentioned contextualisation of prevention of deafblindness is optimistic and idealistic, as it assumes that disability can be eliminated. It is proposed that this contextualisation should be understood in the context where determinants of health such as individual health behaviours and lifestyle, socio-economic status, level of education, employment and working conditions, access to quality health care services and the physical environment are modifiable or ideal (WHO 2010). Even in these ideal or modifiable situations, disability cannot be completely eradicated; however, it can be significantly reduced. The WHO (2010) argued that health promotion does not require costly intervention or elaborate technology; instead, it requires social interventions through investing time and energy in supporting health promotion campaigns. It is also argued in Chapter 7 that earlier preventive health care services should be made available for hearing-impaired children, regardless of limited resources.

9.3.1. Primary prevention

Primary prevention within the context of deafblindness, may, among others, include immunisation campaigns against communicable diseases, genetic counselling, prenatal and postnatal care at the primary health care level and measures to control endemic diseases (WHO 2010). Considering the causes (prenatal viral infections, premature birth, genetic conditions and age-related conditions) and categories of deafblindness (congenital, acquired, congenital, and acquired and age-related), primary prevention has a significant role to play in reducing the incidence of deafblindness.

Targeted immunisation campaigns are effective primary prevention intervention strategies to potentially prevent the congenital causes of deafblindness, such as rubella. Rubella, a rare but mild infection, is the most common prenatal viral infection that can lead to potentially devastating lifelong consequences (Boshoff & Tooke 2012; Gilsdorf 2018). If an expectant mother contracts rubella, she can pass it on to her unborn baby. Rubella is said to cause damage to the eyes, ears and heart of the unborn baby (Boshoff & Tooke 2012), resulting in congenital rubella syndrome. Congenital rubella syndrome is prevalent in LMICs (Boshoff & Tooke 2012; Dammeyer 2015; Jaiswal et al. 2018), although it is completely preventable through effective immunisation programmes. Regarding the prevention of rubella, Boshoff and Tooke (2012) lamented that rubella vaccination is not routinely incorporated in the EPI in LMICs. However, a recent study seems to suggest that Africa's immunisation coverage is successful even though the uptake is low (Mihigo et al. 2018). Based on this, it can be argued that rubella vaccines are now part of the EPI in Africa. These authors argue that vaccination of young females will eradicate congenital rubella syndrome immediately; therefore, the benefits are immediate but only if all females are immunised. The argument presented by these authors is in line with the recommendations of the WHO (2010) promoting immunisation campaigns to prevent disabilities, deafblindness included.

In line with targeted immunisation, in 2019, the SANDoH undertook the country's first national household vaccination coverage survey since 1994 (Burnett et al. 2019). This undertaking was informed by several imperatives, including, but not limited to, the WHO's Global Vaccine Action Plan (2011–2020), with a global target for all countries to reach 90% national coverage of all primary vaccines (Burnett et al. 2019). This survey attests to the initiatives taken by the South African government to align with global trends in immunisation programmes to eliminate health conditions and, ultimately, disabilities. Overall, the initiatives demonstrate the DOH's initiatives in aligning with the SDG initiatives to improve the health status of children beyond survival.

In cases of hereditary causes of deafblindness, the WHO (2010) recommended that families be referred for genetic counselling where concerns about current or future pregnancies may be discussed. Where there is a potential that the next child may have a disability, families can be given relevant information, and the opportunity to make an informed decision is provided. This is reliant on access to health care facilities; therefore, if females do not have readily available access to health care facilities, it will hinder their access to this much-needed health information and education. Health information and educatiocan empower people with disabilities and their families to acquire knowledge and life skills necessary to improve their health outcomes (WHO 2010).

Although the authors recommend genetic counselling as part of primary prevention strategies, they are also cognisant of the South African context. In particular, they acknowledge the sensitivities and complexities related to cultures and religion and how these can empower or disempower females depending on their context and setting. The strong link between culture and religion and decision-making regarding genetic counselling cannot be downplayed (Anderson 2009). For example, cultural and religious beliefs may influence how mothers of unborn babies perceive genetic counselling, especially from a moral lens. In cases where mothers have opted for genetic counselling, cultural and religious beliefs may influence how these mothers react to the results of the genetic tests, whether or not they divulge the findings to other family members and, ultimately, the health-seeking journey (Greenberg et al. 2012). It then becomes imperative that the health care system engages with programmes that will empower women to be able to make informed decisions regarding their health and babies'.

Prematurity is one of the main contributors to acquired deafblindness. For some time, it was believed that excessive oxygen therapy administered to premature babies caused deafblindness. However, current evidence suggests that oxygen levels are only a contributing factor (Batshaw, Pellegrino & Roizen 2007). Premature babies are exposed to increased levels of medications such as antibiotics and diuretics known to be harmful to the auditory system (Moroe & Hughes 2017). These medications are said to cause rupture of the underdeveloped blood vessels in the inner ear, thereby interrupting the flow of blood to the inner ear, which subsequently destroys hair cells. This destruction can lead to sensorineural hearing impairment (Moroe 2021). Additionally, the eyes of premature infants are said to be fragile and vulnerable to injury after birth. If injured, this may result in a condition known as retinopathy of prematurity (ROP) (Higuera 2016). Retinopathy of prematurity is the abnormal growth of blood vessels in an infant's eye, characterised by retarded growth of blood vessels that result in the development of scar tissue and retinal detachment, increasing the risk of vision loss or blindness (Higuera 2016).

According to Fernandez Turienzo et al. (2016), children who survive prematurity-related complications will likely encounter poor health problems and, in severe cases, a lifelong disability, which will result in significant financial costs to health care and the broader society. This poor health outcome presents a case for antenatal care.

Antenatal care is considered the most effective method of improving outcomes in expectant women and their babies (Hollowell et al. 2011). Therefore, access to health care, specifically antenatal care, plays a critical role in significantly reducing prematurity and the subsequent complications that may lead to disabilities such as acquired deafblindness.

In the South African context, Ngxongo (2018) discussed approaches to antenatal care, specifically, the basic antenatal care (BANC) approach. This approach has yielded positive benefits such as facilitating a comprehensive package of and the integration of primary health care services, which include the availability of accessible antenatal care, policies, guidelines and protocols, as well as training and in-service education for primary health care professionals, to name a few (Ngxongo 2018). However, not all primary health care community clinics have been able to successfully implement and sustain the BANC approach (Ngxongo 2018).

Primary prevention plays a critical role in preventing disabilities. As recommended by the WHO (2010), primary health care, prenatal and postnatal care and immunisation campaigns are the backbone in the prevention of disabilities. If primary prevention and health promotion are implemented as intended, the global burden of disease could be lowered by as much as 70% (WHO 2010). The authors of the current chapter argue that although quantitatively, the impact of primary prevention on reducing disability is not known, it cannot be disputed that efforts put towards controlling potential disabilities (e.g. immunisation drives) have positively and significantly achieved the desired outcomes.

As audiologists are potentially the professionals who first identify the presence of a hearing loss and, ultimately, deafblindness, they must be aware of the causes and the risk factors associated with deafblindness. Primary prevention audiology entails raising awareness of the risk factors associated with hearing loss and deafblindness. Moroe (2021) argued that, generally, deafblindness may result from the same conditions that cause hearing impairment, such as CHARGE (coloboma heart defects, atresia choanae, growth retardation, genital abnormalities and ear abnormalities), Usher syndrome and Goldenhar syndrome. Chapter 1 foregrounds the importance of prevention and early detection of hearing loss as part of the scope of practice that South African audiologists need to increase their focus on. Among other strategies, prevention and early detection of hearing loss can be achieved using the High-Risk Register (HRR), also known as targeted screening (Kanji & Khoza-Shangase 2019, 2021). In a study by Kanji and Khoza-Shangase (2012), success in early detection and intervention resulted in the adoption of the HRR despite missing 25%–50% of neonates with hearing loss, particularly when used in isolation. The HRR is useful in identifying children who require monitoring and follow-up screening and in contexts where UNHS is not feasible, such as in LMICs (Kanji & Khoza-Shangase 2012). Khoza-Shangase (2021b) argued that within the South African context, the use of the HRR should be used as an interim step towards UNHS, while efforts are increased to get UNHS mandated as that will come with human resource and equipment planning that is required.

Moreover, as part of health promotion, audiologists participate in activities such as the annual World Hearing Day and other Deaf Awareness campaigns aimed at raising awareness about the causes of hearing impairment. These campaigns provide valuable opportunities to target and include deafblindness in the activities. Therefore, preventive audiology has a crucial role to play in hearing health care and promotion. As disability cannot always be prevented, where a disability is present, secondary prevention should be implemented, the focus of the next section.

9.3.2. Secondary prevention

Secondary prevention aims to control or manage the disease before it manifests clinically (Duplaga et al. 2016; Pandve 2014). Therefore, secondary prevention promotes early detection and intervention through timely screening to detect asymptomatic disease. In the case where a disability is already present, secondary prevention will entail controlling the expected symptoms or progression of the disability. Specifically, preventive audiology plays a crucial role in the early detection and prevention of deafblindness. This is because the ability to hear is a prerequisite or precursor to learning to communicate verbally.

The importance of early detection and intervention cannot be overemphasised. Ideally, early detection and intervention should take place within the first year of life (Khoza-Shangase 2021a; Moroe 2021). Failure to timeously implement early detection interventions may result in missing the critical period of early neurodevelopment, thereby reducing the opportunities to learn, which may negatively impact the QoL for the affected child and their family (Anthony 2016). Consequently, the child with deafblindness may be delayed in communication, cognition, reading and social-emotional development (JCIH 2007).

If EI is not affected, communication may potentially be compromised. Moroe (2021) discussed *three goals* for early detection and intervention in deaf-blind children. The first goal is to open up a new channel of communication and explore the environment. Deafblindness presents severe restrictions on the child's access to communication and language. Most deaf-blind children are unable to experience the nuances of shared language or rely on others to model language for them (DB-LINK 2017). A child with a visual impairment typically relies on their hearing to compensate for visual impairment. Conversely, a child with a hearing impairment relies on their vision to compensate for the hearing impairment (Cappagli et al. 2017; Newton & Moss 2001). For a deaf-blind child, they cannot rely on one sense to compensate for the absence of the other. Consequently, the reception of information necessary for learning, interaction, and overall development is negatively compromised. It is clear that unless deafblindness is detected early and intervention provided timeously, impairment of these senses may potentially result in serious consequences for a developing child.

The second goal of early identification and intervention in this population is to facilitate adequate social-emotional bonding, early communication, language, emergent literacy, access to learning materials, and educational experiences (Anthony 2016). Deaf-blind children typically experience developmental delays in social interaction, independence, engagement, accessing information from their environment, communication, and socio-emotional development (Hartshorne & Schmittel 2016). As a result, their social interactions may seem confusing, purposeless or even fearful, which may restrict their interactions, and emotional bonding and trusting relationships may not be easily formed. Because of these restricted interactions, deaf-blind children may present with challenging behaviours or stereotypical behaviours known as 'blindisms' (Valente, Theurel & Gentaz 2018). These behaviours may include body rocking, head shaking, eye-poking and hand flapping (De Vaan et al. 2013). Deaf-blind children use these behaviours to express their frustration or as attempts at communication. As such, they must be provided with specific instructions on how to manage their interactions with the environment (Hartshorne & Schmittel 2016). Therefore, early detection and prevention of these challenging behaviours are paramount in addressing the communication and emotional needs of deaf-blind children.

The third goal of early detection is to mitigate the multiplicative effects of deafblindness. As deafblindness is a multisensory disability, a multidisciplinary approach to management is recommended. This should entail early referrals to other relevant professionals to ensure timely intervention that maximises and enhances communication, learning and socialisation, particularly in the critical early years.

Locally, evidence suggests that there are no active early identification and intervention programmes specifically for deaf-blind children (Moroe 2021). Moroe (2021) provided *six reasons* for the lack of active early identification and intervention in this regard. Firstly, in line with global trends, the incidence of deafblindness in South Africa is significantly low. Deafblindness is hardly discussed in public arenas, save for minor coverage in public engagements that are characterised by low-societal preparedness and receptiveness to accommodate deaf-blind individuals (Maguvhe 2014). Secondly, deafblindness, in most cases, results from the same conditions causing hearing impairment. Despite this, a focused early detection and prevention programme for deafblindness cease to exist. Screening for deafblindness is traditionally embedded either in EHDI programmes or during ophthalmological assessment. Holte et al. (2006) states that when deafblindness is suspected, ophthalmologic evaluation is warranted to assess oculomotor function, visual acuity, peripheral vision, visual adaptation, colour perception and eye pressures. Currently, in South Africa, it is not clear: (1) at what stage this referral is made, (2) what protocol ophthalmologists use to assess deaf-blind children, and (3) what level of care deaf-blind individuals receive (primary, secondary or tertiary health care level).

Thirdly, health care professionals, such as audiologists, speech therapists, occupational therapists, physiotherapists and ophthalmologists are not adequately trained to detect and provide intervention services to individuals with multisensory impairments. Fourthly, under ideal conditions, early detection and intervention should take place within the first year of life. Global trends indicate that early detection health care programmes for children who are deaf-blind are present in special educational need or disability (SEND) schools for the visually- and hearing-impaired or with special educational needs (Hersh 2013). Deaf-blind learners are not accommodated in special educational needs or disabilities (SEND) schools in South Africa. Consequently, these children are more likely to attend schools for learners with general, special educational needs or disabilities, and not necessarily or specifically deaf-blind schools. Fifthly, there is a dearth of information on the availability of therapists and teachers with expertise in the management of deaf-blind learners. In an ideal context, where there are health care professionals deployed at schools for learners with special educational needs or disabilities, learners with deafblindness would be referred timeously for screening, evaluation and treatment of communication and learning difficulties. Lastly, the FCEI approach in South Africa is still in its infancy (Maluleke, Chiwutsi & Khoza-Shangase 2021). Family-centred early intervention is integral for early detection and intervention, and it is even more so in deaf-blind children (Maluleke, Chiwutsi & Khoza-Shangase 2021). Chapter 8 strongly argues for enabling caregivers as key co-drivers of early detection and intervention within the African context to ensure FCEI, while Chapter 10 argues that any effort geared towards EHDI, including that of family involvement, should carefully also deliberate on the economic evaluation of EHDI programmes within the South African context – placing EHDI on the political advocacy and resource allocation agenda. As the effects of deafblindness cannot be reversed, there is, therefore, a need for tertiary prevention.

9.3.3. Tertiary prevention

Tertiary prevention is defined as the intervention for people who have already developed a disorder or disability, aimed at abating the ramifications of the disorder or disability on the individual's life and that of their family (Khasnabis et al. 2010). At this level of intervention the focus is on (re)habilitative interventions, depending on whether the disability was congenital or acquired. As deaf-blind children are likely to only be identified at school-going age, the Department of Education has a significant role in implementing interventions that are conducive, responsive and promote reasonable accommodation for this population. Khoza-Shangase (2021b) carefully presented deliberations and recommendations around continuity of care for hearing-impaired children that include intervention at schools as a way to maximise EHDI benefits within the resource-constrained South African context. However, before children are referred for school placement they should receive aural habilitation as part of tertiary preventive audiology.

Aural habilitation refers to the plan to improve communication with young hearing-impaired children who have not yet developed spoken language (Minnesota Hands & Voices 2020). Children who are deaf-blind vary widely in the degree of hearing loss and onset age. Therefore, it is important to consider these factors when enrolling them for aural habilitation. Aural habilitation in this population entails the provision of assistive listening devices (including hearing aids and cochlear implants) and the determination of the best communication modality for the child and their family (Nelson & Bruce 2019). Communication modes for this population are outlined by Hersh (2013, p. 447) and include:

- Spoken language.
- Sign language.
- Tactile sign language: A deaf-blind individual holds the other person's wrists and feels their movements as they sign.
- Deaf-blind manual alphabets: Spelling using signs that represent the alphabet. There are two main approaches: The speaker signs the letter onto the listener's flat palm; the listener puts their hand over the speaker's vertical hand and feels the movements of their fingers. Both approaches are quicker than Spartan.
- Tadoma: A deaf-blind individual places one hand on the other person's chin, lips or throat to feel their movements as they speak.
- The deaf-blnd block alphabet (Spartan): A deaf-blind individual draws blocked capital letters on the palm of the other.
- Finger Braille: The individual types six fingers as a Braille keyboard.

If appropriate, these communication modes can be used in conjunction with assistive listening devices. Chapter 8 carefully deliberates on evidence around the choice of communication mode and family considerations thereof. In addition to aural habilitation, reasonable accommodation should also be prioritised for deaf-blind children.

Reasonable accommodation is defined as (UN Committee on the Rights of Persons with Disabilities 2016):

> [*T*]he necessary and appropriate modification and adjustments, not imposing a disproportionate or undue burden where needed in a particular case to ensure persons with disabilities the enjoyment or exercise on an equal basis with others of all human rights and fundamental freedoms. (p. 1)

Simply stated, reasonable accommodation entails implementing effective and practical interventions that enable a person with a disability to work as effectively as their peers without a disability (National Disability Authority 2019). In the case of deafblindness, interventions that enable access to education on an equal footing with their peers are important. The authors of this chapter argue that reasonable accommodation is not synonymous with inclusive education but concede that, where possible, reasonable accommodation can be incorporated within inclusive education.

Inclusive education is not an easy concept to define, but integral to the definition are the: (1) fundamental right to education, (2) principle that values students' well-being, dignity, autonomy, and contribution to society and (3) continuing process to eliminate barriers to education and promote reform in the culture, policy and practice in schools to include all students (Schuelka 2018). Inclusive education purports that students are taught in a mainstream classroom regardless of their dis(ability) (Schuelka 2018). Interestingly, Schuelka (2018) noted that inclusive education does not mean segregation (e.g. placing children in special units or special classrooms) or integration (e.g. integrating children with disabilities in mainstream settings only if they can adjust). Inclusive education recognises that all learners must be taught in the same educational space regardless of their dis(abilities) (Schuelka 2018). Fundamentally, inclusive education seeks to capacitate all children in realising their capabilities, which will contribute to productive and meaningful growth (Hayes & Bulat 2017). While this is a noble and commendable initiative, it sadly does not address the unique needs of deaf-blind children.

The Committee on the Rights of Persons with Disabilities (CRPD) emphasises that no 'one-size-fits-all' formula exists when looking at children with disabilities and those who require reasonable accommodation (Hayes & Bulat 2017). Differently abled students may require very different accommodations owing to the severity of their disability and their personal learning preferences

(UN CRPD 2016). This is particularly true for deaf-blind children. The World Federation of the Deafblind (WFDB) notes that society incorrectly assumes that services meant for hearing- or vision-impaired children are also sufficient for deaf-blind children (WFDB 2018). This statement cannot be further from the truth as deaf-blind children present with unique educational needs; therefore, educational services tailored only for children who are hearing-impaired would not benefit them. Secondly, the WFDB (2018) addressed the importance of having services that are solely meant for children with disability. This is in line with the notion that the effects of deafblindness on developing children are multiplicative. Additionally, it is in line with the definition of deafblindness as (Wolford 2016):

> [*C*]ombined vision and hearing loss causing such severe communication and other developmental and educational needs that the student cannot be accommodated in special education programmes solely for students with deafness or students with blindness or in special education programmes solely for students with multiple disabilities. (p. 1)

Article 24 of the CRPD mandates that member states should ensure that accommodation is provided for persons with disabilities in educational contexts. Section 3c of Article 24 specifically refers to deaf-blind learners and urges member states to deliver education in acceptable and appropriate languages and modes of communication for the individual in an environment that enhances academic success and social development (UN 2006). Similarly, Articles 25 and 26 of the CRPD direct member states to ensure that persons with disability enjoy the best attainable standard of health care, habitation and rehabilitation without discrimination. It further challenges member states to put measures in place that ensure that persons with disabilities attain access to all services that individuals enjoy without disabilities. Khoza-Shangase, Sebothoma & Moroe (2021) suggested that tele-audiology can be utilised in the South African context as part of efforts to enhance inclusivity and equality of children with disability in schools through ICT.

Under the patronage of the CRPD, the implementation of inclusive education at all levels of education is by law a mandate for member states, thus implying that the education for children with disabilities is a human right matter (Biermann 2016). In line with these legal obligations, in South Africa, there are several policies and guideline policies and guidelines that support inclusive education. These include the Department of Education's *White Paper 6* (DoH 2001), the *White Paper on the Rights of Persons with Disabilities* (Department of Social Development 2016) and the *Framework and Strategy for Disability and Rehabilitation* (SADoH 2015). The *White Paper 6* on inclusive education was commissioned in 2001 (DoH 2001), with the mandate of ensuring that learners with disabilities get access to the same quality of education as their counterparts without disabilities so that they have the same educational outcomes. While strides have been made to improve education for learners with disabilities in South Africa, *White Paper 6* has unfortunately not been successful in achieving its desired goal as learners with disabilities continue being excluded from education (Donohue & Bornman 2014). The success of tertiary prevention for deaf-blind children is dependent on their access and inclusion to both health care services and education.

Access should fulfil the dimensions of availability, acceptability, geographical accessibility, financial accessibility and quality (Peters et al. 2008). These dimensions are described in more detail next:

- **Availability:** In the context of health care, availability pertains to 'providing the appropriate type of quality health care to all citizens that require health care, such as health care facilities and programmes with adequate human, financial and physical resources that respond to the needs of people accessing these services' (Peters et al. 2008, p. 162). The same principle applies to education, where availability is explained as the existence of schools and programmes that children with disabilities can access. Member states should therefore ensure that they prioritise the establishment and funding of public and private schools for deaf-blind learners (Tomaševski 2001). This is because these learners have additional needs that cannot be accommodated in schools for learners who are either visually- or hearing-impaired (Maguvhe 2014). The challenges faced by deaf-blind learners include failure to grasp information that would typically be obtained through the use of distance senses of vision and hearing. This suggests that accidental learning that occurs through vision loss is not possible. Ultimately, communication delays and difficulties occur (Dammeyer 2014). These challenges necessitate the need for ongoing rehabilitation services provided at health care facilities and schools by a collaborative team of rehabilitation professionals, such as speech-language therapists, audiologists and occupational therapists (Manga & Masuku 2020). Assistive devices and augmentative and alternative communication devices should also be issued and maintained by qualified health care professionals who are trained to assess the candidacy and benefits for a deaf-blind child.
- **Acceptability:** Acceptability is defined as the compatibility and responsiveness of health care workers to the social and cultural disposition of the users of health care services (Peters et al. 2008). This also applies to educational settings, as stated by Tomaševski (2001). Schools that cater for deaf-blind children must provide the highest standard and quality of education that considers the rights of the learners in an inclusive and supportive environment and that is free from discriminatory and denial barriers. As deaf-blind children are heterogeneous (Dammeyer

2014), a 'one-size-fits-all' classroom or therapy approach would be ineffective. Health and education services should be tailored to the specific needs of deaf-blind individuals (Tomaševski 2001). Reasonable accommodation is therefore key.

- **Adaptation:** Adaptation requires educational planning and teaching methods, and it considers the specific ways that the learner will understand and engage with information and how teaching and learning techniques will be tailored for the needs of that specific learner (Maguvhe 2014). Therefore, professionals' knowledge and skills become crucial, which suggests adequate training and support for educators (Janssen et al. 2002; Maguvhe 2014; Manga & Masuku 2020). Educators should be trained to respond appropriately to the interactive behaviours of deaf-blind children and also on strategies on how to modify the interactive environment to aid and encourage the occurrence of desired interactive child behaviours (Janssen et al. 2002). Training should include information on how to offer communicative aids and choices, removal of distractive stimuli and stimuli not wanted by the child from the environment, tuning activities to the child's sensory, cognitive and motor abilities, and demonstration of appropriate interactive behaviours to the child (Janssen et al. 2002). McLetchie and Riggio (2001) also supported these recommendations and further suggest the following considerations: the use of smaller group sizes, instructional arrangement, involvement of speech and language therapists and audiologists, support for assistive technology, and augmentative and alternative communication.
- **Geographical accessibility:** Geographical accessibility is the 'physical distance or travel time from service delivery point to the user' (Peters et al. 2008). Health care facilities and schools should be available within a reasonable geographical distance to deaf-blind children (Peters et al. 2008; Tomaševski 2001). Children who are deaf-blind should not be disadvantaged from receiving services because of transportation barriers.
- **Financial accessibility:** Financial accessibility pertains to the relationship between the costs of health care services and whether or not people accessing these services can afford them without enduring negative economic consequences (Peters et al. 2008). Financial considerations need to be made for the accommodation needs related to therapeutic interventions, assistive devices, and augmentative and alternative communication. Education and health care should ideally be economically accessible to children with disabilities, including this population (Ramaahlo, Tönsing & Bornman 2018).

Similarly, Tomaševski (2001) used similar dimensions to advocate for the universal coverage of education for all children. This author recommends that reasonable educational accommodation should be available, accessible, acceptable, and adaptable (Tomaševski 2001).

Locally, tertiary prevention for deaf-blind children was discussed against the backdrop of access to education and health care services. South Africa is home to 'three nations': the very wealthy, the missing middle and a large majority of people in South Africa living in poverty (Mpofu & Ndlovu-Gatsheni 2019). Persons with disabilities, including those with deafblindness, are overrepresented in the latter category, where many in these households continue to be marginalised and still subjected to undesirable access to education, health care, energy, sanitation and clean water.

The ongoing marginalisation and deprivation of basic education and health care needs for persons with disabilities is a systemic ramification of apartheid, a system that for decades segregated people across racial lines in South Africa. In this system, black people were subjected to poor quality education and health care in their designated townships or homelands (Mpofu & Ndlovu-Gatsheni 2019). The education and health care system that serve children with disabilities followed similar trends. While most white children with disabilities had fully functional schools, black children with disabilities did not have schools unless special educational need or disability (SEND) schools were introduced, often by missionaries or charity organisations (Khumalo & Hodgson 2001). It was inevitable that these schools had inadequate resources and poorly trained staff as the government did not support them.

South Africa has some of the most comprehensive legislation and policies to facilitate access toersons with disabilities across different entities, including health care and education; however, the policies have been unsuccessful owed to poor implementation and monitoring strategies (Donohue & Bornman 2014).

Data from South African schools for the visually impaired or for learners who need special educational advancement suggest that schools for deaf-blind learners should accommodate deaf-blind learners. (Maguvhe 2014). Reasonable accommodation (in terms of availability, accessibility [geographical and financial], acceptability and adaptability) is not responsive fulfil the needs of deaf-blind learners. Currently, there is a shortage of schools for learners with special educational needs or disabilities (SEND) and even fewer schools cater for deaf-blind learners. Consequently, parents are often turned away from schools or placed on waiting lists because of unavailable spaces. This is further compounded in schools catering to the needs of deaf-blind children, as far fewer schools exist for this population or accommodate these children.

Schools for deaf-blind children also have a shortage of teachers who are adequately trained to teach them (Manga & Masuku 2020). Most available schools are far and not easily accessible to the children and their families.

Maguvhe (2014) lamented that, in South Africa, the curricula for deaf-blind learners are not aligned with the national curricula. As a result of this lack of alignment, schools are bestowing institution-based certification, which potential employers do not recognise. There is, therefore, a need to ensure that the curricula are also in line with the curriculum of the country (Maguvhe 2014).

The aforementioned discussion suggests that South Africa still has a long way to go in addressing the health and educational needs of deaf-blind children.

■ 9.4. Recommendations and solutions

This section outlines the solutions and recommendations for the potential prevention of deafblindness, early detection and the enhancement of the QoL of deaf-blind children and their families in sub-Saharan Africa:

- Considering the causes of deafblindness (e.g. infections and preterm births), it is important to strengthen maternal health care programmes, specifically antenatal clinics in public health care facilities to improve maternal health and reduce mortality and disability. Antenatal clinics and postnatal health care services provide a critical opportunity to implement interventions. This is particularly relevant because the rate of preterm births is higher in LMICs such as South Africa (WHO 2012) than in HICs.
- Maternal health care programmes should include maternal immunisations for mothers during their pregnancy to target potential infections in both the pregnant mother and fetus. Maternal immunisations should ideally be scheduled along with antenatal classes as expectant mothers tend to be more accessible to medical care during the period of antenatal care. Arguably this has been achieved in South Africa, even though this may not be the case in the rest of sub-Saharan Africa. It cannot be taken for granted that all pregnant mothers attend antenatal classes. Therefore, primary health care through the involvement of CHW must encourage pregnant women in communities to attend antenatal classes as this may result in improved quality of care before, during and after pregnancy.
- Health promotion (at the primary health care level as well as at the community level) regarding sexual and reproductive health should cater to both adolescent girls and women. This will empower both girls and women to make informed choices related to family planning strategies as early as possible. Health promotion information will also assist in addressing decisions related to adolescent pregnancies and gaps between births. Health-related information related to unhealthy pre-pregnancy weight, chronic diseases, prevention, screening and management of infectious

diseases such as HIV and AIDS and sexually transmitted infections, substance abuse and poor psychological health need to be included in health promotion and prevention strategies, as these factors have been identified as risk factors for preterm births.

- Care needs to be taken when compiling health literacy information. Adequate health literacy information needs to be provided in a language and formats that can be understood by expectant mothers regardless of their literacy levels. In their health promotion programmes and literacy information, health care workers need to emphasise the importance of promoting healthy nutrition and environmental and occupational health.
- There is also a need for developing countries such as South Africa to implement medical strategies that facilitate improved childbirth practices to limit preterm births.
- Early hearing loss and visual loss with universal and targeted screening are highly recommended to implement prompt intervention in the case of identified cases.
- The authors of this chapter also recommend an interdisciplinary approach to prevent deafblindness in children. This approach is relevant, especially considering the interface between health-, education- and social-related implications of deafblindness for the affected individual and their families. Having recommended this approach, it is imperative to acknowledge that deafblindness is still a disability that is not well-known to most people, including the health care thereof, education and treating clinicians. This is partly because of its low prevalence, so these professionals may not be adequately trained to manage deaf-blind children, thus disadvantaging them. This emphasises the need for awareness, training and support for these professionals who provide acceptable quality services to improve the livelihood of deaf-blind children.
- Even though the value of inclusive education is acknowledged and supported by the authors of this chapter, especially in its quest to ensure education for all children through the accommodation of children with disabilities in school and preventing othering and isolation of these children, this system of education may not be ideal for all children who are visually- and hearing-impaired, considering their specific communication, development and educational needs. The authors believe that some deaf-blind learners may benefit from schools that cater to their specific needs. Schools must be equipped with educators who are trained specifically in deafblindness. Ongoing support from speech-language therapy, audiological intervention, occupational therapists, psychologists and other relevant professionals through the development of individualised educational and rehabilitation plans needs to be provided. Caregiver involvement is imperative in the management process.
- Governments must commit to providing the necessary resources that will make education accessible to deaf-blind children. Strategies for successful

policy implementation and monitoring need to be strengthened to ensure that policies related to access to education for children with disabilities achieve the desired outcomes. Investment must be made in the provision of assistive and augmentative and alternative communication devices.
- There is a need to re-engineer the curricula offered to deaf-blind children if they are going to be meaningful contributors to the country's economy. Maguvhe (2014) specifically recommended that the curriculum must have goals and achievable outcomes for teaching deaf-blind learners.
- Accommodation strategies such as curriculum differentiation that will make learning for children living with deafblindness meaningful need careful deliberation.

9.5. Conclusion

Early detection and intervention of deafblindness during the first year of life are recommended as the gold standard for these children flourish with positive communication, educational and employment outcomes (Anthony et al. 2015). Although the incidence of deafblindness is low, it has implications for the QoL of the child with deafblindness and their family and health promotion initiatives, particularly those relating to the SDGs. While deafblindness, as a disability, cannot be completely eradicated, its incidence and negative impact can be significantly reduced through primary and secondary prevention. This will alleviate the burden of disease in countries that already face access to health care challenging.

To achieve this, it is important to advocate for primary and secondary prevention activities of deafblindness. Evidence suggests that in developing countries, early detection and intervention are yet to be achieved, as detection and intervention for deaf-blind children do not occur until children reach school age. This finding, coupled with factors such as the unique and complex nature of deafblindness, its progression and multiple causes, justifies the intervention of deafblindness across different levels of prevention (Moroe 2021).

Preventive audiology has a significant role to play in potentially preventing deafblindness across all levels of prevention. In primary prevention, preventive audiology can contribute through campaigns that highlight the risk factors associated with deafblindness in babies and children. In secondary prevention, preventive audiology plays a significant role in early detection and intervention in deaf-blind children. Finally, in tertiary prevention, preventive audiology should focus on the provision of aural habilitative services, facilitation of reasonable accommodation access to information and resources for deaf-blind children and their families, as well as timely referral to other professionals. This will contribute to lessening the lifelong and progressive negative effects of deafblindness in babies and young children, with consequent improved QoL for them and their families.

Chapter 10

Economic evaluation of EHDI programmes in South Africa: Putting EHDI on the political advocacy and resource allocation agenda

Ntsako P. Maluleke[a,b]
[a]Department of Speech-Language Pathology and Audiology,
Faculty of Health Sciences, School of Healthcare Sciences,
Sefako Makgatho Health Sciences University,
Pretoria, South Africa
[b]Department of Audiology, Faculty of Humanities,
School of Human and Community Development,
University of the Witwatersrand,
Johannesburg, South Africa

■ 10.1. Introduction

Health economics is the comparative analysis of alternative courses of health care actions with regard to both costs and consequences (Dukhanin et al. 2018). Assessing economic value in health care is not a new concept, but in recent years health economics has been widely used to help prioritise resource allocation for health care and public health care services (Doshi & Willke 2017;

How to cite: Maluleke, NP 2022, 'Economic evaluation of EHDI programmes in South Africa: Putting EHDI on the political advocacy and resource allocation agenda', ed. K Khoza-Shangase, *Preventive audiology: An African perspective*, AOSIS Books, Cape Town, pp. 199–212. https://doi.org/10.4102/aosis.2022.BK209.10

Dukhanin et al. 2018). Health economics bridges the gap between the theory, economics and practice of health care. Its earliest roots date back to 1932, with the formation of the Bureau of Medical Economics by the American Medical Association. However, the first publication of this science as 'health economics' was in 1958 (Jakovljevic & Ogura 2016). Since then, this field has experienced great development and extensive diversification from its earliest roots into the various sub-disciplines available today (Blumenschein & Johannesson 1996; Jakovljevic & Ogura 2016).

Focus on health economics has underscored the need for decision-makers to evaluate health care interventions' health and cost impacts (Lakdawalla et al. 2018) and ensure cost-effective, evidence-based practice where limited health care benefits are maximised (Gage et al. 2006; Kernick 2002). Evaluation of health care has traditionally focused on the cost associated with individual components of care such as inpatient and outpatient health care, as well as pharmaceutical costs, while benefits to health care were generally focused on the short-term outcomes related to acute health care (Mauskopf et al. 1998). Health care costs are, however, interconnected and so consideration of the total health care costs, as opposed to consideration of the individual health care costs, is warranted (Mauskopf et al. 1998; Remme, Martínez-Alvarez & Vassall 2017), given that increasing expenditure in one aspect of health care may decrease expenditure in another aspect of health care and overall health care savings (Mauskopf et al. 1998).

Furthermore, analysis of health care costs focusing only on illness and disease provides a single-sided view of the direct costs without due consideration of the indirect costs, such as lost or diminished productivity and the need for social and educational support (Mauskopf et al. 1998). Good health is a combination of a range of biological, environmental, behavioural and social factors; thus, quality health care service is only one aspect of how good health is achieved (Remme et al. 2017). Thus, decision-makers need all this information to make informed decisions regarding the allocation of scarce health care resources (Mauskopf et al. 1998). A holistic evaluation of health care is in contrast to evaluation frameworks that limit the evaluation to health care services used to allocate resources, compromising patients' QoL (Remme et al. 2017).

Despite the evident value of health economics, there has been a reluctance to embrace this formal approach for health care resource allocation decisions in Europe and the United States (Bate, Donaldson & Murtagh 2007; Gage et al. 2006; Lakdawalla et al. 2018). Davies et al.'s (1994) appraisal of health care technology in the European community revealed that economic evaluation had a relatively low impact on health care policy and decision-making. Similar results were reported by Russell et al. (1996), who revealed that CEA seldom informed health services in the United States. Reasons provided for the low impact of these analyses in health care include difficulties accessing relevant information, the information provided not being in a format that is understandable to non-economists, the information answers questions from a different perspective from that of decision-makers and an insufficient supply of the information in a timely fashion (Bate et al. 2007; Lakdawalla et al. 2018). However, the need remains for a comprehensive outcomes assessment for new health care interventions (Mauskopf et al. 1998).

10.2. Economic evaluation of early hearing detection and intervention programmes

Childhood hearing impairment constitutes one of the most prevalent sensory impairments; consequently, it incurs substantial economic costs to society (Chorozoglou et al. 2018). Future projections estimate that hearing impairment will be the fifth leading cause of the burden of disease globally by 2030 (WHO 2020). The economic impact of unaddressed hearing impairment and subsequent multifaceted and negative effects of the hearing impairment at a personal and societal level render EHDI efforts imperative for children who present with congenital or early-onset hearing impairment. However, public health care interventions such as EHDI services need to demonstrate the magnitude of the benefits relative to the financial cost of the service, especially in LMICs, which are characterised by over-burdened health care systems and resource constraints (Remme et al. 2017). This chapter outlines the most commonly used economic evaluation methods and their application to the field of audiology and EHDI services. Furthermore, it provides recommendations using these methods to garner political and funding support in LMICs such as South Africa.

10.2.1. Economic impact of childhood hearing impairment

Hearing impairment is a significant contributor to the burden of disease, ranking it as the fourth leading contributor to years lived with disability (YLD) globally (Swanepoel & Clark 2018), higher than chronic diseases such as diabetes, dementia and chronic obstructive pulmonary disease (WHO 2020). Figures estimate that 737 (6%) out of the 12 million infants born annually in LMICs such as South Africa are born with a congenital or early-onset hearing impairment (Störbeck 2012). Thus, six newborns per 1000 live births in LMICs are born with a congenital or early-onset hearing impairment, as opposed to two newborns per 1000 live births in HICs (Peer 2015).

The early years during childhood are crucial for optimum speech and language development. Thus, an unaddressed hearing impairment at this age has a negative impact characterised by delays in speech and language development, psychosocial development, cognitive skills development, literacy development, academic achievement, employment and social integration, especially in LMICs (Maluleke, Khoza-Shangase & Kanji 2019; Störbeck 2012; Swanepoel & Hall 2010). However, there is a dearth of population-based longitudinal data that measure the economic impact of hearing impairment (National Academies of Sciences 2016). However, the economic impact of an unaddressed hearing impairment across the lifespan of one individual is estimated at $1 million international, with an annual global cost of $750bn–$790bn for moderate to severe hearing impairment (greater than 35 dB in the better ear) (WHO 2017). Between 63% and 73% of the estimated $750bn–$790bn costs are incurred in LMICs (WHO 2020).

The reported annual global cost of $750bn–$790bn for an unaddressed hearing impairment across the lifespan includes costs associated with health care, educational support, loss of productivity and cost societal costs. However, this amount does not cover the cost of hearing devices (WHO 2020). Furthermore, these costs do not include the cost of providing informal care, preschool and higher education for children with hearing impairment because of a lack of documented literature in these areas. Moreover, there is a lack of country-specific data, especially in LMICs (WHO 2017). These costs are calculated for moderate or higher degrees of hearing impairment, with the conservative assumption that additional costs for educational support for children with hearing impairment are only incurred in children with at least moderately severe hearing impairment (greater than 50 decibels) (WHO 2017). These costs should be understood within the reality that even a mild unilateral hearing loss and or a transient hearing loss can have a negative effect on academic/speech-language development.

Childhood hearing impairment is an aetiologically heterogeneous condition (Olusanya 2012), with estimates suggesting that 50% of congenital hearing impairment has a genetic aetiology (Ahmed, Shubina-Oleinik & Holt 2017). Furthermore, preventable causes such as birth asphyxia, chronic OM, measles and mumps, use of ototoxic medication and exposure to excessive noise contribute to the high prevalence of childhood hearing impairment (Olusanya 2012; WHO 2020). While some aetiologies for childhood hearing impairment are preventable, prevailing socio-economic and weak health care systems in many LMICs render complete elimination or significant reduction of these causes unattainable (Olusanya 2012; Peer 2015). Therefore, complete prevention of both genetic and non-genetic hearing impairment in childhood is unlikely to be achieved in any country (Olusanya 2012).

Consequently, secondary prevention of childhood hearing impairment through EHDI becomes imperative to provide safety nets for those who unavoidably will be hearing impaired (Olusanya 2012). However, South Africa is characterised by an over-burdened health care system where hearing impairment competes with other life-threatening health priorities for the limited resources available (Maphumulo & Bhengu 2019). Thus, childhood hearing impairment is viewed as less urgent and has consequently received lesser financial attention and political will from the DoH (Maluleke, Chiwutsi & Khoza-Shangase 2021a). Furthermore, hearing health care professionals are unable to meet the burgeoning volume of needs while performing at capacity within significant budgeting constraints (Khoza-Shangase & Michal 2014; Swanepoel & Clark 2018). Chapters 2 and 3 explores the capacity versus demand challenges and how these negatively impact service delivery within the South African context.

Without EHDI services, the mean age at identification of congenital or early-onset hearing impairment is two years and three months; following maternal suspicion of the hearing impairment because of significant delays in developmental milestones (Khoza-Shangase & Michal 2014; Maluleke et al. 2019). Preventive efforts such as EHDI are the most cost-effective and high-yielding strategy to combat the negative effects of hearing impairment, especially in resource-constrained LMICs (Leclair & Saunders 2019; Maluleke et al. 2021b). Through EHDI services, the devastating, multifaceted and negative effects of hearing impairment can be mitigated at a personal and societal level (Meinzen-Derr, Wiley & Choo 2011; Vas, Akeroyd & Hall 2017). This affords children with hearing impairment an opportunity and resources to develop speech and language abilities on par with their peers with typical hearing (Maluleke et al. 2019). Early hearing detection and intervention are recognised as the gold standard of care for the assessment and management of early childhood hearing impairment (Olusanya 2012) and are also recognised as an undeniable right for children with hearing impairment and their families (Pribanikj & Milkovikj 2009).

The goal of EHDI is to ensure that all infants are identified as early as possible and for appropriate intervention to commence no later than three-to-six-months-old (Dukhanin et al. 2018; JCIH 2019). This approach falls within the preventive care model of service delivery, providing a platform for improved hearing health care (National Academies of Sciences 2016). Integrating ear-and-hearing health care in such public health approaches is the key to ensuring everyone's sustainable and equitable access to services (Chadha, Kamenov & Cieza 2019). These efforts require sufficient availability of hearing health care professionals as well as hearing health care investment and expansion in LMICs, where children currently have high rates of hearing impairment, with little or no access to hearing health care services (Leclair & Saunders 2019).

Global health care policymakers face difficult financial decisions in balancing severely constrained health care budgets with the rising demand for health care services (Remme et al. 2017). Thus, it is imperative that policymakers are knowledgeable about the economic costs of health problems, including hearing impairment, and the potential costs that might be avoided to plan the best use of their health care budgets (WHO 2017). Thus, this chapter aligns EHDI services with the global agenda of SDGs and economic benefits in an effort to garner the necessary political support for resource allocation.

10.2.2. Aligning early hearing detection and intervention services to the sustainable development goals and economic benefit

The importance of economic value in health care has risen to more prominence in recent years because of the UHC movement (Sell 2019). The world agreed to UHC as a priority (Ghebreyesus 2017). Universal health care coverage is defined as access to key affordable preventive, curative and rehabilitative health care interventions for all (Awoonor-Williams et al. 2016; Shisana et al. 2006) and embraces fairness, equity and benefit with international reach (Cerf 2020). In order to meet the objectives of UHC, numerous HICs and LMICs, including South Africa, are introducing or extending their UHC efforts (Fusheini & Eyles 2016). This process requires governments to define essential service packages guaranteed to all citizens (International Health Partnership 2018).

Designing essential service packages in the era of UHC requires both cost-effectiveness and budget impact information for health care services in different settings (International Health Partnership 2018). Thus, a health care service such as EHDI must be aligned with the SDGs and demonstrate economic benefit to earn the necessary and strong political will to receive allocation of the limited funds, which is currently lacking (Khoza-Shangase 2020; Khoza-Shangase & Michal 2014; Olusanya 2012). Sustainable development goals aim to tackle socio-economic inequities and environmental factors hampering human development (Remme et al. 2017). Various nations committed to 17 interconnected SDGs and the 169 targets that underpin them, to be met by 2030 at the United Nations in September 2015 (Stafford-Smith et al. 2017). The interconnectedness of the SDGs reflects the fact that sustainable development in any country requires multidimensional and multi-sectoral policy interventions (Tangcharoensathien, Mills & Palu 2015). The SDGs are an expansion of the MDGs, which expired in 2015 (Stafford-Smith et al. 2017; Tangcharoensathien et al. 2015). Unlike the MDGs, SDGs reflect a more holistic understanding of the nature of sustainable development and its interaction with human health, environmental protection and social justice (Bennett et al. 2020; Dukhanin et al. 2018).

Similarly, health promotions and addressing health inequities involve the integration of multilevel interventions with an emphasise on enabling healthy environments, re-orientating health services and promoting well-being and healthy choices (Fortune et al. 2018). The SDG 3 calls for governments to ensure healthy living and promote well-being for all at all ages, with a focus on all health conditions (Bennett et al. 2020; Leclair & Saunders 2019). Advancing global child health and well-being involves more than achieving gains towards the under-five and neonatal mortality targets as outlined in SDG 3 (Alfvén et al. 2019). Although mortality indicators are critical for monitoring progress, they do not provide a holistic picture of the burden of disease borne by children, their families and society (Alfvén et al. 2019). Children need to thrive, and their health and well-being need to form the core of what will become society's future human capital and a resource for tomorrow's affluence (Alfvén et al. 2019).

Thus, growing public health care issues such as childhood hearing impairment are significant barriers to the child's ability to thrive. In order to ensure that children with hearing impairment develop into resources and future human capital for tomorrow's affluence, the hearing impairment must be addressed through appropriate efforts in hearing impairment prevention, identification and treatment according to SDG 3 (Leclair & Saunders 2019). Furthermore, the educational repercussions of childhood hearing impairment must be addressed, according to SDG 4, which calls for inclusive and equitable quality education and the promotion of lifelong learning opportunities for all (Leclair & Saunders 2019). Achieving these and various other goals for children with hearing impairment will require hearing health care investment and expansion, especially in LMICs (Leclair & Saunders 2019). Thus, EHDI services need to demonstrate that the extent of additional benefits relative to the degree of additional costs is greatest, subject to identified budget constraints, within LMICs (McNamee et al. 2016), hence the need for the economic evaluation of EHDI services.

10.2.3. Economic evaluation of early hearing detection and intervention

Economic evaluations vary in scope and purpose (Grosse et al. 2018). In an effort to demonstrate the magnitude of additional benefits relative to the magnitude of additional costs, a full economic valuation is warranted. A full economic evaluation assesses the balance of intervention costs with the resultant health outcomes and costs that have been avoided as a result (Grosse et al. 2018).

The SDGs have set much higher and more ambitious health-related goals and targets than the MDGs (Tangcharoensathien et al. 2015). However, confronting choices about how to spend society's limited resources on health care is not an easy task (Neuman 2017; Neumann & Sanders 2017). Although prevention efforts such as EHDI can be the most cost-effective way to maintain the health of the population in a sustainable manner, concerns about the upfront costs and intangibility of outcomes frequently lead to a lack of action and continued investment in increasingly expensive curative approaches (Ghebreyesus 2017; WHO 2014). Within economic evaluations, cost-effective refers to an intervention that improves long-term health and economic outcomes (Grosse et al. 2018).

McNamee and colleagues (2016) argued that there are various ways to conduct an economic evaluation of health interventions; and provide useful evidence about health equity impact and their trade-offs (Cookson et al. 2017). Economic evaluations of EHDI services have typically been partial analyses of the estimated costs of implementing UNHS using different screening technologies; only a smaller number of analyses have attempted to calculate the health and economic benefits of early detection of hearing loss or deafness (Grosse et al. 2018). The most commonly used economic evaluation methods with their application in the field of audiology and EHDI services are discussed next.

☐ 10.2.3.1. Cost-consequence analysis

Cost-consequence analysis (CCA) is an extension of cost-effectiveness analysis (CEA). With CCA, multiple benefits are measured and reported separately (see Table 10.1) (McNamee et al. 2016). It is recommended in complex interventions where outcomes cannot be easily converted to monetary value or reported in one health measure (Sørensen et al. 2020). Cost-consequences analysis only considers intermediate outcomes. Within EHDI, various studies have evaluated the cost of screening and diagnosis per diagnosis achieved (Grosse et al. 2018). What is evident from these studies is that costs are highly variable across studies as a function of multiple factors such as methodological differences, the personnel conducting the screening and the technology used for the screening (Grosse et al. 2018). Thus, in CCA, a series of outcome measures are presented alongside the costs, enabling decision-makers to consider the outcomes most relevant to them (Hartfiel & Edwards 2019). Cost-consequence analysis provides a clear, descriptive summary for decision-makers that is often easier to interpret than cost-effectiveness, cost-utility and cost–benefit analysis (Gage et al. 2006; Hartfiel & Edwards 2019). However, CCA does not provide guidance regarding how the different outcomes should be weighed against each other, especially in cases whereby some outcomes show benefits and some show disbenefits necessitating a decision on the relative value of each outcome (Hartfiel & Edwards 2019).

TABLE 10.1: Example of a cost-consequence tabulation.

Component category	Cost components	Drug A		Drug B	
		Units	Costs	Units	Costs
Direct medical care use/costs	Drug A/B	-	-	-	-
	Other drugs				
	Physician visits				
	Hospital stays				
	Home care				
	Other medical care (e.g. dialysis)				
Direct non-medical care use/costs	Transportation	-	-	-	-
	Crutches and other equipment				
	Paid caregiver time				
Indirect resource use/costs	Time missed from work for patients	-	-	-	-
	Time missed from work for unpaid caregivers				
	Time missed from other activities for patients				
	Time missed from other activities for unpaid caregivers				
Total direct and indirect costs		-	-	-	-
Symptom impact	Patient distress days	-	-	-	-
	Patient disability days				
Quality of life impact	Quality-adjusted life-years decrement	-	-	-	-
	Quality of life profile measure scores				

Source: Mauskopf et al. (1998).

☐ 10.2.3.2. Cost-benefit analysis

Cost-benefit analysis (CBA) measures the benefits of the programme in monetary terms. It adds up all the total costs of an intervention and compares them against its total benefits or outcomes (see Table 10.2) (McNamee et al. 2016; WHO 2017). This method assumes that a monetary value can be associated with all the costs and benefits of a health care intervention, including tangible and intangible returns (Rognoni et al. 2020). Thus, it allows for direct calculation of the net monetary cost of achieving a health outcome (Robertson, Skelly & Phillips 2019; WHO 2016). However, evaluating health outcomes in monetary terms is somewhat controversial, thus limiting the use of this method in health care (WHO 2016). Consequently, this method is prominently used in environment and transport appraisal (McNamee et al. 2016). However, CBA forms part of decision-making in some HICs, such as the United States where CAE and cost-utility analysis (CUA) is not widely used at the policy level (Sharma et al. 2019). Chapter 6 delves into challenges around cost–benefit analysis in audiology, with ototoxicity as a case example.

TABLE 10.2: Costs and benefits.

Organisations incurring resource use/costs	Form of benefits to patients/public
National Health Service	Gains in health
Other public section	Other non-healthy benefits, for example, information and reassurance
Patients and their families	Process benefits, for example, reduced waiting times

Source: McIntosh, Donaldson and Ryan (1999).

10.2.3.3. Cost-effectiveness analysis

Cost-effectiveness analysis (CEA) expresses the costs and consequences of alternative interventions as cost per unit of health outcome (WHO 2014). It quantifies the health gains per given expenditure on a health intervention and can only be measured in comparison with two or more other interventions (Grosse et al. 2018; Verguet, Kim & Jamison 2016). Cost-effectiveness analysis also reflects the relationship between the lifetime monetary costs of an intervention and the resultant health benefits, which can be measured in terms of either the life-years gained (LYG), quality-adjusted life-years (QALYs) or disability-adjusted life years (DALY) averted by an intervention (Saunders, Francis & Skarzynski 2016).

The primary objective of CEA is to maximise societal welfare and universal health care for all (Cookson et al. 2017). CEA's cost items include any resources with an opportunity cost associated with the health care programme. Benefit items include health effects and other impacts on people's well-being. (Lakdawalla et al. 2018; McIntosh et al. 1999). While cost is measured in monetary terms, effectiveness is measured independently and may be measured in terms of clinical outcomes such as LYGs, QALYs or DALYs to account for the QoL outcomes (McGregor 2003).

When comparing interventions during a CEA, the incremental cost-effectiveness ratio (ICER) is often used to express the result (Lakdawalla et al. 2018). The ICER is the difference in costs divided by the difference in health effects (Lakdawalla et al. 2018). Thus, the ICER describes the incremental price of obtaining a unit of health effect from a given health intervention when compared with an alternative intervention (Saunders et al. 2016). The ICER value is used to determine which interventions are cost-effective and are to be included in prioritised health interventions (Remme et al. 2017). However, the ICER value cannot be used to make a recommendation to policymakers without prior decisions by policymakers on what constitutes a health effect or what the cost targets or thresholds are. Cost targets or thresholds are typically based on per capita gross domestic product (GDP) (Lakdawalla et al. 2018). According to WHO's (2014) Choosing Interventions that are Cost-Effective (WHO-CHOICE) project, an intervention that costs less than three times the national annual GDP per capita is considered cost-effective, whereas an intervention that costs less than one times the national GDP per capita is considered highly cost-effective.

Cost-effectiveness analysis is used globally to inform priority settings in health care and public health care settings (Cookson et al. 2017; Dukhanin et al. 2018). Furthermore, it is used to inform decisions on how to maximise health returns from limited resources (Neumann & Sanders 2017). It provides a specific, theoretically well-grounded structure for combining the cost and benefit of an intervention (Doshi & Willke 2017), thus demonstrating the intervention approach providing the most health outcomes possible with available resources (Neumann & Sanders 2017).

Cost-effectiveness analysis is the most common economic evaluation method conducted within the field of audiology and EHDI in particular. Some of the CEAs conducted in EHDI, as obtained during a literature review search, include:

1. cost-effectiveness of neonatal hearing screening programmes in China (Tobe et al. 2013)
2. cost-effectiveness of UNHS compared to no screening (Grosse et al. 2018)
3. cost and outcome of conducting hearing screening programmes using a two-step DPOAE screening protocol (Ramkuma et al. 2018)
4. cost-effectiveness of AABR in universal neonatal hearing screening (Heidari et al. 2017).

Most economic evaluations, as illustrated by the studies outlined above, have been partial analyses that focused on estimating the cost of implementing UNHS using different screening technologies. Saunders and colleagues (2015) compared the cost-effectiveness of deaf education versus cochlear implants for children with severe-to-profound sensorineural hearing loss using DALYs in low-resource environments. However, this study is only one of a few studies that have estimated the potential reduction in the costs of special education services for some children (Grosse et al. 2018). Furthermore, within CEA, there is a dearth of analyses that have attempted to calculate the health and economic benefits of early detection of hearing impairment and its subsequent management. However, if audiologists are to be strong advocates for audiological services, including EHDI, an understanding of and employment of these cost-effectiveness evaluations is warranted (Saunders et al. 2016). Cost-effectiveness analysis is the recommended method of economic evaluation in health care as it is better suited to address the UHC objectives and for allocating scarce health care resources (Culyer & Chalkidou 2019), a required need for the South African context. Furthermore, the WHO strongly advocates for the use of CEA in order to help governments set health care priorities in both HICs and LMICs (Saunders et al. 2016).

10.2.3.4. Cost-utility analysis

Cost-utility analysis (CUA) is a form of CEA that allows for the comparison of different health outcomes in terms of quality-adjusted-life-years (QALYs) (McGregor 2003; McNamee et al. 2016). It is used to compare two different interventions whose benefits may be different; thus, it provides value judgment about increases in the utility (QALYs) associated with different health outcomes (Kaur et al. 2020; McGregor 2003). Utility is a measure of value or preference attached to a health outcome and is linked to QoL measures (Saunders et al. 2016). This is achieved by assigning a utility to any state of health or disability on a scale ranging from 0 (*immediate death*) to 1 (*state of perfect health*). The outcomes of any health intervention can then be calculated as the product of an increase in utility that the intervention may cause and the time in years that it may be enjoyed (McGregor 2003; Steele et al. 2007).

Cost-utility analysis is particularly useful when comparing two different procedures or interventions whose benefits may be different and for which limited resources must be allocated across an entire population. Consequently, interventions that are expected to produce fewer QALYs for any given cost are given lower priority when allocating scarce resources (McGregor 2003). This method of analysis has been used effectively in the field of audiology to demonstrate the cost-effectiveness of cochlear implants, resulting in cochlear implants being funded in both public and private health care sectors (Foteff et al. 2016; Qiu et al. 2017; Saunders et al. 2016).

10.2.3.5. Conjoint analysis

Economic evaluations focusing on the cost of interventions and their outcomes are only one component of many elements involved in health care decision-making. Other important considerations include legal, ethical, cultural and political concerns; pragmatic issues of logistics, feasibility; and, importantly, patients' expectations and preferences (Neumann & Sanders 2017), hence the need for conjoint analysis. Conjoint analysis is an evaluation approach that uses survey methods to elicit trade-offs among attributes and attribute levels to determine respondents' preferences for alternative products (Marshall et al. 2010). It is a method of eliciting stated preferences from patients that goes beyond traditional health care outcome measures to account for non-health outcome attributes in the process of delivery of health care services (Lancsar & Louviere 2008).

The underlying theory of a conjoint analysis is that a product or service can be described by its characteristics or attributes (Ryan & Farrar 2000). This survey method provides an estimation of the relative importance people attribute to various components of health care, measures how individuals are willing to trade between these characteristics and estimates the overall satisfaction they gain from various forms of health service provision (Fitzpatrick et al. 2019). A conjoint analysis offers a mechanism for patients to participate in decision-making and considers how different stakeholders may value outcomes (Bridges et al. 2011; Marshall et al. 2010); thus, helping decision-makers understand the health care service choices of communities, the perspectives of different user segments or the unique preferences of individual patients (Cunningham, Deal & Chen 2010).

In the field of audiology, only a handful of conjoint analyses have been conducted thus far. In one of the studies, Fitzpatrick and colleagues (2019) used conjoint analysis to quantify parents' preference for service attributes for children with mild bilateral or unilateral hearing impairments. In another study, Findlen, Malhotra and Adunka (2019) investigated parent perspectives on multidisciplinary paediatric hearing health care. The complex nature of childhood hearing loss requires a clinical approach that is inclusive of multiple providers from varied disciplines providing well-coordinated health care (Findlen et al. 2019). Thus, conjoint analysis provides a systematic way of evaluating the clinical process and outcomes while taking into account various factors such as costs, benefits and end-user preferences (Findlen et al. 2019).

10.3. Solutions, recommendations and future research

The environment in hearing health care is changing rapidly. These changes have had and will continue to have a profound influence on the audiologist's scope of practice and the service delivery that audiologists provide to their clients. Thus, there is an urgent global need for health care sector decision-makers to evaluate both health and economic impact in considering the adoption and implementation of various health care services (Lakdawalla et al. 2018).

According to WHOs (2014), European regional office:

> Containing or reducing the costs of health care without negative effects on health outcomes requires cost-effective prevention interventions to play a much more substantial role. If health spending is to be reduced or even stabilized, without compromising quality and outcomes, further measures are needed. (p. 11)

Funding for prevention remains a small proportion of overall health care spending but can represent excellent value for money. Gains in both the short and long term, as well as for sectors other than health care, are possible (cf. WHO 2014, p. 15).

Early hearing detection and intervention of childhood hearing impairment are imperative in order to provide safety nets for children who unavoidably will present with hearing impairment (Olusanya 2012). However, despite the widely reported effectiveness of these programmes in HICs, EHDI programmes in LMICs, including South Africa, lack the necessary support from policy and legislature as well as budget allocation. The WHO (2017) recommended the use of the knowledge of the economic costs associated with any health care problem, such as hearing impairment, and the potential costs that might be avoided, as a powerful tool for policymakers in planning the best use of their health care budgets. Thus, to garner political and funding support for EHDI services within resource-constrained LMICs, South Africa must demonstrate the cost-effectiveness of these services with due consideration of the following factors:

1. Aligning EHDI outcomes with the SDGs, especially UHC.
2. Demonstrating substantial effects of EHDI programmes beyond the health care system into interrelated sectors such as education, social services and economic productivity.
3. Careful tailoring of EHDI programmes based on caregivers' preferences of service attributes and what the buyer-patient, payer or society can afford.

Future research in this field could investigate the economic benefits of EHDI services within the South African context.

■ 10.4. Conclusion

Health care costs will continue to receive scrutiny as health care budgets are increasingly squeezed (Mauskopf et al. 1998). However, economic evaluations in health care do not appear to have been an important direct contributor to mandating EHDI services in the United States and other European countries (Grosse et al. 2018). However, policymakers in the United States and other European countries took such analysis into consideration when developing EHDI policies. Thus, economic evaluations that provide stakeholders with an understanding of the costs or budgetary implications of new interventions are very influential, especially in the current climate of budgetary constraints in health care. Cost-effectiveness measures may not be an official policy criterion currently, but if one waits for the availability of evidence of long-term outcomes to conduct these economic evaluations, the opportunity to inform policy decisions and alleviate concerns from legislators about the cost implications of new policies, such as EHDI, may be missed.

Chapter 11

Early detection and management of occupational and environmental noise

Nomfundo F. Moroe
Department of Audiology, Faculty of Humanities,
School of Human and Community Development,
University of the Witwatersrand,
Johannesburg, South Africa

11.1. Introduction

Noise-induced hearing loss (NIHL) is 100% preventable through HCPs. The goal of an HCP is to eliminate the presence of noise as a risk factor, thereby preventing the development of NIHL in people exposed to hazardous noise levels. The principles underpinning HCPs are aligned with health promotion and disease prevention interventions. Therefore, this chapter seeks to demonstrate how disease prevention interventions complement the HCP pillars and the hierarchy of noise control. Furthermore, this chapter discusses the contextual factors contributing to the current status of the implemented HCPs. This is followed by a summary of recent advances in the prevention of NIHL. Lastly, the chapter offers recommendations on the management of NIHL within the African context.

Noise, an unwanted sound (Basner et al. 2014), is a ubiquitous environmental hazard of the modern world (Khan et al. 2010). It emanates from various recreational activities such as concerts, sporting events, lifestyle activities and

How to cite: Moroe, NF 2022, 'Early detection and management of occupational and environmental noise', ed. K Khoza-Shangase, *Preventive audiology: An African perspective*, AOSIS Books, Cape Town, pp. 213–233. https://doi.org/10.4102/aosis.2022.BK209.11

places of worship. Environmental sources include traffic and occupational activities such as construction, mining and manufacturing (Lusk et al. 2016; Oguntunde et al. 2019). According to Jamir, Nongkynrih and Gupta (2014), noise occurs in two major settings, namely, environmental noise and occupational noise. Environmental noise emanates from all sources, excluding noise produced in the industrial workplace (Jamir et al. 2014). The most common sources of environmental noise include traffic noise, loudspeakers, recreational activities and fireworks, to name a few. On the contrary, occupational noise emanating from work-related processes during the execution or performance of one's occupation.

Prolonged exposure to noise is associated with a range of adverse effects including, but not limited to, annoyance, sleep disturbances, impaired cognitive performance and cardiovascular diseases such as hypertension (Dale et al. 2015). Noise-induced hearing loss is also a common disability in noisy occupations (Ding, Yan & Liu 2019). Lusk et al. (2016) argued that the impact extends beyond annoyance. It is a public health hazard with significant negative effects on the health outcomes and economic outcomes of individuals exposed to excessive noise. As such, hazardous noise exposure is ranked a major public health agenda, particularly in LMICs (Yongbing & Martin 2013).

The effects of noise can be grouped into direct/auditory or indirect/non-auditory impacts. The auditory effects (direct impact of exposure) include tinnitus (Delecrode et al. 2012), temporary and permanent threshold shift, and hearing loss (Ryan et al. 2016). Non-auditory effects (resulting from the indirect impact of exposure) include annoyance, masking of warning signals, communication difficulties and increased blood pressure (Basner et al. 2014; Park et al. 2017).

The health effects associated with hazardous noise exposure cannot be overemphasised. As such, Fink (2017) maintained that the safe noise level for the prevention of hearing loss is 70-decibel time-weighted average for a 24-h period, despite the National Institute for Occupational Safety and Health (NIOSH) recommending 85 A-weighted decibels as the minimum exposure level, beyond which the employer is mandated to implement an HCP (Fink 2017).

Hazardous noise exposure can potentially cause NIHL, which is a progressive sensorineural hearing impairment, because of prolonged exposure to excessive noise (Ding et al. 2019). Globally, NIHL is the second most common cause of acquired hearing loss, after presbyacusis (Mostaghaci et al. 2013). In 2017, WHO (2017) reported that globally, 360 million people have severe hearing loss, with close to 1.1 billion young people (aged between 12 and 35 years) having a propensity to develop a hearing loss, a portion of which is because of excessive noise exposure (Chadha & Cieza 2017; Ding et al. 2019).

Noise-induced hearing loss is not life-threatening, even though it is associated with cardiovascular disease. However, the effects of poorly managed hearing loss impact the financial health and well-being of the affected individual, their family, colleagues, employer and the State (Moroe 2018). Fortunately, NIHL is 100% preventable through effectively managed and well-executed HCPs (Le et al. 2017). However, once present, it is irreparable (Arenas & Suter 2014; Kardous 2016). Moroe (2020a) described an HCP as a theory and evidence-based intervention built from seven non-linear but interacting pillars that act both independently and interdependently. These pillars are active in that their effectiveness is influenced by the engagement of different stakeholders during the formulation, implementation and evaluation of HCPs. Furthermore, the pillars are fragile and are embedded in multiple social systems that may include personal, interpersonal and environmental factors that may be outside of intervention efforts. Lastly, HCPs are open systems that feedback on themselves (Moroe 2018).

A comprehensive and effective HCP comprises seven pillars, namely, periodic noise exposure monitoring, engineering controls, administrative controls, personal hearing protection, audiometric evaluations, employee or management education and training and record-keeping (Hong et al. 2013). The goal of an HCP is to eliminate the presence of noise as a risk factor, thereby preventing the development of NIHL in people exposed to hazardous noise. Therefore, an HCP is designed and implemented according to the hierarchy of noise control which, in turn, is aligned with health promotion and disease prevention levels and strategies as depicted in Figure 11.1.

Health promotion is concerned with empowering people to exercise control over their health outcomes (Olukemi 2019). Prevention, on the contrary, is concerned with 'measures to not only prevent the occurrence of disease but to also arrest progression and reduce consequences' (Duplaga et al. 2016:478). The need for prevention cannot be overemphasised. Prevention is stratified into five levels, given as follows:

1. **Primordial prevention:** Interventions aimed at preventing the penetration of risk factors into the population (Pandve 2014a).
2. **Primary prevention:** Interventions concerned with precluding the onset of a disease or injury through risk reduction by either modifying exposures that potentially cause a disease or the enhancement of resistance to a disease agent (Duplaga et al. 2016; Pandve 2014a).
3. **Secondary prevention:** Interventions concerned with controlling or managing the disease before it manifests clinically (Duplaga et al. 2016).
4. **Tertiary prevention:** Aims to decrease the adverse effects of the disease and optimise the QoL of the affected individual (Duplaga et al. 2016; Pandve 2014a).
5. **Quaternary prevention:** This entails taking action to identify workers at risk of over-medicalisation and protecting them from new, untested medical remedies while recommending interventions that are ethically sound (Pandve 2014b).

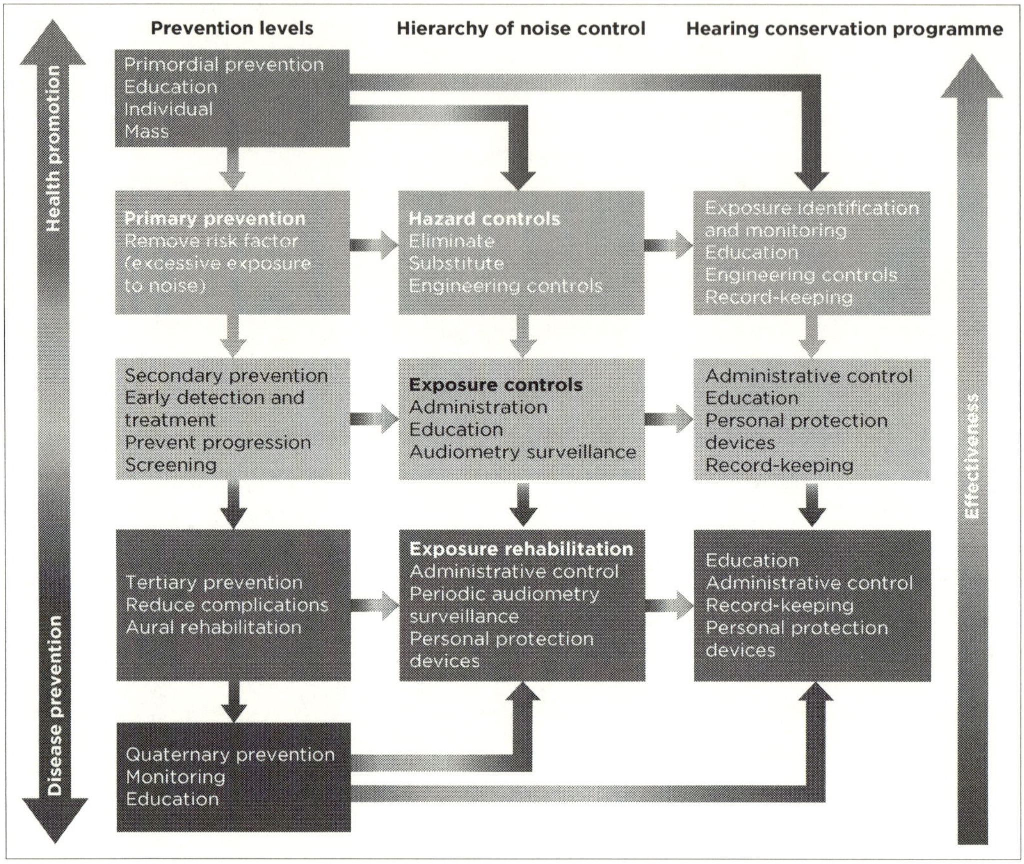

FIGURE 11.1: Diagram depicting the synergy of the components of noise-induced hearing loss prevention.

Correspondingly, preventive occupational audiology in the form of an HCP encompasses these five levels.

In discussing prevention and HCPs in this chapter, it should be noted that the pillars of an HCP will not be discussed in a specific pattern. For instance, applying administrative controls such as rotating workers from a noisy area to a quieter area at the secondary level is aimed at delaying the development of ONIHL; at the tertiary level, the aim is to minimise the progression and the impact of excessive noise on an employee who has already suffered hearing loss. Additionally, the interventions that will be presented in this chapter are more in line with occupational noise exposure as these industries have legislations in place which govern their practises and response to health and safety in the workplace. Education, however, is applicable as a pillar that cuts across all levels of prevention and hierarchies of controls, and this will be illustrated in the discussion.

11.1.1. Primordial prevention

Primordial prevention is concerned with interventions aimed at preventing the penetration of risk factors into the population (Pandve 2014a). This involves the implementation of interventions and education to avert health risk factors through individual and mass education on environmental, economic, social and behavioural attributes and cultural patterns of living. Therefore, primordial prevention is concerned with broader health determinants beyond personal exposure to risk, which is the focus of primary prevention (Pandve 2014a).

Concerning environmental and occupational noise, primordial prevention focuses on education, which is one of the pillars of an HCP, to conscientise people about noise, both the exposed and the unexposed. Hearing loss is an invisible disability (Tye-Murray 2009), and its effects are delayed and only realised when the damage has already occurred. Therefore, educating the general population on the effects of noise will potentially contribute towards health promotion that encourages people to take control of their ear-and-hearing health care actively. According to Victor Hugo, as cited by Elahi (2006), 'No cause can succeed without first making education its ally'. At the individual level, education can focus, for instance, on the impact of environmental noise, particularly on the use of personal listening devices and the impact of traffic noise on hearing. There is a growing concern about the increased exposure to recreational noise in settings such as nightclubs, bars, cinemas, concerts, live sporting events, fitness classes and even churches (WHO 2015). There is an increase in the use of recreational devices such as personal music players and video game consoles that emit sounds commonly operated at unsafe volumes (WHO 2015). Keppler, Dhooge and Vinck (2015) argued that the maximum equivalent continuous output levels of personal music players (PMPs) range between 97 dBA and 103 dBA for earbuds (insert earphones) and supra-aural headphones, respectively, while sound intensity levels at concerts and clubs can amount to 105 dBA and 112 dBA, respectively. These concerns are also echoed by Tung and Chao (2013), who lamented that in modern living environments, in addition to the general use of personal listening devices and going to clubs and concerts, many teenagers have developed a habit of using personal listening devices while reading, taking public transport or while sleeping.

Traffic noise is the biggest contributor to environmental noise. Reportedly, vehicular traffic contributes to approximately 55% of total urban noise (Vijay et al. 2015). Traffic noise adversely affects people exposed, with the biggest impact being on drivers. Interestingly, drivers are exposed to both environmental and occupational noise in that vehicles are a source of traffic/environmental noise and the source of occupational noise for them. Consequently, drivers are exposed to many physical and physiological stresses such as traffic noise, vibration, temperature fluctuations, ergonomic problems and safety risks such as accidents (Ansari et al. 2016), over and above communication difficulties. Kirchner et al. (2012) argued that the inability to hear poses a safety concern, as drivers' hearing may be compromised and they may miss warning signals such as sirens, thereby increasing the risk of accidents. Therefore, education can go a long way in raising awareness among drivers and those affected by environmental noise about the dangers of excessive noise exposure. Furthermore, education can promote early detection of hearing loss where drivers can routinely undergo hearing assessments to monitor their hearing. Lastly, over and above the effects of environmental noise, people exposed to high levels of occupational noise face two big threats: the loss of employment and exposure to excessive noise for many hours each day over several years.

Education can raise awareness on risk factors associated with hazardous noise exposure at a mass or population level. These risk factors are grouped into non-modifiable and modifiable factors. Non-modifiable factors include age (Kerketta, Gartia & Bagh 2012), race (Pyykkö et al. 2007) and sex (Pratt et al. 2009), while modifiable factors include smoking (Fabry et al. 2010), ototoxic agents (Kirchner et al. 2012) and ototoxic drugs used to treat diseases like HIV, AIDS, TB and cancer (Khoza-Shangase 2020a). Furthermore, education at this level can address auditory and non-auditory effects of hearing loss (Delecrode et al. 2012). Auditory effects are caused by the direct impact of noise, and these may include temporary and permanent threshold shifts resulting in hearing loss (Hind et al. 2011; Pienkowski 2017; Ryan et al. 2016), while non-auditory effects result from indirect impact of exposure to excessive noise. These effects may manifest through annoyance, masking of warning signals, communication difficulties and increased blood pressure (Basner et al. 2014; Omer Ahmed 2012; Park et al. 2017).

It is important to raise awareness about the risk factors and effects of excessive exposure as the general population may not be aware of their susceptibility or the relationship between noise exposure and some medical conditions with which they may present. Education can promote collaboration between the general population and audiologists. This may create an environment where people can be made aware of the need to attend hearing evaluations and promote World Hearing Days as well as Deafness Awareness Weeks. A key benefit would be to promote and highlight the role of audiologists in the preservation of hearing across one's lifespan. Education can also provide the population with communication strategies and address stigma associated with hearing loss. Occupationally, audiologists can be involved in teaching and training workers to adhere to the pillars of an HCP. More specifically, education can focus on the use of hearing protection devices (HPDs) when in noisy areas, compliance to audiometry screening and assessments, medical surveillance, monitoring changes to hearing patterns and reporting of comorbidities that may render a worker susceptible to hearing loss and/or more significant hearing loss. Last, but not least, education at this prevention level can serve to sensitise the general population and individuals exposed to occupational and environmental noise to their rights. This encourages policymakers to develop regulations and permissible noise levels that are environmentally and occupationally friendly. Therefore, if the goal of primordial prevention is to prevent or stop the appearance of risk factors at a population level (Pandve 2014a), education needs to be prioritised at all levels of prevention.

11.1.2. Primary prevention

Primary prevention is concerned with precluding the onset of a disease or injury through risk reduction by either modifying exposures that potentially cause the disease or the enhancement of resistance to a disease agent (Duplaga et al. 2016; Pandve 2014a). Therefore, in preventive occupational audiology, primary prevention entails implementing comprehensive evidence and theory-based HCPs to reduce the risk of exposure in industries prone to excessive noise production such as mining, construction and the military (Feder et al. 2017).

According to the hierarchy of noise control, elimination is the primary preventive intervention in precluding the onset of ONIHL. However, noise is ubiquitous in these industries because of the machinery used. Chaudhary (2017) argued that noisy machinery is often a necessary component of certain work processes, and while machines can be made safer, they cannot be eliminated. Where elimination is not feasible, noisy machinery can be substituted or replaced. Substitution is the second most effective intervention for controlling risk factors by swapping one risk for another. Noisy machinery can be replaced with less noisy equipment, a strategy known as 'buying quiet'. Buying quiet is an initiative aimed at buying quieter equipment as a measure to control noise at the source (Gumede et al. 2014). This is a long-term investment and is potentially arduous and costly (Bruce 2007; Suter 2012), although research shows that the benefits may far outweigh the perceived cost. As far as effective intervention for controlling risk factors is concerned, the next level of intervention is isolation. Isolation entails separating the risk factor in time or space from the people at risk through containment or enclosure, i.e., keeping the hazard 'in' and the worker 'out' or vice versa (Chaudhary 2017).

The most effective isolation strategy is mechanisation. This is a process that involves the substitution of manual tasks with machinery, with the machines becoming the interface between humans and the task (Gumede 2018). Gumede (2018) asserted that mechanisation promotes and has the potential to improve competitiveness, health and safety, profitability and improvements that have varying impacts on different stakeholders. This is particularly true for workers who may lose their jobs to mechanisation. As such, Gumede (2018) cautioned that while in the medium to long term, mechanisation will yield benefits, it potentially has a negative impact on the labour complement and on the communities in which these companies operate. In instances where the aforementioned primary prevention interventions – elimination, substitution and isolation – are not feasible, the next point of call is engineering controls.

Engineering controls are defined as 'a physical modification made to the source of noise or the permanent physical environment around the source of the noise' (The Georgia Tech 2019–2020). According to Bruce (2007, p. 33), engineering controls guarantee 'permanence, effectiveness with or without worker/supervisor compliance, less absenteeism, easier communication, lower worker compensation costs, and reduced legal costs'. Implementing engineering controls involves four principles (The Georgia Tech 2019–2020):

1. **Sound insulation:** Prevents the transmission of noise by the introduction of a mass barrier through the use of materials that have high-density properties such as bricks, concrete and metal.
2. **Sound absorption:** Using a porous material that acts as a 'noise sponge' by converting the sound energy into heat within the material. Common sound absorption materials include open-cell foams and fibreglass.
3. **Vibration damping:** Applicable for large vibrating surfaces. The damping mechanism works by extracting the vibration energy from the thin sheet and dissipating it as heat. A common material is sound-deadened steel. This control is applicable to large vibrating surfaces.
4. **Vibration isolation:** Prevents transmission of vibration energy from a source to a receiver by introducing a flexible element or a physical break. Common vibration isolators are springs, rubber mounts, cork, etc.

The above-mentioned interventions are all aimed at eliminating the onset of ONIHL.

11.1.3. Secondary prevention

Secondary prevention is concerned with controlling or managing the disease before it manifests clinically (Duplaga et al. 2016). This involves implementing interventions that identify and treat pre-clinical pathological changes to manage disease progression (Pandve 2014a). In practice, secondary prevention promotes early detection and intervention through timely screening to detect asymptomatic disease with the aim of improving health outcomes. At this stage, the aim is to prevent a rapid progression of the disease in spite of exposure to the risk factors. In preventive occupational audiology, secondary prevention entails monitoring for early detection and treatment of ONIHL. This requires the implementation of administrative controls, audiometric surveillance, education, the use of PPE and good record-keeping.

According to the hierarchy of noise controls, administrative controls are the next option when elimination, substitution and engineering controls are not feasible. Administrative controls are interventions implemented to reduce risk by minimising the time of exposure to noise (Bauer & Babich 2006). This involves rotating workers from noisy to quieter areas. While this description of administrative controls is too simplistic, Bauer and Babich (2006) argued that administrative controls are not readily implemented because of a lack of trained workers for efficient job rotation, union contract issues and safety concerns. If applied appropriately, administrative controls are an effective tool to change work practices, management policies or worker behaviour (Verbeek et al. 2014), to promote early detection and intervention by ensuring timeous screening for the early development of hearing loss in workers exposed to hazardous noise. Early detection of ONIHL is carried out through audiometry surveillance, which is essentially workplace hearing tests, using pure-tone audiometry as the gold standard (HearSafe Solutions 2018).

Audiometric surveillance is a legal requirement and is legislated as part of compliance in the *South African Occupational Health and Safety Act 85 of 1993)*. The Occupational Safety and Health Act requires that all workers exposed to noise that is more than 85 dBA in intensity be screened for ONIHL (Mostaghaci et al. 2013). Audiometric testing can reveal hearing loss at an early stage (Leshchinsky 2018). Additionally, audiometry creates an opportunity to educate employees on the latent effects of noise exposure and promotes awareness of hazardous noise present in everyday activities (Leshchinsky 2018). This practice promotes the routine use of HPDs in everyday situations (Schulz 2014). Audiometry, including extended high-frequency audiometry and otoacoustic emissions as tools for early detection and diagnosis, helps to identify changes in hearing before clinically significant hearing loss develops (Mostaghaci et al. 2013).

The effectiveness of audiometric surveillance as a preventive strategy lies in monitoring the standard threshold shift (STS) – a 10 dB or more change in the average hearing threshold at 2 000 Hz, 3 000 Hz and 4 000 Hz (Mostaghaci et al. 2013). In the presence of an audiogram depicting hearing within normal limits, a positive STS is critical in identifying workers who may be susceptible to the hazardous effects of noise (Ross et al. 2010). Therefore, it is imperative that a baseline audiogram, which is the first audiogram performed before an individual commences employment or within 30 days of commencement of employment, is conducted to serve as a reference baseline for all subsequent periodic audiometry evaluations to monitor improvement or STS (McDaniel et al. 2013).

Audiometric surveillance as a pillar cuts across two prevention levels – secondary and tertiary prevention levels. As a secondary prevention tool, surveillance is concerned with monitoring the STS through periodic hearing evaluation. Internationally, the Occupational Safety and Health Administration

(OSHA) and the NIOSH legislations mandate that employees exposed to occupational noise should undergo periodic hearing assessments to monitor and establish that no shift has occurred in the pure-tone threshold. OSHA defines an STS as an average increase of 10 dB or more at 2 KHz, 3 KHz and 4 KHz in one or both ears, while NIOSH defines it as an average increase of 15 dB or more at 500 Hz, 1 KHz, 2 KHz, 3 KHz, 4 KHz or 6 KHz in one or both ears (Brungart et al. 2019). In South Africa, STS is calculated at 2, 3 and 4 KHz (Musiba 2020). Conducting audiometric surveillance is undertaken to identify a permanent threshold shift in the STS. A permanent shift is suggestive of a potential hearing loss, depending on the degree of the shift from the baseline audiogram. As a secondary preventive measure, monitoring the STS is a way of early identification where the individual's STS is tracked for any sign of a shift. When a permanent shift is noted, EI strategies should be implemented. These can be in the form of administrative controls, as discussed earlier, or the provision and use of HPDs, education and awareness training. Within the South African context, the legislation mandates that an STS of >2 dB but < 5 dB is prioritised to halt the progression of STS from reaching a 10 dB shift across all the relevant frequencies. Therefore, monitoring the STS becomes crucial as preventive strategies can be subsequently implemented.

In the event that a permanent STS reaches a 10 dB shift, the second arm of audiometric surveillance is activated: tertiary prevention. Tertiary prevention will be discussed in detail later in this chapter. In relation to tertiary prevention, audiometric surveillance is conducted to quantify hearing loss for compensation purposes by calculating the percentage of loss of hearing (PLH) (Bronkhorst & Shutte 2013). To calculate the PLH, the individual's hearing thresholds and a baseline audiogram are used as a reference value against which the hearing loss is measured (Bronkhorst & Shutte 2013). The PLH is calculated at 500 Hz, 1 KHz, 2 KHz, 3 KHz and 4 KHz per ear according to the quality of hearing in each ear. After calculating the PLH, the test with poorer hearing is said to be the baseline audiogram and will be used as the reference point for future audiograms and to monitor the hearing threshold for monitoring and compensation purposes (Bronkhorst & Shutte 2013). To determine a PLH shift, the baseline PLH is subtracted from the PLH of routine screening audiometry. If a difference of a PLH shift of >10% is suspected, an audiologist must carry out diagnostic baseline audiometric testing. Where a PLH shift of >10% is confirmed, the case is referred to the occupational medical practitioner or otorhinolaryngologist to establish the definitive cause of the hearing loss (Bronkhorst & Shutte 2013). If the hearing loss is confirmed to be work-related, the case should be reported to the Compensation Commissioner or the applicable insurance fund for compensation purposes (Bronkhorst & Shutte 2013). This stage is considered the tertiary preventive stage as hearing loss already exists. At this level, the aim is to minimise the impact of the hearing loss on the affected individual. This is accomplished through aural rehabilitation (AR), which will be discussed in detail later in this chapter. From this discussion, the role of audiometry surveillance as a preventive tool cannot be overemphasised. If implemented carefully and routinely, this pillar can effectively be used as an early identification tool and an EI tool if a hearing loss is suspected, and where a hearing loss is confirmed, it can be successfully used to facilitate compensation and AR.

Hearing protection devices are the least effective component of the hierarchy of controls. However, evidence suggests that HPDs are routinely used to reduce excessive noise exposure and lower the incidence of ONIHL (Brown et al. 2015). Globally, evidence indicates a heavy leaning on HPDs in the workplace (Bruce 2007; Bruce & Wood 2003; Hong et al. 2013; Ntlhakana, Kanji & Khoza-Shangase 2015; Suter 2012). Arguments have been put forward highlighting the challenges with using HPDs. These concerns include reduced audibility and distorted acoustic information, as well as discomfort when worn for longer periods (Brown et al. 2015; Ntlhakana et al. 2015). Beamer, McCleery and Hayden (2016) submitted that HPDs can be effective when used in conjunction with all the other pillars of an HCP. The author of this chapter argues that education can lay a firm foundation for the use of HPDs. If employees are informed about the benefits of using PPE, and if administrative and engineering controls are well implemented, the risks can be significantly reduced. A comprehensive record-keeping system with buy-in from all stakeholders will ensure that employees' hearing health can be monitored to facilitate timely and early identification and intervention.

11.1.4. Tertiary prevention

Tertiary prevention aims to decrease the adverse effects of the disease and optimise the QoL of the affected individual (Duplaga et al. 2016; Pandve 2014b). At this level of prevention, the focus is on rehabilitative interventions that may include vocational rehabilitation to retain workers after injury. Related to preventive audiology, intervention will focus on AR. Aural rehabilitation is defined as a range of services aimed at reducing the adverse effects that a hearing loss has on the individual's participation and enjoyment of their daily activities, thus improving their QoL. It is a process where individuals who have sustained a hearing loss are provided with intervention and training to minimise the impact of the hearing loss (Brodie, Smith & Ray 2018).

Aural rehabilitation seeks to help workers get used to their hearing loss, explore appropriate hearing amplification devices and improve conversation and communication in general (Brodie et al. 2018). Therefore, AR incorporates counselling, sensory management, as well as auditory training and instruction, with the goal of minimising the negative psychosocial effects of hearing loss, improving self-management and increasing the efficacy of assistive technology (Coco, Ingram & Marrone 2019). Through the education pillar, counselling can focus on three aspects - informational counselling, personal adjustment counselling and support groups. Informational counselling focuses on providing education to the person with a hearing loss on available treatment interventions. Personal adjustment counselling addresses the person's psychological, social and emotional acceptance of hearing loss and occupational prospects. Where possible, community groups can be established to offer ongoing support (Sweetow 2018).

Aural rehabilitation can also focus on the use of assistive listening devices, hearing aids or cochlear implants, as well as on environmental modification and vocational counselling to identify and implement specific accommodations or modifications for workplace settings (Sweetow 2018). In an occupational setting, specifically, AR entails implementing administrative controls, particularly rotating workers from a noisy area to a quieter area. Additionally, the use of HPDs will have to be monitored. Workers fitted with hearing aids will need to be educated on the possibility of their hearing becoming progressively worse if continued exposure to excessive noise occurs. Most importantly, these workers need to be monitored with good record-keeping being critical in the tracking of workers' progress. Tertiary prevention is concerned with minimising the impact of hearing loss and improving the quality of the worker's life. It, therefore, follows that audiologists have a critical role to play in providing AR services that are responsive to the needs of workers who have sustained hearing loss on duty.

11.1.5. Quaternary prevention

Quaternary prevention entails taking action to identify workers at risk of over-medicalisation and protecting them from new, untested medical remedies while recommending interventions that are ethically sound (Pandve 2014b). Khoza-Shangase (2020b) asserted that NIHL is influenced by health conditions and illnesses such as HIV, AIDS and TB. Other authors have investigated the link between NIHL and blood pressure and hypertension (Kuang, Yu & Tu 2019; Liu et al. 2016; Wang et al. 2018), cardiovascular disease (Ding et al. 2019; Li et al. 2019; Xua & Francis 2019) and diabetes (Ashkezari et al. 2018; Soares et al. 2018; Yadav & Yadav 2018). Furthermore, individuals without a history of hearing loss may acquire hearing loss because of the ototoxic nature of the drug regimen used to treat HIV, AIDS and TB (Khoza-Shangase 2020a). Therefore, it is important for audiologists to keep a detailed record of the risk factors, medical history, and hearing status of individuals exposed to excessive noise.

A paucity of evidence exists in record-keeping in the mining industry. Record-keeping is critical in the workplace as it promotes and maintains accountability, commitment and consistency (Byrne 2005; Khoza-Shangase et al. 2020). Considering that ONIHL develops gradually and over time, the importance of keeping accurate records of each employee is critical and cannot be overemphasised. Records can be used to determine an employee's exposure to noise, thereby allowing for effective and accurate programme evaluation, which is important for programme sustainability. Accurate record-keeping allows for easy identification of challenges and therefore lays the ground for relevant changes (Byrne 2005). Proper record-keeping facilitates the implementation of effective and appropriate individual conservation programmes, where employees' multiplicative factors such as concomitant exposure to other toxins – and co-occurrence of TB and HIV with ototoxicity – are considered in employees' HCP plans (Khoza-Shangase 2020b). Additionally, proper record-keeping facilitates accurate comparative analysis of employee thresholds for compensation purposes when employees are eligible for compensation. Lastly, responsible sound record-keeping identifies responsive research agendas to inform relevant evidence-based information to be accessed by management in order to enhance the mines' HCPs (Byrne 2005; Ntlhakana et al. 2022).

■ 11.2. Preventive environmental and occupational audiology in the South African context

In South Africa, HCPs were formally implemented over two decades ago, after the declaration of the 1996 Mine Health and Safety Act (President's Office 1996). Thereafter in 2003, the South African Mine Health and Safety Council (MHSC) comprising representatives from the State, labour and employers, implemented the 2003 MHSC milestones, which were aimed at targeting the elimination of ONIHL in this sector. These milestones were two-pronged and targeted two imperatives. The first milestone aimed to ensure that by December 2008, there would be no deterioration in hearing greater than 10% in occupationally exposed individuals. The second milestone stated that, by December 2013, the total noise emanating from the installed equipment would not exceed a sound pressure level of 110 dB (A) (Edwards & Kritzinger 2012). In 2013, the milestones were evaluated and refined to make them more specific and measurable. Subsequently, in 2014, revised milestones were promulgated. The first milestone stated that by December 2016, no employee's standard thresholds will exceed 25 dB from the baseline when averaged over 2000 Hz, 3000 Hz and 4000 Hz in one or both ears. The second milestone focused on machinery, the source of noise, and stated that by December 2024, the amount of noise produced by the equipment must not exceed a sound pressure level of 107 dB (A) (MHSC 2014).

The aforementioned 2003 MHSC milestones were not achieved, hence the revised 2014 milestones that are still in effect. Looking at the 2003 milestones, arguably, preventive occupational audiology has not been completely successful in the South African mining sector. The author of this chapter submits that preventive occupational audiology has been unsuccessful because of:

1. the framing of the milestones
2. the absence of occupational audiologists
3. the quadruple burden of disease currently faced by South Africa as a LMIC
4. the complex nature of HCPs.

11.2.1. Framing of the milestones

Firstly, arguably, the manner in which the milestones are framed significantly reflects some weaknesses. These weaknesses could potentially explain why HCPs have failed in the mining industry. A close look at the milestones reveals that the targets focused on only two aspects of hearing conservation: hearing deterioration (audiometry surveillance/administrative controls) and noise reduction at source (engineering controls). Undoubtedly, these two pillars are critical and integral in controlling hazardous noise in the workplace. However, they address matters at the managerial level and exclude key stakeholders such as mineworkers who are directly affected by hazardous noise. Arguably, education of and buy-in from the mineworkers serves as a preventive measure which is a key to the success of any intervention involving the miners. Therefore, there ought to be careful deliberation around the role of mineworkers during the setting of targets, if HCPs are to succeed.

Secondly, the manner in which the targets are sequenced raises concerns - hearing deterioration before the noise source is misaligned with the goal. Reducing noise at the source and engineering controls should precede reducing the deterioration of hearing loss, which is an administrative control. Noise is the risk factor and therefore falls under primary prevention. Currently, these milestones seem to promote secondary prevention over primary prevention, thereby undermining the hierarchy of controls in the prevention of ONIHL.

Thirdly, looking at the time frames for achieving these milestones, it is anticipated that reducing exposure to the individual will be achieved prior to reducing noise at the source. In reality, reducing noise at the source should be prioritised over exposure to the individuals, because if noise is controlled at the source, exposure to the individual is greatly reduced.

11.2.2. Absence of occupational audiologists

A perusal of documents on the role of occupational audiologists in South Africa revealed a role limited to audiometric surveillance and compensation of hearing loss (De Koker n.d.; De W Oosthuizen 2006). Furthermore, this role can be undertaken by non-audiologists, such as audiometricians. This undermines the importance of preventive occupational audiology as occupational audiologists undergo specialised and specific training on preventive occupational audiology. A study conducted by Moroe and Khoza-Shangase (2018) identified the following factors as contributing to the limited role of occupational audiologists in preventive occupational audiology:

1. There is a scope-context misalignment of the caseload expected for occupational audiologists.
2. Occupational audiologists are juniorised and their responsibilities are executed by non-audiologists who do not have adequate training on the impact and latent effects of ONIHL. This is done to reduce costs as audiologists are deemed costly.
3. There is a poor appreciation of the role of occupational audiologists in the workplace.
4. Occupational audiologists are not adequately trained or well equipped with the skills and expertise needed to execute their preventive audiology duties. This limited role also has implications for assessing the risks versus the benefits of preventive occupational audiology (Khoza-Shangase & Moroe 2020).

11.2.3. Burden of disease

South Africa is an LMIC grappling with a quadruple threat of burden of diseases, fewer job opportunities, political unrest and economic instability (Leboea 2017). Particularly in the mining sector, the high incidence of this challenge continues to present barriers to the management of ONIHL (Strauss et al. 2012). However, this challenge is not prioritised by the SADoH or the mining sector, despite its devastating effects. Arguably, ONIHL is overshadowed by the high prevalence of diseases such as HIV, AIDS and TB prevalent in the mining sector (Basu et al. 2009; Khoza-Shangase 2020a; Stuckler et al. 2011, 2013). Additionally, ONIHL is an invisible disease that develops gradually over a period of years (Patel et al. 2001; Tye-Murray 2009). Compared with HIV and AIDS, ONIHL is not life-threatening; however, its impact on the economy is devastating.

According to the World Bank, in South Africa alone, the prevalence of TB in the mining sector is estimated to be between 2500 and 3000 cases per 100,000 individuals, which is 10 times the WHO threshold for health emergencies and three times the incidence rate of the general population (Cullinan 2018). Furthermore, miners are three to four times more likely to be infected with HIV and AIDS (Stuckler et al. 2011). Bhunu, Mushayabasa and Smith (2012) asserted that in the presence of an HIV infection, the probability of acquiring TB increases. Therefore, the co-infection of HIV, AIDS and TB implies that affected mineworkers may be on treatment for HIV and AIDS and/or TB (Khoza-Shangase 2010, 2020a). Workers, who are on treatment for HIV, AIDS or TB, if exposed to prolonged excessive noise, are at significant risk of greater clinical hearing loss because of the synergistic effects of noise and ototoxic medications. This may increase the prevalence, onset and progression, nature, as well as the degree and configuration of ONIHL in the affected population (Khoza-Shangase 2010). Recently, Khoza-Shangase (2020a) provided evidence confirming that miners previously treated for TB have poorer high-frequency hearing thresholds compared with workers without a history of TB. The synergistic effects of noise and ototoxic medications highlight the importance of strategic HCPs that consider ototoxicity (Khoza-Shangase 2020b). This requires monitoring through proper record-keeping and possibly the use of otoprotective/chemo-protective agents to promote hearing conservation in at-risk workers infected with HIV, AIDS and TB.

11.2.4. Complex nature of hearing conservation programmes

Hearing conservation programmes implemented in the South African mining industry are currently not achieving the desired results. Over and above the aforementioned reasons, HCPs are complex interventions (Moroe 2018). This complexity can be attributed to the fragile nature of the pillars largely influenced by the active engagement and feedback from various stakeholders involved in their formulation and implementation. Furthermore, the fact that HCPs are 'built from multiple interacting components, which act both independently and interdependently' from each other also attests to their complex nature (Shiell et al. 2008). In summary, the complexity of HCPs can be summarised as follows (Moroe 2018):

Hearing conservation programmes are:

- evidence and theory-based interventions
- active and able to achieve their effect through the active involvement and engagement of individuals
- comprised of long journeys
- non-linear in their implementation chains and can even go into reverse
- fragile and embedded in multiple social systems
- are prone to be borrowed
- are open systems that feedback on themselves

South Africa, although an LMIC faced with all the challenges associated with LMICs, has sound and evidence-based HCPs, which are very capable of eradicating NIHL caused by both environmental and occupational sources of noise. Furthermore, as demonstrated in the preceding discussion, the HCPs implemented in South Africa are in line with health promotion and disease prevention and take into account the hierarchy of controls in preventing NIHL. These HCPs would benefit from recent advances in the early detection and management of NIHL.

11.3. Recent advances in early detection and management of occupational and environmental noise

> We live in an era of unprecedented technological advancement that impacts every aspect of our lives, from the way we shop and travel to the way we communicate with friends and family. These trends are resulting in new methods and tools that change the way safety professionals and industrial hygienists prevent hearing loss. (Brauch 2017, p. 1)

With regard to prevention and early detection of ONIHL, advances have led to the use of smartphones and low-cost sensors, and this has subsequently prompted government agencies to promote and implement HCPs to facilitate worker safety and optimal health outcomes (Brauch 2017).

To explore recent advances in the prevention of occupational noise, Moroe and Khoza-Shangase (2020) conducted a systematic review of literature in the last 10 years. The results of the review yielded the following advances: use of metrics, pharmacological interventions and hair cell regeneration, artificial neural networks, audiology assessment measures, noise monitoring advances and conceptual approaches to HCPs. These approaches are presented in Table 11.1 in relation to preventive levels, the hierarchy of noise control and the HCPs. The following chapter, Chapter 12, plunges deeper into these advances, contextualising them to the African context for the achievement of zero ear and hearing harm, specifically within the mining industry.

The analysis of the advances in intervention listed in Table 11.1 shows that all the prevention levels, the hierarchy of controls and the pillars of the HCPs are represented. This is encouraging in that it suggests that innovation and new advances are aligned with health promotion and NIHL prevention. There seems to be a preference for primary and secondary prevention in these advances. This is not surprising as the hierarchy of controls and the pillars are concentrated around the primary and secondary prevention levels. This also suggests that there is a focus on prioritising the reduction of the impact and progression of hearing loss. Arguably, if the concerns around the implementation of HCPs in South Africa were to be addressed, the goal of health promotion and prevention for measures to not only prevent the occurrence of disease, such as risk factor reduction, but also to arrest its progression and reduce its consequences once established may be achieved.

TABLE 11.1: Summary of recent advances in the prevention of noise-induced hearing loss.

Authors, date and country	Research title	Recent advance	Prevention level	Hierarchy of control	Hearing conservation pillar
Davies et al. (2012); China	'The use of the kurtosis metric in the evaluation of occupational hearing loss in workers in China: Implications for hearing risk assessment'	**Metrics** A set of quantitative tools used to assess, monitor, improve or evaluate compliance and success of programmes to set and track goals of the implemented programme (Sullivan et al. 2004)	Primordial prevention Primary prevention	Hazard control Exposure control Exposure rehabilitation	Exposure monitoring Engineering controls Administrative controls
Moroe et al. (2019); South Africa	'A proposed preliminary model for monitoring HCPs in the mining sector in South Africa'		Secondary prevention Tertiary prevention		Audiometry surveillance Education and training
Al-Dayyeni et al. (2018); United States	'Investigations of auditory filters based excitation patterns for assessment of noise-induced hearing loss'		Quaternary prevention		Personal protective equipment Record-keeping
Choi et al. (2014); Republic of Korea	'Therapeutic effects of orally administrated antioxidant drugs on acute noise-induced hearing loss'	**Pharmacological interventions** Approaches developed for the prevention or treatment of NIHL through the use of antioxidant drugs to restore the balance between antioxidant defence and the formation of free radicals in the cochlea (Choi & Choi 2015)	Quaternary prevention	Exposure control	Record-keeping
Choi et al. (2015); Republic of Korea	'Noise-induced neural degeneration and therapeutic effect of antioxidant drugs'				Education and training
Mukherjea et al. (2012); United States	*The design and screening of drugs to prevent acquired sensorineural hearing loss*				Audiometry surveillance
Oishi et al. (2011); United States	*Emerging treatments for noise-induced hearing loss*				Administrative controls
Santaolalla et al. (2013); Spain	'Inner ear hair cell regeneration: A look from the past to the future'				
Tieu et al. (2013); United States	'Current pharmacologic otoprotective agents in or approaching clinical trials: how they elucidate mechanisms of noise-induced hearing loss'				
Zheng et al. (2017); United States	'Cochlear hair cell regeneration after noise-induced hearing loss: Does regeneration follow development?'				

Table 11.1 continues on the next page→

TABLE 11.1 (cont.): Summary of recent advances in the prevention of noise-induced hearing loss.

Authors, date and country	Research title	Recent advance	Prevention level	Hierarchy of control	Hearing conservation pillar
Aliabadi et al. (2015); Iran	'Prediction of hearing loss among the noise-exposed workers in a steel factory using an artificial intelligence approach'	**Artificial neural network** Artificial neural networks are analytical techniques that simulate the learning processes of the human cognitive system and the neurological functions of the brain by processing data like biological neurons in the brain (Deng, Chen & Pei 2008)	Primary prevention	Hazard control	Engineering control
Aliabadi et al. (2013); Iran	'An empirical technique for predicting noise exposure level in the typical embroidery workrooms using artificial neural networks'				
Rehman et al. (2012); Malaysia	'Predicting noise-induced hearing loss and hearing deterioration index in Malaysian industrial workers using gradient descent with adaptive momentum algorithm'				
Sabanci et al. (2017); Turkey	'Noise source determination by using artificial neural network in a metal workshop'				
Badri (2010); Jordan	'Development of neural networks for noise reduction'				
Bakay et al. (2018); United Kingdom	'Hidden hearing loss selectively impairs neural adaptation to loud sound environments'	**Audiology assessment measures**	Secondary prevention	Level 2 – Exposure control	Record-keeping
Lobarinas et al. (2017); United States	'Evidence of 'hidden hearing loss' following noise exposures that produce robust TTS and ABR wave-I amplitude reductions'				Education and training
Plack et al. (2014); United Kingdom	'Perceptual consequences of 'hidden' hearing loss'				Audiometry surveillance
Plack et al. (2016); United Kingdom	'Towards a diagnostic test for hidden hearing loss'				Administrative controls

Table 11.1 continues on the next page→

TABLE 11.1 (cont.): Summary of recent advances in the prevention of noise-induced hearing loss.

Authors, date and country	Research title	Recent advance	Prevention level	Hierarchy of control	Hearing conservation pillar
McTague et al. (2013); United States	'Impact of daily noise exposure monitoring on occupational noise exposures in manufacturing workers'	**Noise monitoring interventions**	Secondary prevention	Level 2 – Exposure control	Record-keeping
					Education and training
					Audiometry surveillance
					Administrative controls
Michael et al. (2011); United State	'Role of continuous monitoring in a hearing conservation programme'				
Rabinowitz et al., (2011); United States	'Effect of daily noise exposure monitoring on annual rates of hearing loss in industrial workers'				
Williams et al. (2012); United States	'Usability of a daily noise exposure monitoring device for industrial workers'				
Bayley et al. (2013); United States	'Wireless headset noise exposure dosimeter'				
Moroe et al. (2018); South Africa	'Occupational noise-induced hearing loss in South African large-scale mines: Exploring HCPs as complex interventions embedded in a realist approach'	**Conceptual approaches** Synthesis of available evidence used to explain the phenomenon of occupational noise and HCPs, with the goal of mapping out actions required in the course of elimination of excessive exposure to noise in the workplace (Moroe & Khoza-Shangase 2020)			
Brereton et al. (2016); United Kingdom	'Buy quiet as a means of reducing workplace'	**Buying quiet** An initiative focused on adopting and promoting the use of quieter machines as a strategy to control noise at the source (Gumede et al. 2014)	Primary prevention	Level 1 – Hazard controls	Engineering controls

Source: Moroe and Khoza-Shangase (2020).

Key: ABR, auditory brainstem response; HCP, hearing conservation programme; NIHL, noise-induced hearing loss; TTS, temporary threshold shift.

■ 11.4. Conclusion

There is no disputing that prevention is better than cure, and timely intervention can be less costly and more effective than providing services later in life (Gardner 2019). Environmental and occupational noise exposures have a negative effect on the community at large, as well as on people exposed to occupational noise. It is commendable that HCPs currently implemented incorporate evidence and theory-based interventions in the management of noise as a risk factor. However, as this chapter has illustrated, there are still some factors that impact the success of health promotion and prevention of environmental and occupational NIHL, particularly within LMICs like South Africa. Within the South African context, it is, therefore, important that environmentally, at a national level:

- A need is created to raise awareness of the impact of noise on the QoL and the well-being of the community at large. Noise is not easily avoidable, so it is important that the general population be made aware of the negative effects of excessive exposure to it.
- Awareness should be raised about the need to include hearing acuity screening when other medical screening is conducted. The general population may not be aware of the risk factors as well as the auditory and non-auditory effects of exposure to excessive noise.
- Studies should be conducted on the prevalence of recreational noise among youth and young adults. There is an increase in the use of personal listening devices, particularly among the youth; therefore, there is a need to alert this population about the dangers of hazardous noise as this may have implications for their occupational choices in the near future.
- Awareness should be raised about the role of audiologists in the prevention of hearing loss from birth to death, targeting at-risk groups such as drivers who are exposed to excessive environmental as well as occupational noise.
- The general population gets empowered about regulations and permissible environmental noise levels.

Occupationally, there is a need for industries to ensure the following:

- Hearing conservation programmes implemented in the workplace are responsive to the needs of the population being exposed to excessive noise and ensure that they are implemented accordingly.
- Education and record-keeping are included at every level of prevention.
- Hearing conservation programmes are implemented as a strategy to prevent the development of NIHL and not the management of NIHL.
- Employees are empowered to get buy-in for the successful implementation of HCPs.

The aforementioned recommendations require central and key involvement of audiologists, with South African audiologists needing to advocate for their role in the prevention of NIHL and the implementation of HCPs.

Chapter 12

Occupational noise-induced hearing loss and preventive audiology: Using contemporary evidence to achieve zero-ear harm in South African mines

Katijah Khoza-Shangase
Department of Audiology, Faculty of Humanities,
School of Human and Community Development, University of the Witwatersrand,
Johannesburg, South Africa

12.1. Introduction

Sufficient global evidence indicates that, through timeous, efficient and committed collaboration between relevant stakeholders, NIHL is highly predictable and preventable (Le et al. 2017; Metidieri et al. 2013; Moroe & Khoza-Shangase 2020; Moroe et al. 2018). Despite this evidence, Le et al. (2017) argued that NIHL is probably worse than currently assessed and, therefore, may be a bigger problem than it is currently acknowledged globally. These authors believe that worldwide deliberations among ear-and-hearing health care practitioners on the prevalence, treatment and prevention of NIHL are important. Although prevention and protection are the initial defence

How to cite: Khoza-Shangase, K 2022, 'Occupational noise-induced hearing loss and preventive audiology: Using contemporary evidence to achieve zero ear harm in South African mines', ed. K Khoza-Shangase, *Preventive audiology: An African perspective*, AOSIS Books, Cape Town, pp. 235–251. https://doi.org/10.4102/aosis.2022.BK209.12

positions, this is not to ignore the promising treatment and preventive options in pharmaceutical agents, for example, the use of neurotrophins, antioxidants and steroids as otoprotective treatments (Campbell et al. 2011; Henderson & Tanaka 2009; Le Prell, Hammill & Murphy 2019; Moroe & Khoza-Shangase 2020). As ear-and-hearing health care practitioners, audiologists have an important and central role to play in advocating for the prevention of ONIHL as this forms part of their scope of practice, particularly in LMICs where diverse priorities compete for attention within a resource-constrained environment. This chapter deliberates on contemporary evidence aimed at the prevention of ONIHL at all levels of prevention from primary to tertiary levels, expanding on what Chapter 11 has covered.

In a systematic review by South African researchers where exposure to occupational noise in LMICs was explored, Moroe et al. (2018) found significant gaps in evidence that have local relevance and are responsive to the context, which could be used to drive preventive audiology initiatives in this field. In this systematic review that was performed in line with the Cochrane collaboration guidelines and Preferred Reporting Items for Systematic Reviews and Meta-Analysis, publications indicating developments in the management of ONIHL in the African mining industry between 1994 and 2016 were analysed. The review revealed that ONIHL prevalence is still high in this context, regardless of reports of HCPs implementation in most mines. Moreover, reviewed evidence suggests that the mining industry is fully cognisant of this epidemic but has had limited success in curbing it (Dekker et al. 2011; Edwards et al. 2015; Edwards & Kritzinger 2012; Musiba 2015; Ntlhakana, Khoza-Shangase & Nelson 2020a, Ntlhakana, Nelson & Khoza-Shangase 2020b).

The review findings further revealed a significant paucity of studies on the management of ONIHL in Africa, with the limited available data revealing four key findings. Of the four key findings, firstly, research conducted tended to focus on a few but not all the pillars of HCPs as recommended in the literature (Amedofu 2007; Amedofu & Fuente 2008; Hong et al. 2013). Moroe et al. (2018) argued that for HCPs to be efficient and sustainable, all seven pillars must be cohesively and comprehensively addressed. These pillars include employee/management education and training, administrative controls, engineering controls, periodic noise exposure monitoring, audiometric evaluations, personal hearing protection and efficient record-keeping (Amedofu 2007; Hong et al. 2013; Khoza-Shangase, Moroe & Edwards 2020; Moroe et al. 2018). Analysis of the studies indicated that studies within this African context focused mainly on four pillars and investigated these in a piecemeal fashion. Pillars that seem to enjoy research focus are personal hearing protection, administrative controls, engineering controls, and education and training, while pillars such as periodic noise exposure monitoring, audiometric evaluations and record-keeping have received less attention, to the detriment of the evidence base for best practice in this context. For example, the Workplace Safety Health Council (WSHC) (2014) cautioned how overlooking the monitoring of periodic noise exposure significantly impacts the whole HCP as workers exposed to hazardous noise levels in the work environment are identified from this pillar. Therefore, WSHC (2014) recommended that noise monitoring be conducted once every 3 years or each time mechanical modifications are effected.

Moroe et al. (2018) argued that effective record-keeping is crucial for the maintenance of accountability. Because ONIHL has a gradual and progressive development nature, appropriate and efficient record-keeping is key, as records can be referred to for tracking and monitoring the employees' exposure to noise and the impact of that noise on the employees. These authors believe that this efficient record-keeping facilitates efficacious HCP evaluation and alteration as required, ensuring programme sustainability if effective or programme alterations if ineffective, in the same way as done in other preventive monitoring programmes such as ototoxicity monitoring (Amedofu 2007; Khoza-Shangase & Masondo 2020; Khoza-Shangase, Moroe & Edwards 2020).

Good record-keeping also facilitates accurate, individualised conservation and monitoring programmes in employees who have compounding risk factors such as simultaneous exposure to other toxins such as ototoxicity from treatments for TB and HIV and simultaneous chemical/solvents exposure. Furthermore, it plays a vital role in the comparative analysis of workers' hearing thresholds from longitudinal assessments for compensation purposes; should prevention measures fail (Ntlhakana et al. 2020a; Ntlhakana et al. 2021), then records of leading indicators are needed. Good record-keeping also facilitates accurate research that provides evidenced-based recommendations that can enhance HCPs (Khoza-Shangase 2020). A gap in research on HCPs would lead to limited application of best practices guided by relevant evidence. However, Ntlhakana et al. (2022) warned that this record-keeping must adhere to ethical principles and the South African *Protection of Personal Information Act* (PoPIA 2020).

Secondly, of the four key findings, the studies reviewed comprised small sample sizes. Additionally, there were shortcomings with the data collection methods adopted. Of the studies that adopted interviews, surveys and retrospective record reviews as data collection methods, the greatest number of participants included in the studies was 200. These limited sample sizes have a significantly negative impact on the generalisability of the findings of these studies to the general ONIHL population. This limitation becomes particularly challenging in a largely diverse context like South Africa where socio-economic, linguistic and cultural diversity have been argued to have a significant influence on health-seeking and health intervention adherence behaviours (Flood & Rohloff 2018; Khoza-Shangase & Mophosho 2018, 2021).

Thirdly, in the review, ONIHL was not viewed as a complex problem requiring complex interventions, but rather an extraction of certain factors for research purposes was done, with the neglect of others that are just as important in HCPs. Lastly, of the four key findings, clear evidence of the rising prevalence of ONIHL in African countries was found, thereby intensifying the need for more studies on its assessment and management in the mining sector. Consequently, Moroe et al.'s (2018) review highlighted the need for preventive measures in ONIHL to be reflected on by the occupational health care industry and practitioners as an imperative effort toward achieving zero ear harm within LMICs, like South Africa. From a knowledge generation and sharing perspective, one also questions if these identified gaps are purposefully created and sustained within this industry to maintain the *status quo*, which is profit driven and ensures capital profits at the expense of the health and safety of its workers (Moroe & Khoza-Shangase 2018). Moroe and Khoza-Shangase (2018) bemoaned how researchers have been driven to perform studies on challenges faced by this industry precisely because the South African mining industry has been commonly slated for its inadequate health and safety record as well as its excessive numbers of mortalities while making significant profits. Interest in conducting research in the mining industry is, however, not without challenges.

One of the key documented challenges to conducting research in South African mines is access. In their study on access to South African mines for research, Moroe and Khoza-Shangase (2018) found three factors that served as barriers to access, which one can argue demonstrates that such spaces appear to specifically block access to independent reviews and evaluations. The three factors highlighted in this study are: (1) lack of listing of contact details of key personnel on the mines' websites; (2) protracted response time for access to research data between the time initial contact is made and the time in which the mine responds; and (3) unwillingness by the mines to allow independent and external access to data on their management of ONIHL as well as advancements made in HCPs in different mines. Moroe and Khoza-Shangase (2018) concluded that denied access to researchers by mines adds to the inability to come up with efficient and efficacious HCPs through best practice, a practice which is guided by evidence that is relevant to the African context. Objective evidence that is established by external and independent parties to the mines is critical for best practice as mines, on their own, are not objective players in such evidence creation because of a potential inevitable conflict of interest. For HCPs to be successful, impartial evidence, regardless of how it portrays the mining industry's reputation, is required. It is only when such objective evidence base is carefully and transparently scrutinised that material and effective management strategies can be considered and employed, with evidence-driven strategic planning arrived at by regulatory bodies such as the HPCSA and the South African MHSC.

The MHSC (2016) took a clear position on 'every mine worker returning from work unharmed every day: Striving for zero harm' as one of its fundamental objectives in its operations. Despite this council articulating this goal in its policies and adherence efforts by the South African Chamber of Mines, Moroe et al. (2018) argued that the council has failed in as far as achieving zero harm in as far as ear-and-hearing health care of mineworkers is concerned. Current evidence presented by these authors reveals that approximately 73.2% of South African miners are exposed to hazardous noise at levels greater than the legislated occupational exposure limit of 85 dB, regardless of the implementation of HCPs (Edwards et al. 2011; Khoza-Shangase et al. 2020; Strauss et al. 2014), with an overreliance on HPDs as the first-line preventive measure (Bruce 2007; Bruce & Wood 2003; Hong et al. 2013; Ntlhakana, Kanji & Khoza-Shangase 2015; Moroe et al. 2018; Suter 2012; Yaakobi & Putter-Katz 2020).

Ntlhakana et al. (2015) highlighted a concern about this overreliance on HPDs as the primary preventive measure for ONIHL, regardless of their well-documented weaknesses. Evidence has indicated that HPDs are most effective in the prevention of ONIHL when utilised as part of other measures in a comprehensive HCP, but not in isolation (Berger, Franks & Lindgren 1996; Brink et al. 2002; Davies, Marion & Teschke 2008; Edwards et al. 2015; Ntlhakana et al. 2015; Rabinowitz et al. 2007; Rashaad Hansia & Dickinson 2010; Seixas et al. 2011; Toivonen et al. 2002). The South African Department of Minerals and Energy (DME 2003) is opposed to HPDs being used as a first line of defence, but rather fervently advocates the use of personal protection devices as the last option if engineering administrative controls and audiometric evaluation are impractical, unavailable or fail to produce the desired effects.

This overreliance on HPDs was also evident in Moroe et al.'s (2018) systematic review as most of the studies reviewed concentrated on HPDs. These authors further highlighted that there were difficulties linked to the use of HPDs such as irritation and adverse effects of noise attenuation on job-related communication. Several other authors (Ntlhakana et al. 2015; Suter 2012; Tak, Davis & Calvert 2009) supported the fact that these challenges negatively influence the workers' compliance and adherence to HPDs use, which has significant consequences for companies' HCPs as it means that employees, whose HPDs are uncomfortable to wear, will be in danger of ONIHL as there will be no other effective protective measures in place to protect them from noise-related injuries. Moroe et al. (2018) also concluded that although HPDs decrease the level of hazardous noise reaching the ear, they should not be utilised in isolation, and certainly not as a primary prevention strategy, particularly as there are numerous other influencing factors requiring attention in a comprehensive HCP, factors such as concomitant exposure to other toxins.

Concomitant exposure to other toxins, as well as to diseases that are risk factors for hearing loss such as TB, HIV and AIDS, exacerbates the ONIHL problem (Edwards 2013; Edwards & Franz 2009; Khoza-Shangase 2020a, 2020b). In relation to these exacerbating factors, current evidence highlights a critical lacuna in global HCPs addressing the risk that these conditions add to the burden of ONIHL within the mining sector. In the South African context, toxins and diseases such as TB are highly prevalent in mining communities, raising questions on the receptiveness, as well as pre-emptive nature of HCPs in preventing ONIHL within this population (Khoza-Shangase 2020a, 2020b). Careful consideration of the influence that such diseases can have on otology and audiology in any context is essential because some of them may lead to hearing loss either as a primary, secondary/opportunistic effect or as a side effect of treatment received. The implications for an employee diagnosed with such a disease who is also simultaneously exposed to hazardous noise levels are significant, requiring consideration in the formation, execution and monitoring of the HCP that that employee is placed under.

12.2. Current status of occupational hearing loss and hearing conservation programmes in Africa and solutions

Evidence from studies into the efficacy of management of ONIHL within the South African mining industry reveals significant gaps that warrant intensive and systematic intervention by both the research and the clinical community to achieve successful management of this occupational health condition. For successful HCPs, comprehensive and well-integrated planning that recognises the complex multi-component nature of the required interventions, with coverage of all seven pillars, is crucial (Moroe et al. 2018). These types of interventions are what Moroe (2018) and Khoza-Shangase et al. (2020) advanced and should be viewed as *Complex Interventions*, thus allowing for realistic implementation and outcomes expectations.

Complex interventions are interventions developed from numerous interrelating parts, which may operate both independently and interdependently (Medical Research Council 2000; Moore et al. 2015). Behaviours and their parameters and practices of organising them form part of these components of complex interventions, with the outputs of these interacting components and behaviours having an impact at individual, organisational and population levels (Datta & Petticrew 2013). Evidence indicates that complex interventions have commonly been undertaken for health improvement goals either at individual, organisational or population level in several fields including public service administration where reforms, regulations and assessments are done (Pawson et al. 2005), as well as in medical and public health research (Moore et al. 2015), including HCPs (Moroe 2018).

Against this backdrop, Khoza-Shangase and Moroe in 2020 Guest Edited a special issue collection titled *Occupational hearing loss in Africa: An interdisciplinary view of the current status*. This Special Issue comprehensively covers contemporary Afrocentric evidence that closes the identified lacuna in occupational audiology with relevance and responsiveness to the African context. The Afrocentric nature of the evidence presented allows for best practice in the assessment and management of ONIHL or meeting the elimination of OHL targets within the African continent, which was the goal of the Special Issue. Driven by the objectives of preventive audiology, the Special Issue, therefore, examined the challenges confronted by the occupational health fraternity in dealing with ONIHL within the African mining industry and explored potential solutions to achieve zero ear harm. Manuscripts in this collection focus on five sub-themes that are either directly or indirectly associated with the main theme of OHL including (1) policy and legislation in the management of occupational noise; (2) contextual factors, barriers and facilitators influencing the implementation of HCPs; (3) other toxins contributing to OHL; (4) monitoring and evaluation factors in occupational noise; and (5) recent advances in the management of occupational noise – as depicted in Figure 12.1 and presented in the section that follows.

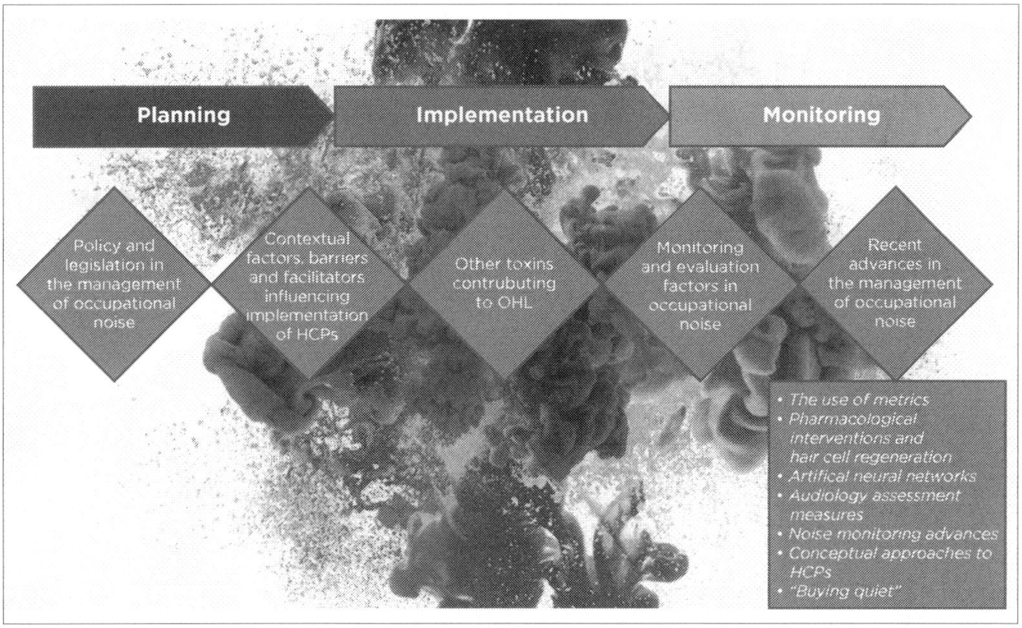

Key: HCPs, hearing conservation programmes; OHL, occupational hearing loss.

FIGURE 12.1: Current status of OHL and hearing conservation programmes in Africa and solutions at planning, implementation and monitoring stages.

12.2.1. Policy and legislation in the management of occupational noise

Manning and Pillay (2020) comprehensively explored the role of regulatory authorities in *A Critical Analysis of Current South African Occupation Health Law and Hearing Loss*. In Manning and Pillay's paper, a detailed study of contemporary South African occupational health law and how this relates to hearing loss is conducted. The authors utilised experience and critical science as methodological devices to conduct a review of legal texts, comprising South African primary and secondary laws, as well as unpublished (non-peer-reviewed) grey literature. These were thematically analysed, aided by a semantic approach, with a critical interpretation of data utilising the Bill of Rights as a central analytical framework.

This review yielded four themes that describe the South African occupational health law and OHL: '(1) separate and unequal regulatory frameworks; (2) monologic foregrounding of noise; (3) minimisation of vestibular disorders; and (4) dilution of ototoxic agents' (Pillay & Manning 2020, p. e1). The authors argue that their findings indicate that a severely split up legal framework of occupational health and safety in South Africa maintains an 'excessive noise hearing loss' theory that negatively impacts the equal protections and benefits rights of all employees - and not just prioritising those exposed only to excessive noise. This position is in agreement with the complex intervention argument advanced earlier in this chapter. Pillay and Manning (2020) concluded that the South African occupational health and safety law needs to be synchronised such that the scope of hearing protection legislation is extended to incorporate the inclusive range of recognised ototoxic hazards within this context, such as chemicals. This is particularly important as sufficient evidence exists that has established a relationship between solvents and central auditory processing disorders (Fuente & McPherson 2007; Fuente, McPherson & Hickson 2013; Gopal 2008; Lobato et al. 2014), as well as vestibular dysfunction (Hodgkinson & Prasher 2006; Ödkvist et al. 1982) in this population. Arguments advanced in Pillay and Manning's paper, although couched within South Africa as a case study, have generalisable implications for LMICs.

12.2.2. Contextual factors, barriers and/or facilitators influencing implementation of hearing conservation programmes

Key to the identified contextual factors influencing the implementation of HCPs within the African context are the well-documented capacity versus demand challenges with a significant incongruence between the number of people requiring audiological services and available audiologists

(Khoza-Shangase & Moroe 2020a; Khoza-Shangase, Moroe & Neille 2021). Khoza-Shangase and Moroe (2020a) reviewed South African HCPs in the Context of Tele-Audiology while exploring if tele-audiology can be efficiently utilised within a complex intervention such as HCPs. The established value of tele-audiology as a model of ear-and-hearing health care delivery in resource-constrained settings is well argued by these authors and they offer valuable contextually-responsive recommendations on how tele-audiology could be fruitfully utilised within the African mining context. Because of the significant capacity versus demand difficulties in LMICs, and the necessity to expand and extend audiologists' involvement in the management of ONIHL as part of their scope of practice; these authors, supported by Khoza-Shangase (2019), recommend that training institutions, the profession of audiology and policymakers thoroughly explore tele-audiology as an additional platform to deliver ear-and-hearing health care services in these contexts. The advent of COVID-19, with its social distancing requirements, made this imperative an urgent need for continuity of service delivery (Khoza-Shangase et al. 2021).

Tele-HCPs have been investigated as one of the foremost suggestions to expand audiologists reach within LMIC contexts. This is in the context of evidence indicating the limited application of tele-audiology within this context; but with nuanced data analysis indicating that in the last 10 years, strong evidence in the utilisation of this platform of service delivery within occupational audiology has indicated potential growth. Khoza-Shangase and Moroe (2020a) concluded that because of the large capacity versus demand challenges in LMICs, as well as the importance of preventive care and universal ear care coverage, tele-audiology needs to be carefully considered for service delivery. The use of tele-audiology with task-shifting, where paraprofessionals meet the HPCSA's minimum standards and regulations, with overall programme management by audiologists, will facilitate planning, implementation and monitoring of successful HCPs within this context. The use of tele-audiology within the South African context to address the capacity versus demand challenges has been extensively covered in Chapter 2 and Chapter 3.

The other important contextual factor covered in the Special Issue involves risk versus benefit evaluations in ONIHL and HCPs. In this viewpoint publication that uses the South African context, Khoza-Shangase and Moroe (2020b) raised critical strategic indicators and key variables that require the attention of audiologists and the rest of the occupational health when conceptualising HCPs that yield positive outcomes within the South African mining context. Even though this manuscript uses the South African mining sector as a context, the discussion and recommendations offered can be generalised to other LMICs. Khoza-Shangase and Moroe (2020b) lamented the fact that, within both research and clinical communities, vigilance around ONIHL, which entails the active involvement of audiologists in the South African mining industry's HCPs, has been sparse. Clinically, in South Africa, these authors highlighted the fact that the role has been given to mid-level workers and paraprofessionals who are not uniformly trained to meet minimum standards and regulations, in a non-tactical, non-methodical and non-comprehensive manner. These authors further argued that this situation is exacerbated by the prevailing accountability uncertainty where, external to the mines, accountability rests with more than one body, where the mining industry regulatory body appears more prominently, with tacit or peripheral regulation by the HPCSA and the SANDoH. The limited participation and contribution of audiologists towards risk and benefit evaluation of HCPs in the development and monitoring processes and their lack of engagement with ear health and safety policy and regulations construction and promulgation processes within this context can explain this exclusion of audiologists in this important task. Regulatory authorities are crucial in ensuring compliance and holding employers responsible for the Khoza-Shangase and Moroe (2020b) eradication of ONIHL as an occupational health injury, while advocating for the principal role that audiologists should occupy during the risk–benefit evaluation of HCPs.

12.2.3. Other toxins contributing to OHL

Current evidence within the African context highlights the importance of viewing ONIHL as complex and occurring in the realm of other toxins. Pillay (2020, p. 1) answered the diagnostic question: 'what is known about occupational ototoxic chemicals with or without noise exposure in South Africa?', by conducting a qualitative mapping study of published peer-reviewed and grey literature from 1979 to 2019. Findings in this study indicate that research in this area is primarily centred around the Gauteng gold mining sector, with significant emphasis on ototoxicity for the treatment of TB and HIV. The focus of research in the province of KwaZulu-Natal is mainly on commerce and industry, with the inclusion of both the formal and informal sectors. When grey literature is analysed, findings indicate a lack of State policies that mention chemical ototoxicity as an influencing factor towards OHL. Reviewed evidence paints a clear picture of OHL being conceived to be caused only by noise exposure and not by other toxins. Pillay (2020) concluded that increasing attention towards chemical exposures as other toxins to monitor in OHL is starting to be gained in South Africa and highlights that HCPs, even in their complex multi-layered and multi-causal nature, should consistently fulfil the interests of the workers and not economic interests of the employers. Consequently, laws and regulations should consider occupational ototoxic chemicals as part of the risk factors for OHL within HCPs.

The other toxins included in the Special Issue that also require careful consideration are medications used to treat diseases such as TB, HIV and AIDS. Khoza-Shangase (2020a) reminded the reader that ONIHL does not occur in a vacuum where comorbid conditions such as HIV and AIDS, and TB do not exist. It is, therefore, important to consider how the burden of disease impacts the manifestation and management of ONIHL if zero ear harm is to be achieved by HCPs in contexts where the burden of disease requiring treatment with ototoxic medications exists, such as South Africa. Recently, Khoza-Shangase (2020a) found that South African gold miners with a history of TB treatment present with more severe high-frequency hearing thresholds than those without this history. These findings revealed the significance of considered HCPs that individualise comorbid conditions and their treatments, including incorporating ototoxicity monitoring in those employees with this additional risk factor. Furthermore, these findings raise the value of exploring the benefit of using otoprotective/chemo-protective agents for preventive care in the South African mining population.

The incidence of middle ear pathologies in adults within the mining industry (Sebothoma 2020) substantiates the case that over and above chemical exposure, conditions such as TB and HIV should be considered as compounding factors in OHL. The influence of these conditions on ontological function and audiological presentation should not be ignored nor minimised as sufficient evidence has indicated that these conditions can lead to hearing loss either as themselves (primary cause), as the effect of their secondary or opportunistic infections, or iatrogenically (side effect of treatment options for that condition). For HCPs to be successful for employees presenting with these conditions while exposed to noise in the workplace, the potential complex interactive effects of all the risk factors must be taken into consideration in the planning, execution and continuous assessment and monitoring of the HCPs (Khoza-Shangase et al. 2020). Despite the limited evidence on middle ear pathologies in mineworkers, Sebothoma (2020) reported that the available literature reporting on varying middle ear pathologies is enough to highlight a need for further investigations into this ear and hearing manifestation in this population. With the high incidence of HIV and AIDS in this population, and the well-established relationship between HIV and AIDS and middle ear pathologies (De Jong, Luder & Gross 2019; Khoza & Ross 2002; Khoza-Shangase 2020; Obasikene et al. 2014; Sebothoma & Khoza-Shangase 2018, 2020), an increased focus on this aspect of preventive audiology within South African mines is necessary. Chapter 5 recommends that this be done through adopting a programmatic approach as a clinical framework within the mining industry's Striving for Zero Harm Programme, under the South African Department of Labour – or similar programmes in other LMICs.

12.2.2.1. Monitoring and evaluation factors in occupational noise

As far as monitoring and evaluation factors in occupational noise within the African context are concerned, issues of patient factors such as the influence of age on ONIHL need careful consideration (Grobler et al. 2020). The focus on the employees is further highlighted by Mapuranga, Maziriri and Letshaba (2020), where the importance of how factors such as noise exposure at work as well as the employees' predisposition to hearing impairment, as well as job performance, can be significantly influenced by occupational noise. In their study conducted on manufacturing small and medium enterprises (SME) workers, Mapuranga et al. (2020) found that occupational noise has a positive and significant effect on attitudes towards noise exposure and observed vulnerability to hearing loss in this group. Moreover, these authors indicate that their findings showed that attitudes towards occupational noise exposure and the measurable vulnerability to hearing loss also have a positive and significant effect on the workers' job performance. These findings are essential to consider during the planning, implementation, monitoring and evaluation of HCPs initiatives. Positive attitudes can positively influence employees' active ownership of, as well as full involvement and adherence to HCPs.

Moroe (2020) further argued that such findings become relevant when occupational health practitioners' (OHPs) views on training methods adopted for training mineworkers on ONIHL are considered. In her study, Moroe (2020)'s findings revealed a complete lack of awareness by OHPs on the training methods used with this population, thus impacting the mineworkers' knowledge about ONIHL and its resultant outcomes. However, OHPs do recognise the influence that factors such as educational and literacy levels, language and financial resources have on the training. Thus, Moroe (2020) asserted that, for effective awareness campaigns and sustainable HCPs, health literacy needs to be prioritised within the South African mining industry. The conceptualisation and implementation of this plan must take into cognisant workforce diversity, which can include factors such as education, language, culture and financial resources.

Audiologists, as central members of the OHPs, is further underscored by Ntlhakana et al. (2020b) in their study involving secondary electronic data review of one South African mine. The objective of this review was to establish risk factors for ONIHL that the mine's hearing conservation practitioners viewed as essential for meeting the South African 2014 HCP milestones, as well as to establish how mineworkers presenting with these risk factors were managed. For these identified factors to be useful in a HCP, they would have to be well amalgamated into the mine's proactive data management system (PDMS). Findings, which can be generalisable to the greater South African mining context, revealed considerable gaps in the mine's data management systems, with the mine's PDMS demanding careful consideration for it to be able to facilitate early identification of ONIHL. The attention that the mine's PDMS requires entails inclusion and integration of risk factors for ONIHL beyond just noise exposure levels and demographic profile data, such as burden of disease factors with the ototoxic treatments taken by miners. Key to these factors are TB and HIV and their medical management, as these are significant risk indicators for ONIHL within the South African context where these conditions have high prevalence.

Lastly, under monitoring and evaluation factors, the classification of audiograms in the prevention of NIHL (Musiba 2020) and the application of a feedback-based noise monitoring (FBBM) matrix (Moroe et al. 2020) are considered. Musiba (2020) identified various strategies of audiograms classifications based on changes to hearing thresholds from baseline findings. Musiba (2020) identified two main differences in these classification methods: (1) the frequency, as well as the size of the hearing threshold change, that is applied to establish hearing loss and (2) the plan of intervention referral pathway adopted once a hearing loss is identified, hence the author's recommendation of earnest deliberation on the use of the UK Health and Safety Executive (UKHSE) scheme for categorisation of audiograms. This scheme is argued to be an unsophisticated tool that not only provides thresholds but also offers guidance on management plan following identification of the ONIHL.

Accurate, comprehensive and efficient data capturing, organisation and utilisation are critical to any efficient programme application and monitoring. Khoza-Shangase (2020, p. e2) maintained that such efficient data management is dependent on utilisation of 'accredited sensitive and valid measures as well as classification and criteria; with the data allowing matrix and models to be utilised in a complex manner to plan, execute and monitor primary preventive programmes such as HCPs'. For example, Moroe et al. (2019) responded to the failure of achieving the desired outcomes of HCPs within the South African mining sector by proposing the utilisation of a FBBM model as an instrument for monitoring and managing ONIHL. This model, a conversion of the risk management framework from ISO 31000 (Department of Finance, Australia 2016), is described as a basic static feedback model that has direct real-world functions in decision-making regarding HCPs for all relevant stakeholders within the mining industry such as mine workers, administrators and policymakers. The model is made up of five subsystems:

1. baseline or reference point
2. control unit that comprises of laws, policies and regulations that govern practice, as well as the set milestones
3. actuator, whose function is to guarantee adherence to set policies and regulations
4. implementation phase via the worker exposed to noise
5. assessment or evaluation stage.

Furthermore, the nature of the model, its recognition of policies relating to the management of ONIHL in the mining industry, as well as the fact that it comprises of all the pillars of HCPs allows for it to be utilised as part of an EI and management strategy for ONIHL in the mines. The contextual relevance and responsiveness of this model were tested when Moroe et al. (2020) put it into action, with findings revealing its value in the early prediction of ONIHL, which leads to better precision in implementing preventive audiology strategies as part of the health and safety goals of mines. These preventive strategies would range from primordial to tertiary-level initiatives within the sector, as described in Chapter 1 of this book.

Moroe et al.'s (2020) application of the FBBM matrix as a predictive tool illustrates how big data in South African mines can be used through a basic static feedback model to calculate, monitor and offer measurable information to the mineworkers, the employers and administrative leaders for HCPs planning and implementation. Therefore, Moroe et al. (2020) recommended the utilisation of this FBBM model as part of HCPs within South African mines.

☐ 12.2.2.2. Recent advances in the management of occupational noise

In a systematic review by Moroe and Khoza-Shangase (2020), the value of LMICs keeping abreast with a contemporary evidence base from HICs on advances in HCPs is highlighted. These authors argue that, although LMICs might not be sufficiently equipped to be on par with international application of these recent advances, attempts should be made to examine the possible implications of these for HCPs in their respective countries where ONIHL is still highly prevalent. The examination of these advances within LMICs should include feasibility and efficacy studies in these contexts to confirm that they are contextually relevant and responsive to facilitating the success and sustainability of implementation within their HCPs.

The recent international advances that require careful scrutiny for the African context and other LMICs have been presented under seven areas:

1. **The use of metrics:** With accurate data collection using sensitive measures, as well as efficient data capturing and management, metrics, as an advancement, can be utilised for efficient HCPs that are predictive in nature, affording enhancement of early detection of ONIHL and thus success in preventive audiology.
2. **Pharmacological interventions and hair cell regeneration:** International availability of pharmacological interventions whose goal is to prevent the onset and development of NIHL, as well as those that can reverse or treat NIHL in the form of hair cell regeneration, requires attention by LMICs.
3. **Artificial neural networks:** These have been hailed as one of the best artificial intelligence methods that can be utilised in HCPs because of their ability to save and use empirical data because they mirror the human cognitive system as well as the brain's neurological functions in learning (Aliabadi et al. 2013).

4. **Audiology assessment measures:** Measures with high sensitivity and specificity for ONIHL to allow for early detection of hearing changes at micro levels, that is prior to the hearing loss becoming a 'measurable' threshold shift are reviewed. Such measures are key for positive outcomes to be achieved in efficient preventive audiology programmes.
5. **Noise monitoring advances:** All initiatives aimed at enhancing the application of the noise exposure pillar of HCPs are reviewed. For example, patented devices aimed at eliminating noise in the workplace through accurate and continuous monitoring of noise in the workplace are presented.
6. **Conceptual approaches to HCPs:** Because of the acknowledged complexity of ONIHL, the methodologies adopted to manage it require common phenomenological approaches where activities aimed at eliminating excessive exposure to noise are mapped out, with complex interventions by Moroe (2018) put forward as one recent advance.
7. **'Buying quiet':** Although '*buying quiet*' as one of the strategies within HCPs is not a recent development, Moroe and Khoza-Shangase (2020) argued that collaboration between companies that manufacture machinery used in mines and mine owners to develop and procure quieter equipment is a new paradigm shift with a high cost-benefit that can force the industry to invent and produce quieter products.

Serious reflection on these findings by the South African HCPs stakeholders is required because learning from HICs can be of benefit to LMICs for them to be able to achieve hazardous noise elimination targets as well as prevent ONIHL. The same arguments are advanced by Madahana et al. (2020) when they present specific lessons learned from HICs on engineering noise control for mines. These authors offer one key recommendation that encourages the South African mining industry to document and publish recent advancements in effective techniques utilised for engineering noise control. These authors recommend a comprehensive scoping of the context exercise within South African mines, where machinery and production processes that generate excessive noise are identified and documented for effective engineering noise control to be implemented on them. Furthermore, difficulties encountered during engineering noise control applications should also be identified to address excessive noise generation and exposure comprehensively in South African mines.

All these authors offer critical review and analysis of global advances and lessons while simultaneously critiquing their feasibility as well as potential efficacy within the South/African mining industry, thus affording the reader with an opportunity to engage with them with an Afrocentric eye for contextually relevant and responsive application.

Evidence reviewed above has methodically focused on subjects including challenges and solutions to implementation of HCPs within LMICs – with a specific focus on Africa; the influence of context on implementation of HCPs;

policy and law in occupational health and HCPs; as well as assessment, management and monitoring of ONIHL within HCPs; in this pioneering Special Collection on OHL in Africa in the almost 100 years history of the audiology profession in South Africa. The current context provided by these papers and recommendations for preventive audiology in ONIHL emphasise the following fundamental issues:

1. the value of applying what is documented in texts, policies, laws and regulations into practice
2. the importance of adopting a collaborative working model with all relevant stakeholders in HCPs, where the role of the audiologists becomes more centrally located rather than peripherally as is currently the practice
3. the importance of keeping up-to-date with recent developments from HICs on ONIHL and HCPs, as well as cautious application of these advancements considering contextual relevance and responsiveness
4. the significance of situational analysis in programme implementation so as to ensure best practice
5. the complex nature of OHL with the value of addressing it within complex interventions (Khoza-Shangase et al. 2020).

■ 12.3. Conclusion

A dearth of contextually relevant and responsive evidence exists in ONIHL and HCPs within the African context. Current evidence reveals significant gaps in all aspects of occupational audiology, with findings highlighting a need for increased focus in this area as part of preventive audiology initiatives in LMICs, like South Africa. This chapter gathered and compiled contemporary peer-reviewed Afrocentric evidence in identified areas in occupational audiology, with the goal to contextualise the OHPs, including audiologists, to the ONIHL and HCPs landscape in the African continent. Findings are described and discussed while implications for the field of audiology, engineering and occupational audiology within the African context are raised for both research and teaching, as well as clinical practice.

With the current evidence still signifying the high prevalence of OHL in LMICs such as South Africa, serious criticism can be levelled against the mining industry in these regions, particularly because hearing loss is recognised to be a more severe burden in LMICs than in HICs. Such a burden becomes even more pronounced in resource-constrained countries like South Africa where socio-economic inequality is a documented challenge, and therefore, an OHL can serve as a barrier to accessing employment and a restriction to the type of employment an individual with this disability can secure (Thorne 2006). It, therefore, becomes vital to paint a clear picture of OHL and HCPs in LMICs so that strategic planning can yield positive outcomes in as far as curbing and eliminating this occupational health challenge. Taking lessons from evidence and practice in HICs while ensuring Afrocentric application of those lessons is key to successful implementation and monitoring of preventive audiology strategies within this context to achieve zero ear harm. Gaps in African context evidence that have been highlighted in this chapter call for deliberate and concerted efforts to introduce what Mignolo (2005) termed epistemic disobedience, where knowledge privileges people's lives over disciplines, and in this case over profits, and where the epistemic privilege of HICs is not seamlessly accepted as the norm.

Chapter 13

Machine learning models: Predictive tools for occupational noise-induced hearing loss in the South African mining industry

Liepollo Ntlhakana
Department of Audiology, Faculty of Humanities,
School of Human and Community Development,
University of the Witwatersrand,
Johannesburg, South Africa

Katijah Khoza-Shangase
Department of Audiology, Faculty of Humanities,
School of Human and Community Development, University of the Witwatersrand,
Johannesburg, South Africa

13.1. Introduction

Occupational noise-induced hearing loss is considered one of the global burdens that affects workers across various occupational settings (Moroe et al. 2018; Nelson et al. 2005). Although preventable, this type of hearing loss continues to be reported with its consequent negative implications within the

How to cite: Ntlhakana, L & Khoza-Shangase, K 2022, 'Machine learning models: Predictive tools for occupational noise-induced hearing loss in the South African mining industry', ed. K Khoza-Shangase, *Preventive audiology: An African perspective*, AOSIS Books, Cape Town, pp. 253-266. https://doi.org/10.4102/aosis.2022.BK209.13

South African context, despite HCPs having been implemented (Balfour-Kaipa 2014a; Chamber of Mines 2016). According to WHO, ONIHL remains a significant public health challenge and is endemic in many occupational settings worldwide where hazardous noise exposure is a problem (WHO 2020). In the United States, ONIHL is the second most reported occupational disease and injury across various industries (Masterson et al. 2016a; Mazlan & Yahya 2015). In the African continent, ONIHL is highly prevalent in the mining, agriculture and construction industries (Chen Kou-Huang, Su Shih-Bin & Kow-Tong 2020) and is the third most reported occupational disease in South African mines (Balfour-Kaipa 2014a; Moroe et al. 2018). This type of hearing loss is estimated to be the most predominant disabling condition found in more than 10% of the global population and more in working individuals in LMICs, with the sub-sector of mining being the most affected (Nelson et al. 2005; WHO 2010; Zhou et al. 2021). Therefore, there is a need to identify associated risk factors, predict early onset of ONIHL from secondary big datasets that already exist from various industries' HCP repositories and reduce the ONIHL prevalence rates in these occupational contexts.

Hearing conservation programmes are used to identify new trends and to monitor existing and previous trends drawn from the company's databases that cause employees' health hazards, where noise exposure is the leading cause (Ntlhakana, Khoza-Shangase & Nelson 2020a). Hearing conservation and noise exposure surveillance reports differ for different regions and occupational settings; however, there are primary variables that make up a hearing conservation surveillance programme. These variables include exposure dose (dBA), occupation, sample initial date and duration, and audiometry data for individual workers (Ntlhakana et al. 2020a, Ntlhakana, Nelson & Khoza-Shangase 2020b). Therefore, hearing conservation surveillance programmes provide the prevalence of the disease (ONIHL) and the success of the companies' HCPs at preventing hearing loss. The South African mines have been able to provide ONIHL prevalence rates and progress made on their HCPs in their annual and audit reports (Balfour-Kaipa 2014b; MHSI 2017), although this has not always been independently established to eliminate conflict of interest that is likely when the employer is both the referee and the player.

Occupational noise-induced hearing loss is a preventable sensorineural type of hearing loss whose onset and development are gradual and progressive because of the frequency of exposure to noise and the intensity level of occupational noise the worker is exposed to (Feuerstein & Chasin 2009). Noise sources known to cause ONIHL are continuous or intermittent in nature. Individuals exposed to these types of noises experience an increase in hearing loss during the first 10 to 15 years of exposure (Feuerstein & Chasin 2009). According to the *South African Compensation for Occupational Injuries and Diseases Act, 1993 (Act No. 130 of 1993)* (COIDA) gazetted circular Instruction

171 of 2001, a continuous, damaging, excessive noise exposure is defined as a noise level ≥ 85 dBA, averaged over an eight-hour period (8 h/TWA), with this being the type of noise that could potentially lead to ONIHL (Government Gazette, 1993). In South Africa, evidence-based literature on excessive noise exposure levels has been well-documented for employees in the mining (all commodities), textile (Bronkorst & Schutte 2013) and construction industries, although it is not limited only to these two industries (De Jager 2017). Consequently, the reported leading cause of ONIHL in various industries within the South African context is excessive occupational noise exposure.

Damage caused by excessive noise exposure to the auditory system occurs in stages, with the initial effect being a temporary threshold shift (TTS) that lasts for 16 h–48 h, accompanied by tinnitus (Feuerstein & Chasin 2009). However, because of the cumulative effect brought by the nature of occupations, the second stage ensues, referred to as a permanent threshold shift (PTS) (Masterson et al. 2016b). The relationship between TTS and PTS is dependent on the extent of damage to the outer hair cells (OHCs), damage that is irreversible but preventable (Masterson et al. 2016b), as comprehensively discussed in Chapter 11 and Chapter 12.

The South African mining industry views ONIHL as a public health and a complex occupational health problem that is also influenced by genetic, demographic, and environmental factors (Khoza-Shangase & Moroe 2020a; Strauss et al. 2014). The complexity is brought about by the diverse nature of modifiable and non-modifiable risk factors associated with ONIHL, with the consequent development of a permanent disability. Occupational exposures specifically emitted during mining processes in the South African mines, for example, the different types of noises emitted by various mine equipment at different exposure levels, as well as concomitant dust and chemical exposure, increase miners' risk for ONIHL (Edwards et al. 2011; Pillay 2020).

Previous studies conducted on HCPs in the South African mines have explored the complex nature of HCPs, for example, interactions between occupational exposures and health hazards (Khoza-Shangase 2020a, 2020b; Strauss et al. 2012), risk management tools used by the mines to control and reduce occupational exposures and prevent health hazards (Moroe et al. 2019; Ntlhakana et al. 2022), as well as the role of various disciplines of the hearing conservation practitioners in HCPs (Moroe 2020). Other health risks, such as treatments for tuberculosis and HIV, that affect miners' auditory system have been reported previously (Brits et al. 2012; Khoza-Shangase 2020a), but have been found to not be routinely and comprehensively recorded in the mines' HCP reports (Ntlhakana et al. 2020a, 2020b). The fact that this type of hearing loss (ONIHL) is associated with various risk factors, is ranked highly in conditions affecting miners, is problematic and shows that HCP strategies used by the South African mines remain inadequate and inefficient at predicting and preventing ONIHL (Moroe & Khoza-Shangase 2020; Ntlhakana et al. 2022). Therefore, HCPs employed in the South African mines should consider inclusive and comprehensive big data recording, which would allow for the early risk identification and prediction of ONIHL through using artificial intelligence (AI) and machine learning (ML).

Helm et al. (2020) asserted that as advancements in data aggregation and deep learning algorithms rapidly occur, AI and ML are primed to radically change health care practice. With contemporary fast technological developments and exponential rises in exceptionally large data sets ('big data'), 'AI has transitioned from mere theory to tangible application on an unprecedented scale' (Helm et al. 2020:69), with it having become deeply entrenched within many parts of society and often operating in the background of our everyday personal electronic devices. ML is considered a subset of AI and displays experiential 'learning' related to human intelligence, while also possessing the ability to learn and advance its analyses through the application of computational algorithms (Naylor 2018). Because of the big data that form part of HCPs, the use of ML tools and models to predict early risks associated with ONIHL is essential for the prevention of ONIHL.

The application of ML models in predicting ONIHL is a relatively new concept that requires evidence-based research to measure HCP effectiveness in the South African mining industry. Ntlhakana et al. (2022), in their study on ethical challenges encountered when using ML to predict ONIHL in platinum miners in South Africa, found that miners' audiometry and occupational hygiene data were available and accessible for research in the mine's HCP, but the medical surveillance records were not accessible in the same datasets. The mines seem to be applying different ethical principles as advocated by the HPCSA (2016) guidelines and protection of personal information as per≈the *Protection of Personal Information Act No. 4 of 2013* (PoPIA 2013) when recording, using, and sharing audiometry and occupational exposure datasets as opposed to medical surveillance datasets. This practice rendered the mines' HCP records incomplete and fragmented, which hindered holistic assessment and management of miners' hearing health care and accurate prediction and prevention of OHL through ML. Ntlhakana et al. (2022) concluded that although the HPCSA ethical principles and the PoPIA guidelines (confidentiality and privacy) used to protect data access and sharing of miners' medical and personal information were relevant, there appeared to be incongruence between data protection and privacy and a lack of clear communication around big data access for clinical care and research. Also, there appears to be a lack of clarity and consistency around data storage and access, which in turn hinders the efficiency of ML systems. Therefore, clarity around miners' data capturing, storage, management and sharing is required, and these authors recommend that the mines should employ ML systems with integrated codes for medical surveillance data, medical ethics and data sharing permission rights for research purposes (Ntlhakana et al. 2022). This chapter deliberates on the rationale and opportunities for ML models as predictive tools for the early identification and prevention of ONIHL within the South African context, with a recommendation that the factors that determine an appropriate and reliable design of an ML model to predict ONIHL be consistently considered. These factors include characteristics of occupational exposures, worker factors and types of ML systems used to collect and analyse data, all of which should be internally and externally validated to allow for the provision of more reliable predictions, especially when working with big data (Zhao et al. 2019).

13.2. Prevalence of occupational noise-induced hearing loss

Nelson et al. (2005) reported the prevalence of ONIHL to range between 7% and 21% across various countries and industries. There is a 14% estimated prevalence of OHL in the United States, comprising of adults exposed to excessive noise in different industrial sectors, from 2011–2012 (Howard & Hoffman 2017). The sub-Saharan countries have the highest prevalence rates at more than 30%, particularly in the mining industry (Grobler et al. 2020; Nelson et al. 2005), possibly because of numerous reasons such as inconsistent, ad hoc and inefficient implementation of HCPs (Moroe et al. 2018). Little evidence exists in sub-Saharan countries reflecting recent prevalence rates across various industries, such as mining, construction, agriculture and textile, to name a few. This reality is a significant lacuna in evidence as reference reports on the prevalence rates and intervention planning are based on old evidence.

A few studies which have provided prevalence rates of ONIHL in the 2000s in the agriculture and mining industries include:

- Masaka (2009) reported a prevalence rate of 27.4% for Zimbabwean underground nickel miners.
- Chadambuka, Mususa and Muteti (2013) reported 37% prevalence for underground miners in Zimbabwe.
- Kitcher et al. (2014) reported prevalence of 24.8% for market mill workers in Ghana.
- Musiba (2015) reported prevalence of 47% on Tanzanian open-pit and underground miners.
- Strauss et al. (2012) reported a 30% prevalence rate for the South African gold miners.

These studies' findings provide some insight into the burden of ONIHL within the African continent across various occupational settings. However, the varied prevalence ranges from 24.8% to 47% should be noted, and sample size differences in the studies they are based on considered during their interpretation. For example, some of these rates were based on small (Musiba 2015) to big data (Strauss et al. 2012), but the ONIHL diagnosis was based on similar assessment criteria and methods (e.g. calculations drawn from averaged high-frequency thresholds of 1000 Hz – 4000 Hz) (Agarwal et al. 2015). Although these studies used secondary data to report on the estimated prevalence of ONIHL, they also provided ONIHL epidemiology which improved researchers' understanding of HCPs outcomes.

The WHO (2020) and previous studies on causes of ONIHL have cited excessive noise exposure levels as the main cause of ONIHL – when considering other possible exposures such as chemical agents' exposure, and have thus recommended the implementation of HCPs, with guidelines for industries to report on noise reduction strategies they apply to mitigate ONIHL (Nelson et al. 2005; WHO 2020). South African industries have adopted these guidelines and implemented HCPs where excessive noise exposure (≥ 85 dBA) is present, particularly in the mining industry (Mine Health & Safety Inspectorate - MHSI 2017). The various South African mining commodities that have submitted their compliance reports to the Department of Mineral Resources and Energy (DMRE) have shared their collected, analysed and reported HCP data, which has allowed for research to be conducted for the establishment of prevalence data of ONIHL in South African mines, as well as determination of the efficacy of HCPs (MHSI 2017; Moroe 2018; Strauss et al. 2012). Furthermore, strategies employed by South African mines to reduce noise emitted by the mines' equipment have been reported, with additional noise reductions expected as some mines continue to report excessive noise exposure levels at levels higher than 100 dBA (MHSI 2017).

Literature reviewed thus far indicates the global burden of ONIHL at more than 20% (Masterson et al. 2016a). In a study conducted on the global burden of ONIHL, Masterson et al. (2016a) used data from the US NIOSH, with data by occupational category and economic sector from various work settings and economic activity rates in each WHO sub-region. These data were used to estimate the prevalence of adult hearing loss (Masterson et al. 2016a). Although data used were prior to the year 2000, the authors were able to show the DALYs, that is, over 4 million DALYs attributed to occupational noise exposure stratified by age, gender and sub-region to confirm their estimates. The conclusion made from this study was that occupational noise exposure (≥ 85 dBA) was the leading cause of adult-onset OHL. The Centre for Disease Control (CDC) conducted a similar comparative study using data from NIOSH (2003–2012), focusing on various industries in the United States, where noise is a problem, with a 2.53 DALYs per 1 000 workers exposed to noise (Masterson et al. 2016a). Mentioned in these studies were limitations around recent and complete data from LMICs, with some industries presenting insufficient noise exposure measurements. Significant to note in these studies were limitations around challenges in accessing occupational noise exposure data for research and risk analysis purposes globally, and hence, researchers need to conduct studies with available data for the estimation of the health impact of occupational exposures. Within the South African context, Moroe and Khoza-Shangase (2018b) reported on similar challenges with accessing data for research purposes to guide HCPs with contextually relevant and contextually responsive evidence.

13.3. Trends in occupational noise-induced hearing loss

Occupational noise exposure is not the only risk factor that causes OHL and ONIHL. Other risk factors such as the worker's age and sex, smoking, exposure to mine dust, chemicals used during some of the mining processes, HIV, tuberculosis and ototoxic treatments for these conditions, and other medical conditions such as diabetes and hypertension have also been associated with ONIHL worldwide (Grobler et al. 2020; Khoza-Shangase 2020a; Kuang, Yu & Tu 2019; Masterson et al. 2016a; Pillay 2020). Therefore, these other risk factors should be considered within HCPs when assessing hearing health risks of workers if the purpose is to prevent all types of OHL. Chapters 11 and 12 carefully and comprehensively reflect on using current evidence to achieve zero ear harm in South Africa and on strategies towards early detection and management of occupational and environmental noise, with careful cognisance of the various levels of preventive care.

So far, there is a dearth of evidence from the South African mining industry context that explores the multifactorial influences of OHL, as well as strategies adopted to comprehensively mitigate against this occupational health condition. Previous South African studies within the mining context have explored causes associated with ONIHL in silos, with limited literature on the combined effects and estimated deterioration in hearing loss that has considered all the risk factors (Khoza-Shangase, Moroe & Edwards 2020). Reasons for this lacuna of evidence proffered by researchers include that HCPs data provided by the mines are incomplete, non-systematic and inconsistent, thereby providing inaccurate prevalence rates of ONIHL, with very little demographic and medical history profiling done to assess the influence of these factors on the hearing loss presentation (Grobler et al. 2020; Khoza-Shangase 2020b; Moroe et al. 2018; Ntlhakana et al. 2022). Despite this shortcoming, HCPs have been able to describe miners' hearing function, establish other risk factors associated with ONIHL, analyse the miners' audiometry data to provide estimated prevalence rates of ONIHL and, to some extent, provide some understanding of trends in ONIHL specific to the South African mining context (Grobler et al. 2020; Khoza-Shangase 2020a; Ntlhakana et al. 2020a, 2020b; Pillay 2020; Sebothoma 2020; Strauss et al. 2012).

Audiological assessments used for the diagnosis of ONIHL follow two protocols that include hearing screening, where early identification and tracking of the hearing function occurs, and diagnostic audiometry which confirms the onset, type, severity, laterality and symmetry of ONIHL (Ntlhakana et al. 2020a). The screening and diagnostic audiometry procedures show protocols followed within the audiometry pillar of HCPs, and they also demonstrate how the company (mines) manages workers (miners) at risk for developing ONIHL (Franz & Phillips 2001; Moroe et al. 2019, 2020). Although screening audiometry establishes whether there is a problem or not very early on in the process and the diagnostic audiometry results in monetary compensation for ONIHL, both these measures are equally important because they allow for both detection and intervention to occur – and if conducted properly, they facilitate the achievement of prevention (Khoza-Shangase & Moroe 2020b; WHO 2020).

Within the South African context, audiometry protocols followed are in line with international standards, and South African mines follow protocols guided by the South African Mine Health and Safety Council (SAMHSC), which requires reporting of ONIHL according to the NIHL Regulations 171. This reporting is for compensation purposes (Feuerstein & Chasin 2009; South Africa 2001). The fact that audiometry protocols used by the South African mines' hearing conservation practitioners have been consistent with international standards is reassuring; however, inconsistencies found in the miners' audiometry records were problematic and cited as one of the main reasons associated with inefficient HCPs within the South African context (Ntlhakana et al. 2020a), alongside the restricted role that audiologists play in decision-making in the South African HCPs (Moroe & Khoza-Shangase 2018a). In a study by Moroe and Khoza-Shangase (2018a), the authors noted the absence of audiologists in audiometry medical surveillance decision-making and their influence in HCP targets set out by the mining companies. There could be reasons for the mines not to include audiologists as part of their HCP strategic partners, such as employment contracts and conditions which may need to be explored by the individual mining companies. According to the HPCSA statistics on the number of registered audiologists in South Africa, there were approximately 3 266 registered audiologists in 2020, which places significant limitations on appropriate ar-and-hearing health care coverage countrywide (Pillay et al. 2020). Therefore, careful planning around audiometry records for programmes that aim to achieve accurate prediction of miners' hearing function that includes the application of ML models is important for this context – even where task-shifting has occurred and audiologists serve as programme managers. Such models require accurate and complete audiometry and medical records that allow for the implementation of efforts toward early identification and prevention of OHL (Ntlhakana et al. 2022).

This chapter recommends the use of data accessed from ML systems to predict and prevent ONIHL in South African mines. Machine learning focuses on computer programmes that have an application of AI to access data, automatically learn from that data, and provide systems that can improve from experience (learned data) without being explicitly programmed (Expert AI 2020; Ntlhakana et al. 2022). South African mines already have medical surveillance data available on risk factors, which are stored in the mines' ML systems. These include occupational exposures, diagnosis of comorbid medical conditions and ototoxic treatments used for medical conditions such as cancer, HIV and TB, as well as the miners' audiometry data. However, research and clinical care enhancement opportunities exist to explore synergies between all the occupational exposures, medical conditions and ototoxic treatments as concomitant secondary effects that cause ONIHL. There is also an opportunity for audiologists to engage in interdisciplinary practice where they collaborate with other hearing conservation practitioners, biostatisticians, computer programmers, software developers and other researchers interested in the field of HCPs (Khoza-Shangase et al. 2020) to improve the understanding of ML systems used to predict and prevent ONIHL.

Machine learning is used to make accurate predictions of ONIHL and has provided opportunities for using large complex datasets to solve both linear and non-linear problems in science studies (Moroe et al. 2020; Zhao et al. 2019). The fact that ML can generate rules from existing data to predict unknown data (health risks) is an attractive feature that has been used in the health care sector, occupational health included, to determine treatment options for patients. The prediction of hearing loss in workers from different industries using different models has been explored by some international researchers (Rehman, Nawi & Ghazali. 2012; Zhao et al. 2019). The following ML models have been used: multilayer perceptron (MLP), adaptive boosting (Adaboost), support vector machine (SVM), random forest, modified back propagation neural network and gradient descent with adaptive momentum (GDAM) (Rehman et al. 2012; Zhao et al. 2019). Researchers were able to obtain predictive levels of between 78.6% and 80.1% (Zhao et al. 2019) and 98% (Rehman et al. 2012), indicating that all the models were highly accurate at predicting ONIHL for workers exposed to diverse types and levels of noises. Similar analysis methods may be explored further by hearing conservation practitioners in LMIC contexts, including South African mines, to investigate the multifactorial risks associated with ONIHL which miners present with within HCPs.

■ 13.4. Occupational hearing loss complexities

The complex nature of occupational diseases such as ONIHL, pulmonary TB, and silicosis in the mining industry have been documented extensively in the literature, with evidence on how these continue to affect miners even with strict monitoring programmes in place (Hermanus 2007; Khoza-Shangase 2020a; Moroe 2018; Nelson et al. 2005; Ntlhakana et al 2020b, 2022; WHO 2010). However, there is little information available on the synergies within these programmes and synergistic influences of these conditions and medications used to treat them with noise exposure on the auditory system, or their potential as determinants of ONIHL risks. Such evidence is important to collect using ML systems already used by the mines to improve risk assessment tools utilised in surveillance programmes and, in turn, improve health service planning (Hermanus 2007; Ntlhakana et al. 2022).

A recent South African study within the mining context showed the use of miners' audiometry data as a measure of HCP effectiveness (Grobler et al. 2020). Grobler et al. (2020) used audiometry data accessed from the mines' computer systems to determine the association between hearing loss and age over time for gold miners at Anglo Gold Ashanti in South Africa. Findings indicated that combined effects of noise exposure and age contributed to hearing loss over time. In this study, the authors found that miners exposed to noise (N = 4399) had a hearing loss deterioration of 3.5 dB, which was more than that of those who were not exposed to noise (N = 2211; 2.9 dB), over a period of 4 years (Grobler et al. 2020). This study focused on the miners' age, noise exposure levels and pure-tone air-conduction low- and high-frequency averages obtained from audiograms, to track the miners' hearing deterioration from baseline over a period of time and also estimated future hearing deterioration, which may lead to ONIHL (Grobler et al. 2020). However, in this study, other occupational exposures (chemicals, dust) and health risk factors such as TB, HIV, diabetes and cancer were not included. Therefore, data accessed from the mines' computer systems, for this study, despite the limitations highlighted, have the potential to be explored further because miners' medical surveillance and occupational exposure data were reportedly available in the mines' ML systems.

Ntlhakana et al. (2020a), in another South African study, showed miners' estimated hearing deterioration over time. These authors used accessed secondary data that contained platinum miners' age, sex, occupations, noise exposure levels, baseline audiometry and annual audiometry with PLH to estimate hearing deterioration (Ntlhakana et al. 2020a). The authors found that miners with a 0% baseline PLH score had a 20% predicted risk of ONIHL and a 45% predicted risk if they had a 40% baseline PLH. The authors concluded that the mine's current secondary data may be utilised to detect miners at risk of developing ONIHL at baseline. This study revealed an alternative way of predicting miners' hearing deterioration through an analysis method that is comparable to the recommended ML analysis method (logistic regression). Such analysis methods could arguably improve hearing health services to miners and, therefore, the efficiency of HCPs.

According to the SAMHSC, the level of hearing deemed acceptable for miners exposed to occupational noise is ≤25 dBHL, and this is based on preserving hearing for conversational speech (Resources 2016). Miners with hearing thresholds that exceed 25 dBHL are diagnosed with hearing loss, and immediate intervention and investigation of related causes should be reported to the DMRE (Resources 2016). Similarly, in the United States, the NIOSH defines a worker's hearing loss as an average hearing level of 25 dB or less (better) but at the frequencies 1 000, 2 000, 3 000 and 4 000 Hertz (Hz). The South African mines refer to the averaged hearing deterioration as STS, and this was accommodated by the new NIHL Regulation 839, which states that fresh baselines should be conducted for all miners. The regulation instructs that STS that accrues from baseline and exceeds 10 dB and is > 25 dB in both ears should be reported to the DMRE (Resources 2016). Table 13.1 illustrates the degree of hearing loss where unilateral and or bilateral STS greater than 25 dBHL should be reported to the DMRE. This strategy, as stated in Regulation 836, allows the mines' hearing conservation practitioners to estimate miners' hearing deterioration and identify those at risk of developing ONIHL early without the application of complex statistical analysis (Resources 2016). Yet, there is an opportunity for all miners' data available on the mines' ML systems to be analysed using complex statistical methods to improve hearing health services (efficient HCP) and prevent any type of OHL.

In a study by Moroe et al. (2020), the authors investigated the implementation of a feedback-based noise monitoring model (FBNMM) as a tool for predicting ONIHL and monitoring and managing HCPs at one platinum mine in South Africa. Findings from this study showed that the FBNMM tool positively predicts ONIHL early for miners exposed to noise (n = 210) and should be used within a complex mine's HCP. The authors conceptualised a model that included the miners' hearing thresholds, noise exposure levels, noise exposure duration, age and the use of HPDs to predict the miners' hearing loss over time using big data (Moroe et al. 2020). Although other occupational exposures (chemicals and dust) emitted during the platinum mine processes were not included in the FBNMM, the authors have shown evidence of other

TABLE 13.1: Hearing as a function of averaged standard threshold shifts.

STS (dBHL)*	Degree of hearing
−10–25	Normal
26–45	Mild
46–55	Moderate
56–70	Moderately severe
71–90	Severe
>90	Profound

Source: Katz et al. (2009); Resources (2016).
Key: dBHL, hearing loss in decibels.
*Range of hearing function.

predictive models that may be compared to the recommended ML model aimed at improving the implementation of HCPs as part of preventive audiology, as argued in Chapter 1 of this book.

So far, no known South African studies have been conducted to establish whether the newly set NIHL milestones (2016) have been effective in facilitating the prevention of hearing loss among miners. Only a few studies have reported trends in miners' hearing loss, and some have predicted the miners' risk for ONIHL by including some of the risk factors that affect the miners' hearing health (Grobler et al. 2020; Khoza-Shangase 2020a; Moroe et al. 2020; Ntlhakana et al. 2020b). There are gaps in the literature regarding the analysis methods used to estimate hearing deterioration and associated risk factors that cause hearing deterioration, which has limited the understanding of ONIHL among hearing conservation practitioners. (Ntlhakana et al. 2022; Seixas et al. 2012). However, the availability of electronic HCPs data presents opportunities for further research, such as the use of complex analysis methods to improve hearing health care services for miners at risk of developing ONIHL within the South African context. In addition, the use of regression analysis from existing ML systems' data allows for the construction of reliable models to predict ONIHL and, in turn, prevent ONIHL early on, with further opportunities for the use of AI in HCPs.

■ 13.5. Solution and recommendations

This chapter explores logistic regression methods to use in predicting and eventually preventing ONIHL in South African miners. Machine learning algorithms are new analysis methods in predicting hearing problems from large complex datasets and have revealed successful outcomes in solving non-linear and linear problems in science studies (Moroe et al. 2019, 2020; Zhao et al. 2019). Advances in health care have seen benefits in domains such as computer vision, automatic speech recognition and natural language processing, all drawn from the existing health care data (Zhao et al. 2019). Regardless of these developments, the direct utilisation of ML in health care has many challenges that arise from the need for health care providers to pursue personalised predictions through data that are created and administered via the electronic medical system, where data collection's primary purpose is to support patient medical care rather than enable future analysis - in research. In South Africa, in industries where noise is a challenge, HCPs' data exist mainly to manage the workers' risk to prevent hearing loss, with an emphasis on audit reports and the hierarchy of prevention and identification of hearing loss trends (SANS10083:2013). Therefore, the current HCPs data and miners' ONIHL records are the low-hanging fruit that can be analysed using ML models for efficient HCPs implementation and monitoring.

Although more work has been done in predicting ONIHL from the South African miners exposed to diverse noises, a dearth of research on ML systems still exists. A review of the opportunities for ML in predicting ONIHL for the South African miners will allow hearing conservation practitioners to realise potential benefits for further data analysis and the need to collaborate with ML researchers from other departments and faculties to come up with complex interventions for ONIHL as a complex occupational health condition (Khoza-Shangase et al. 2020). Some of the opportunities drawn from previous studies in this chapter include the following:

- The determination of how to prevent miners' ONIHL is possible where data in ML systems can play a fundamental role in incorporating key medical conditions in HCPs to ensure that, where required, individualised HCPs are implemented (Khoza-Shangase 2020b).
- The emphasis on electronic medical records, which record the process of medical surveillance and audiometry delivery and operational requirements such as tracking of the miners' hearing function.
- The miners' medical data are heterogeneous and come in a variety of forms that can be used to understand the miners' overall hearing health within a standardised system that ensures the collation of all relevant medical risk factors in all HCPs.
- The capitalisation on existing logistic regression models used by researchers on the miners with ONIHL.
- The advances in tele-audiology increase data capturing via ML systems through automated hearing screening/testing methods allowing for ease of comparative analysis against existing audiometry data (SANS 10083:2013). Automated hearing screening also reduces the workload burden of the occupational health nurse (OHN) while at the same time allowing for easy access to and timeous analysis of data by ML systems.
- Integrating fragmented medical and audiological surveillance records for the miners as these are currently kept in different data sources in most South African mines, which has led to a lack of communication and coordination that has affected the management of miners at risk of developing ONIHL.
- Exploring new ways of data use and analysis, such as the FBNMM (Moroe et al. 2019, 2020), to guide the management of miners at risk of developing ONIHL based on more evidence-based research from a variety of algorithms.
- The phenotyping of miners with ONIHL remains critical within the South African mines. Miners' parameters have already been classified for miners with ONIHL and those without; however, this process needs to be continuously updated to reflect characteristic changes in the South African miners, and these variables need to inform the ML systems used continuously.

- Internal and external validation of data from the mines is important and creates robust models. This two-way validation allows hearing conservation practitioners to collaborate with ML researchers to explore new methods of data analysis in predicting ONIHL for South African miners.

By highlighting existing data ML opportunities in this chapter, audiologists, occupational health nurses, occupational medical practitioners and occupational hygienists are encouraged to consider new ways of approaching HCPs and future collaborations - ways that aim to advance data capturing, data storage and data analysis, so that HCPs implemented are evidence-based and responsive to the context. The national health care coverage prioritises programmes intended for preventable medical conditions; therefore, efficient HCPs that are aimed at prevention should be integrated into the NHI planned by the South African government to facilitate universal ear-and-hearing health care coverage that forms part of universal health care coverage.

13.6. Conclusion

Because of the high prevalence rates of ONIHL recorded in South African mines and how the availability of the mines' HCPs electronic data and availability of the miners' electronic medical and audiometry surveillance records have not been exhaustively analysed in order to predict ONIHL for South African miners, opportunities to explore ML analysis methods exist. A dearth of evidence on the use of new research analysis and clinical methods such as ML algorithms in South African mines raises the need for hearing conservation practitioners to explore these methods. The availability of medical surveillance data that provides risk factors associated with OHL requires hearing conservation practitioners to further analyse these data to accurately predict future hearing loss cases, where all possible influencing factors have been taken into consideration, not just in the assessment but also in the preventive interventions provided within this context. There is a need to consider ML models to improve accurate testing and estimations of occupational health risks caused by all risk factors. For this to happen, deliberations around standard data capturing protocols need to occur to ensure that all relevant data are captured and kept in user- and research-friendly formats that would allow for contextually relevant interventions as well as holistic data analysis to occur. The use of ML models to predict ONIHL on HCPs data accessed from the South African mines can allow for ease in comparative analysis of findings in mines across the country, with improved access to data by independent reviewers for objective analysis devoid of conflict of interest. Such objective reviews would facilitate the planning of HCPs that are evidence-based and guided by best practices. It is important that these systems adhere to ethical principles and PoPIA.

References

Chapter 1

Alexander, KE, Brijnath, B & Mazza, D 2015, 'Parents' decision-making and access to preventive healthcare for young children: Applying Andersen's Model: Health expectations', *An International Journal of Public Participation in Health Care and Health Policy*, vol. 18, no. 5, pp. 1256–1269. https://doi.org/10.1111/hex.12100

American Speech-Language-Hearing Association (ASHA) 1988, *Prevention of communication disorders*, Position Statement, viewed 25 October 2019, <www.asha.org/policy>.

Association of Faculties of Medicine of Canada – AFMC Primer 2013, *AFMC primer on population health: A virtual textbook on public health concepts for clinicians*, viewed 10 July 2019, <https://phprimer.afmc.ca/Part1-TheoryThinkingAboutHealth/Chapter4BasicConceptsInPreventionSurveillanceAndHealthPromotion/Thestagesofprevention>.

Avnstorp, MB, Homøe, P, Bjerregaard, P & Jensen, RG 2016, 'Chronic suppurative otitis media, middle ear pathology and corresponding hearing loss in a cohort of Greenlandic children', *International Journal of Pediatric Otorhinolaryngology*, vol. 83, pp. 148–153. https://doi.org/10.1016/j.ijporl.2016.01.017

Bankaitis, AE & Schountz, T 1998, 'HIV-related ototoxicity', *Seminars in Hearing*, vol. 19, pp. 155–163. https://doi.org/10.1055/s-0028-1082965

Borysiewicz, L 2009, 'Prevention is better than cure', *Clinical Medicine (London, England)*, vol. 9, no. 6, pp. 572–583. https://doi.org/10.7861/clinmedicine.9-6-572

Commission on the Social Determinants of Health (CSDH) 2008, *Closing the gap in a generation: Health equity through action on the social determinants of health: Final Report of the Commission on Social Determinants of Health*, World Health Organization, Geneva.

Dale, LM, Goudreau, S, Perron, S, Ragettli, MS, Hatzopoulou, M & Smargiassi, A 2015, 'Socioeconomic status and environmental noise exposure in Montreal, Canada', *BMC Public Health*, vol. 15, no. 1, a205. https://doi.org/10.1186/s12889-015-1571-2

DeAntonio, R, Yarzabal, JP, Cruz, JP, Schmidt, JE & Kleijnen, J 2016, 'Epidemiology of otitis media in children from developing countries: A systematic review', *International Journal of Pediatric Otorhinolaryngology*, vol. 85, pp. 65–74. https://doi.org/10.1016/j.ijporl.2016.03.032

Delatycki, MB 2012, 'The ethics of screening for disease', *Pathology*, vol. 44, no. 2, pp. 63–68. https://doi.org/10.1097/PAT.0b013e32834e8496

Ding, T, Yan, A & Liu, K 2019, 'What is noise-induced hearing loss?', *British Journal of Hospital Medicine*, vol. 80, no. 9, pp. 525–529. https://doi.org/10.12968/hmed.2019.80.9.525

Edwards, A, Khoza-Shangase, K & Moroe, NF 2020, 'Occupational hearing loss in Africa: An interdisciplinary view of the current status', *South African Journal of Communication Disorders*, vol. 67, no. 2, pp. 1–3. https://doi.org/10.4102/sajcd.v67i2.700

Ehn, M, Anderzén-Carlsson, A, Möller, C & Wahlqvist, M 2019, 'Life strategies of people with deafblindness due to Usher syndrome type 2a – A qualitative study', *International Journal of Qualitative Studies on Health and Well-Being*, vol. 14, no. 1, a1656790. https://doi.org/10.1080/17482631.2019.1656790

Fitzgibbons, J, Beswick, R & Driscoll, CJ 2021, 'Contextualisation of risk factors for hearing impairment', eds. K Khoza-Shangase & A Kanji, *Early detection and intervention in audiology: An African perspective*, Wits University Press, Johannesburg, pp. 89–116. https://doi.org/10.1080/14767058.2019.1658732

Gérvas, J, Starfield, B & Heath, I 2008, 'Is clinical prevention better than cure?', *The Lancet*, vol. 372, no. 9654, pp. 1997–1999. https://doi.org/10.1016/S0140-6736(08)61843-7

Getz, L, Sigurdsson, JA & Hetlevik, I 2003, 'Is opportunistic disease prevention in the consultation ethically justifiable?', *BMJ*, vol. 327, pp. 498–500. https://doi.org/10.1136/bmj.327.7413.498

Govender, M & Paken, J 2015, 'Practices employed by audiologists in the management of adult patients with multidrug-resistant tuberculosis in South Africa', *South African Family Practice*, vol. 57, pp. 363–372. https://doi.org/10.1080/20786190.2015.1085222

Guo, JJ, Pandey, S, Doyle, J, Bian, B, Lis, Y & Raisch, DW 2010, 'A review of quantitative risk-benefit methodologies for assessing drug safety and efficacy-report of the ISPOR risk-benefit management working group', *Value in Health: The Journal of the International Society for Pharmacoeconomics and Outcomes Research*, vol. 13, no. 5, pp. 657–666. https://doi.org/10.1111/j.1524-4733.2010.00725.x

Health Professions Council of South Africa (HPCSA) 2018, *Audiological management of patients on treatment that includes ototoxic medication: Guidelines*, viewed 10 March 2020, <https://www.hpcsa.co.za/Uploads/SLH/Guidelines%20for%20Audiological%20Management%20of%20Patients%20on%20Treatment%20that%20includes%20Ototoxic%20Medications.pdf>.

Kanji, A & Khoza-Shangase, K 2018, 'Objective hearing screening measures: An exploration of a suitable combination for risk-based newborn hearing screening', *Journal of the American Academy of Audiology*, vol. 29, no. 6, pp. 495–502. https://doi.org/10.3766/jaaa.16155

Kanji, A & Khoza-Shangase, K 2021, 'Risk factors for hearing impairment in neonates in South Africa: Scoping the context for newborn hearing screening planning', *The Journal of Maternal-Fetal & Neonatal Medicine*, vol. 34, no. 13, pp. 2107–2116. https://doi.org/10.1080/14767058.2019.1658732

Khoza-Shangase, K 2010, 'Is there a need for ototoxicity monitoring in patients with HIV/AIDS?', *African Journal of Pharmacy and Pharmacology*, vol. 4, no. 9, pp. 574–579.

Khoza-Shangase, K 2017, 'Risk versus benefit: Who assesses this in the management of patients on ototoxic drugs?', *Journal of Pharmacy and Bioallied Sciences*, vol. 9, no. 3, pp. 171–177. https://doi.org/10.4103/jpbs.JPBS_17_17

Khoza-Shangase, K 2020, 'Pharmaco-audiology vigilance in the treatment of adult patients with HIV/AIDS: Ototoxicity monitoring protocol recommendation', *Infectious Disorders-Drug Targets* (Formerly *Current Drug Targets-Infectious Disorders)*, vol. 20, no. 1, pp. 33–42. https://doi.org/10.2174/1871526518666181016102102

Khoza-Shangase, K 2021, 'Confronting realities to early hearing detection in South Africa', eds. K Khoza-Shangase & A Kanji, *Early detection and intervention in audiology: An African perspective*, Wits University Press, Johannesburg, pp. 66–88. https://doi.org/10.18772/22021026567

Khoza-Shangase, K & Kanji, A 2021, 'Best practice in South Africa for early hearing detection and intervention', eds. K Khoza-Shangase & A Kanji, *Early detection and intervention in audiology: An African perspective*, Wits University Press, Johannesburg, p. 264. https://doi.org/10.18772/22021026567

Khoza-Shangase, K, Lecheko, L & Ntlhakana, L 2020, 'The impact of medical interventions for reducing ototoxicity during treatment for multi-drug resistant tuberculosis', *Acta Otorrinolaringológica Española*, vol. 71, no. 6, pp. 349–357. https://doi.org/10.1016/j.otorri.2019.12.003

Khoza-Shangase, K & Masondo, N 2020, 'What are the current audiological practices for ototoxicity assessment and management in the South African healthcare context?', *International Journal of Environmental Research and Public Health*, vol. 17, no. 7, a2613. https://doi.org/10.3390/ijerph17072613

Khoza-Shangase, K & Moroe, NF 2020, 'Risk versus benefit: Should not audiologists assess this in the context of occupational noise-induced hearing loss in the mining industry?', *South African Journal of Communication Disorders*, vol. 67, no. 2, a671 pp. 1–9. https://doi.org/10.4102/sajcd.v67i2.671

Khoza-Shangase, K & Stirk, M 2016, 'Audiological testing for ototoxicity monitoring in adults with tuberculosis in state hospitals in Gauteng, South Africa', *Southern African Journal of Infectious Diseases*, vol. 1, no. 1, a89 pp. 1–6. https://doi.org/10.1080/23120053.2016.1128143

Kolo, ES, Salisu, AD, Yaro, AM & Nwaorgu, OGB 2012, 'Sensorineural hearing loss in patients with chronic suppurative otitis media', *Indian Journal of Otolaryngology Head & Neck Surgery*, vol. 64, no. 1, pp. 59–62. https://doi.org/10.1007/s12070-011-0251-5

Le, TN, Straatman, LV, Lea, J & Westerberg, B 2017, 'Current insights in noise-induced hearing loss: A literature review of the underlying mechanism, pathophysiology, asymmetry, and management options', *Journal of Otolaryngology - Head and Neck Surgery,* vol. 46, no. 1, pp. 1–15. https://doi.org/10.1186/s40463-017-0219-x

Lusk, SL, McCullagh, M, Dickson, VV & Xu, J 2016, 'Position statement: Harmful effects of environmental noise exposures', *Nursing Outlook*, vol. 64, no. 4, pp. 395–396. https://doi.org/10.1016/j.outlook.2016.06.001

Maluleke, NP, Khoza-Shangase, K & Kanji, A 2019, 'Communication and school readiness abilities of children with hearing impairment in South Africa: A retrospective review of early intervention preschool records', *South African Journal of Communication Disorders*, vol. 66, no. 1, pp. 1–7. https://doi.org/10.4102/sajcd.v66i1.60

Martins, C, Azevedo, LF, Ribeiro, O, Sá, L, Santos, P, Couto, L, Costa-Pereira, A & Hespanhol, AP 2013, 'A population-based nationwide cross-sectional study on preventive health services utilization in Portugal - What services (and frequencies) are deemed necessary by patients?', *PLoS One*, vol. 8, no. 11, a81256. https://doi.org/10.1371/journal.pone.0081256

Martin, WH, Sobel, J, Griest, SE, Howarth, L & Yongbing, SHI 2006, 'Noise-induced hearing loss in children: Preventing the silent epidemic', *Journal of Otology*, vol. 1, no. 1, pp. 11–21. https://doi.org/10.1016/S1672-2930(06)50002-9

Metidieri, MM, Rodrigues, HFS, Oliveira Filho, FJMBD, Ferraz, DP, Almeida Neto, AFD & Torres, S 2013, 'Noise-induced hearing loss (NIHL): Literature review with a focus on occupational medicine', *International Archives of Otorhinolaryngology*, vol. 17, pp. 208–212. https://doi.org/10.7162/S1809-97772013000200015

Minovi, A & Dazert, S 2014, 'Diseases of the middle ear in childhood', *GMS Current Topics in Otorhinolaryngology, Head and Neck Surgery*, vol. 13, a114. https://doi.org/10.3205/cto000114

Moeller, MP 2000, 'Early intervention and language development in children who are deaf and hard of hearing', *Pediatrics*, vol. 106, no. 3, a43. https://doi.org/10.1542/peds.106.3.e43

Moroe, NF 2020, 'Occupational noise-induced hearing loss in the mining sector of South Africa: Perspectives of occupational health practitioners on how mineworkers are trained', *South African Journal of Communication Disorders*, vol. 67, no. 2, pp. 1–6. https://doi.org/10.4102/sajcd.v67i2.676

Moroe, NF, Khoza-Shangase, K, Madahana, MCI & Nyandoro, OTC 2020, 'Feedback-based noise management matrix in action', *South African Journal of Communication Disorders*, vol. 67, no. 2, pp. 1–9. https://doi.org/10.4102/sajcd.v67i2.678

Moroe, N, Khoza-Shangase, K, Kanji, A & Ntlhakana, L 2018, 'The management of occupational noise-induced hearing loss in the mining sector in Africa: A systematic review - 1994 to 2016', *Noise & Vibration Worldwide*, vol. 49, no. 5, pp. 181–190. https://doi.org/10.1177/0957456518781860

Moynihan, R, Doust, J & Henry, D 2012, 'Preventing overdiagnosis: How to stop harming the healthy', *BMJ (Clinical Research Ed.)*, vol. 344, e3502. https://doi.org/10.1136/bmj.e3502

Nieman, CL, Reed, NS & Lin, FR 2018, 'Otolaryngology for the internist: Hearing loss', *Medical Clinics*, vol. 102, no. 6, pp. 977–992. https://doi.org/10.1016/j.mcna.2018.06.013

Ntlhakana, L, Khoza-Shangase, K & Nelson, G 2020a, 'Occupational noise-induced hearing loss in platinum miners: What do the data tell us?', *Occupational Health Southern Africa*, vol. 26, no. 1, pp. 8–14. https://doi.org/10.17159/2411-9717/1318/2021

Ntlhakana, L, Nelson, G & Khoza-Shangase, K 2020b, 'Estimating miners at risk for occupational noise-induced hearing loss: A review of data from a South African platinum mine', *South African Journal of Communication Disorders*, vol. 67, no. 2, pp. 1–8. https://doi.org/10.4102/sajcd.v67i2.677

Ntlhakana, L, Nelson, G, Khoza-Shangase, K & Dorkin, E 2022, 'Occupational hearing loss for platinum miners in South Africa: A case study of data-sharing practices and ethical challenges in the mining industry', *International Journal of Environmental Research and Public Health*, vol. 19, no. 1, p. 1. https://doi.org/10.3390/ijerph19010001

Olusanya, B & Newton, V 2007, 'Global burden of childhood hearing impairment and disease control priorities for developing countries', *The Lancet*, vol. 369, no. 9569, pp. 1314–1317. https://doi.org/10.1016/S0140-6736(07)60602-3

Olusanya, BO 2005, 'Can the world's infants with hearing loss wait?', *International Journal of Pediatric Otorhinolaryngology*, vol. 69, no. 6, pp. 735–738. https://doi.org/10.1016/j.ijporl.2005.03.024

Paken, J, Govender, CD, Pillay, M & Sewram, V 2016, 'Cisplatin-associated ototoxicity: A review for the health professional', *Journal of Toxicology*, vol. 2016, a1809394. https://doi.org/10.1155/2016/1809394

Pandve, H 2014, 'Changing concept of disease prevention: From primordial to quaternary', *Archives of Medicine and Health Sciences*, vol. 2, no. 2, pp. 254–256. https://doi.org/10.4103/2321-4848.144366

Rossetti, L 2004, *Communication intervention: Birth to three*, 2nd edn, Thomson Learning, s.l.

Sackett, DL 2002, 'The arrogance of preventive medicine', *Canadian Medical Association Journal*, vol. 167, pp. 363–364.

Sá, L, Ribeiro, O, Azevedo, LF, Couto, L, Costa-Pereira, A, Hespanhol, A, Santos, P & Martins, C 2016, 'Patients' estimations of the importance of preventive health services: A nationwide, population-based cross-sectional study in Portugal', *BMJ Open*, vol. 6, no. 10, a011755. https://doi.org/10.1136/bmjopen-2016-011755

Sebothoma, B & Khoza-Shangase, K 2018, 'A comparison between video otoscopy and standard tympanometry findings in adults living with human immunodeficiency virus (HIV) in South Africa', *South African Journal of Communication Disorders*, vol. 65, no. 1, pp. 1–7. https://doi.org/10.4102/sajcd.v65i1.591

Sebothoma, B & Khoza-Shangase, K 2020, 'Middle ear pathologies in adults living with human immunodeficiency virus: A systematic review', *Annals of Otology, Rhinology & Laryngology*, vol. 129, no. 8, pp. 821–828. https://doi.org/10.1177/0003489420909847

Sebothoma, B, Khoza-Shangase, K, Mol, D & Masege, D 2021, 'The sensitivity and specificity of wideband absorbance measure in identifying pathologic middle ears in adults living with HIV', *South African Journal of Communication Disorders*, vol. 68, no. 1, pp. 1–7. https://doi.org/10.4102/sajcd.v68i1.820

Sharma, N, Jaiswal, AA, Banerjee, PK & Garg, AK 2015, 'Complications of chronic suppurative otitis media and their management: A single institution 12 years' experience', *Indian Journal of Otolaryngology and Head & Neck Surgery*, vol. 67, no. 4, pp. 353–360. https://doi.org/10.1007/s12070-015-0836-5

Shickle, D & Chadwick, R 1994, 'The ethics of screening: Is "screeningitis" an incurable disease?', *Journal of Medical Ethics*, vol. 20, no. 1, pp. 12–18. https://doi.org/10.1136/jme.20.1.12

Stucki, G, Cieza, A & Melvin, J 2007, 'The international classification of functioning, disability and health: A unifying model for the conceptual description of the rehabilitation strategy', *Journal of Rehabilitation Medicine*, vol. 39, no. 4, pp. 279–285. https://doi.org/10.2340/16501977-0041

Thorne, PR 2006, *Best practice in noise-induced hearing loss management and prevention: A review of literature, practices and policies for the New Zealand context*, viewed 17 August 2020, <https://dspace.nal.gov.au/xmlui/bitstream/handle/123456789/481/Best%20practice%20in%20noise%20%20induced%20hearing%20loss%20management%20and%20prevention.pdf?sequence=1&isAllowed=y>.

Thorne, PR, Ameratunga, SN, Stewart, J, Reid, N, Williams, W, Purdy, SC, Dodd, G & Wallaart, J 2008, 'Epidemiology of noise-induced hearing loss in New Zealand', *The New Zealand Medical Journal*, vol. 121, no. 1280, pp. 33–44.

Tshifularo, M, Govender, L & Monama, G 2013, 'Otolaryngological and head and neck manifestations in HIV-infected patients seen at Steve Biko Academic Hospital in Pretoria, South Africa', *South African Medical Journal*, vol. 103, no. 7, pp. 464–466. https://doi.org/10.7196/SAMJ.6786

Tsintis, P & La Mache, E 2004, 'CIOMS and ICH initiatives in pharmacovigilance and risk management: Overview and implications', *Drug Safety*, vol. 27, no. 8, pp. 509–517. https://doi.org/10.2165/00002018-200427080-00004

Vajpayee, M, Negi, N & Kurapati, S 2013, 'The enduring tale of T cells in HIV immunopathogenesis', *Indian Journal of Medical Research*, vol. 138, no. 5, pp. 682–699.

Villa, PC & Zanchetta, S 2014, 'Auditory temporal abilities in children with history of recurrent otitis media in the first years of life and persistent in preschool and school ages', *CoDAS*, vol. 26, no. 6, pp. 494–502. https://doi.org/10.1590/2317-1782/20142014008

Wilson, JMG & Jungner, G 1968, *Principles and practice of screening for disease*, viewed 03 February 2020, <https://www.who.int/ionizing_radiation/medical_radiation_exposure/munich-WHO-1968-Screening-Disease.pdf?ua=1>.

Woolf, SH & Stange, KC 2006, 'A sense of priorities for the healthcare commons', *American Journal of Preventive Medicine*, vol. 31, no. 1, pp. 99–102. https://doi.org/10.1016/j.amepre.2006.03.010

World Health Organization (WHO) 2014, *The case for investing in public health*, World Health Organization, Geneva.

World Health Organization (WHO) 2018a, *Prevention of blindness and deafness*, World Health Organization, Geneva.

World Health Organization (WHO) 2018b, *Addressing the rising prevalence of hearing loss*, World Health Organization, Geneva.

World Health Organization (WHO) 2020, *Health promotion and disease prevention through population-based interventions, including action to address social determinants and health inequity*, World Health Organization, Geneva.

World Health Organization (WHO) 2021, *Hearing screening: Considerations for implementation*, World Health Organization, Geneva.

Yongbing, S & Martin, W 2013, 'Noise-induced hearing loss in China: A potentially costly public health issue', *Journal of Otology*, vol. 8, no. 1, pp. 51–56. https://doi.org/10.1016/S1672-2930(13)50007-9

Yoshinaga-Itano, C 2004, 'Levels of evidence: Universal newborn hearing screening (UNHS) and early hearing detection and intervention systems (EHDI)', *Journal of Communication Disorders*, vol. 37, no. 5, pp. 451–465. https://doi.org/10.1016/j.jcomdis.2004.04.008

Zaman, K & Al Mamun, KA 2017, 'An evaluation of smartphone apps for preventive healthcare focusing on cardiovascular disease', *2017 4th International conference on advances in electrical engineering (ICAEE)*, Dhaka, Bangladesh, September 28–30, pp. 531–536.

Chapter 2

American Academy of Audiology 2008, *The use of telehealth/telemedicine to provide audiology services*, viewed 15 March 2019, <http://audiology-web.s3.amazonaws.com/migrated/TelehealthResolution200806.pdf_5386d9f33fd359.83214228.pdf>

American Speech-Language-Hearing Association 2005, *Audiologists providing clinical services via telepractice: Technical report*, viewed n.d., <https://www.asha.org/policy/TR2005-00149.htm>

Aron, ML 1984, 'An introduction', eds. ML Aron & L Le Roux, *Proceedings of the SASLHA conference on community work*, Johannesburg, South Africa, September, 1984, n.p.

Aron, ML 1986, 'A review report of the Diploma in Speech and Hearing Therapy (Community Work)', unpublished mimeograph, University of the Witwatersrand, Johannesburg.

Aron, ML 1987, 'Community-based rehabilitation for communication disorders', *Unpublished paper presented at SASLHA's National Conference*, September, Johannesburg.

Aron, ML 1989, 'Implementation of community speech and hearing work in disadvantaged areas', *Unpublished paper presented at the 21st Congress of the International Association of Logopaedics and Phoniatrics*, Prague, August.

Baine, SO, Kasangaki, A & Baine, E 2018, 'Task shifting in health service delivery from a decision and policy makers' perspective: A case of Uganda', *Human Resources for Health*, vol. 16, no. 1, p. 20. https://doi.org/10.1186/s12960-018-0282-z

Benson, N 2020, 'Teleaudiology amid COVID-19: Optimizing available equipment', *The Hearing Journal*, vol. 73, no. 10, pp. 10–13. https://doi.org/10.1097/01.HJ.0000719784.51319.87

Biagio, L, Swanepoel, DW, Adeyemo, A, Hall, JW & Vinck, B 2013, 'Asynchronous video-otoscopy with a telehealth facilitator', *Telemedicine and e-Health*, vol. 19, no. 4, pp. 252–258. https://doi.org/10.1089/tmj.2012.0161

Biagio, L, Swanepoel, DW, Laurent, C & Lundberg, T 2014, 'Video-otoscopy recordings for diagnosis of childhood ear disease using telehealth at primary health care level', *Journal of Telemedicine and Telecare*, vol. 20, no. 6, pp. 300–306.

Blecher, M, Daven, J, Kollipara, A, Maharaj, Y, Mansvelder, A & Gaarekwe, A 2017, 'Health spending at a time of low economic growth and fiscal constraint', *South African Health Review*, vol. 2017, no. 1, pp. 25–39.

Bolton, P 2019, 'Global mental health and psychotherapy: Importance of task-shifting and a systematic approach to adaptation', eds. DJ Stein, JK Bass & SG Hofmann, *Global mental health and psychotherapy: Adapting psychotherapy for low-and-middle-income countries*, Academic Press, Washington, DC, pp. 11–24.

Carter, L, Horrigan, J & Hudyma, S 2010, 'Investigating the educational needs of nurses in telepractice: A descriptive exploratory study', *Canadian Journal of University Continuing Education*, vol. 36, no. 1, pp. 1–20. https://doi.org/10.21225/D5RP4B

Christopher, N, Edward, T, Sabrina, BK & Agnes, N 2013, 'The prevalence of hearing impairment in the 6 months – 5 years HIV/AIDS-positive patients attending paediatric infectious disease clinic at Mulago Hospital', *International Journal of Pediatric Otorhinolaryngology*, vol. 77, no. 2, pp. 262–265. https://doi.org/10.1016/j.ijporl.2012.11.013

Coco, L 2020, 'Teleaudiology: Strategies, considerations during a crisis and beyond', *The Hearing Journal*, vol. 73, no. 5, pp. 26–28. https://doi.org/10.1097/01.HJ.0000666404.42257.97

Dawood, N, Mahomed Asmail, F, Louw, C & Swanepoel, DW 2020, 'mHealth hearing screening for children by non-specialist health workers in communities', *International Journal of Audiology*, vol. 60, suppl. 1, pp. 23–29. https://doi.org/10.1080/14992027.2020.1829719

Edirippulige, S, Armfield, NR & Smith, AC 2012, 'A qualitative study of the careers and professional practices of graduates from an e-health postgraduate programme', *Journal of Telemedicine and Telecare*, vol. 18, no. 8, pp. 455–459. https://doi.org/10.1258/jtt.2012.gth107

Fabry, D 2010, 'Applications of telehealth for hearing care', *Audiology Today*, vol. 6, pp. 18–24.

Fagan, JJ & Jacobs, M 2009, 'Survey of ENT services in Africa: Need for a comprehensive intervention', *Global Health Action*, vol. 2, no. 1, pp. 1–7. https://doi.org/10.3402/gha.v2i0.1932

Farmer, P, Frenk, J, Knaul, FM, Shulman, LN, Alleyne, G, Armstrong, L, Atun, R, Blayney, D, Chen, L, Feachem, R, Gospodarowicz, M, Gralow, J, Gupta, S, Langer, A, Lob-Levyt, J, Neal, C, Mbewu, A, Mired, D, Piot, P, Reddy, KS, Sachs, JD, Sarhan, M & Seffrin, JR 2010, 'Expansion of cancer care and control in countries of low and middle income: A call to action', *The Lancet*, vol. 376, no. 9747, pp. 1186–1193. https://doi.org/10.1016/S0140-6736(10)61152-X

Fitzgibbons, J, Beswick, R & Driscoll, CJ 2021, 'Contextualisation of risk factors for hearing impairment', eds. K Khoza-Shangase & A Kanji. *Early detection and intervention in audiology: An African perspective*, Wits University Press, Johannesburg, p. 89. https://doi.org/10.18772/22021026567

Flood, D & Rohloff, P 2018, 'Indigenous languages and global health: Comment', *The Lancet*, vol. 6, no. 2, pp. 134–135. https://doi.org/10.1016/S2214-109X(17)30493-X

Folmer, RL, Saunders, GH, Dann, SM, Griest, SE, Porsov, E, Fausti, SA & Leek MR 2012, 'Guest editorial: Computer-based hearing loss prevention education program for veterans and military personnel', *Journal of Rehabilitation Research and Development*, vol. 49, no. 4, pp. vii–xvi. https://doi.org/10.1682/jrrd.2012.02.0028

Fulton, BD, Scheffler, RM, Sparkes, SP, Auh, EY, Vujicic, M & Soucat, A 2011, 'Health workforce skill mix and task shifting in low-income countries: A review of recent evidence', *Human Resources for Health*, vol. 9, no. 1, pp. 1–11. https://doi.org/10.1186/1478-4491-9-1

Ghebreyesus, TA 2017, 'All roads lead to universal health coverage', *The Lancet Global Health*, vol. 5, no. 9, pp. 839–840. https://doi.org/10.1016/S2214-109X(17)30295-4

Gordon, T, Booysen, F & Mbonigaba, J 2020, 'Socio-economic inequalities in the multiple dimensions of access to healthcare: The case of South Africa', *BMC Public Health*, vol. 20, no. 1, pp. 1–13. https://doi.org/10.1186/s12889-020-8368-7

Govender, SM & Mars, M 2018, 'The perspectives of South African academics within the disciplines of health sciences regarding telehealth and its potential inclusion in student training', *African Journal of Health Professions Education*, vol. 10, no. 1, pp. 38–43. https://doi.org/10.7196/AJHPE.2018.v10i1.957

Grogan-Johnson, S, Meehan, R, McCormick, K & Miller, N 2015, 'Results of a national survey of preservice telepractice training in graduate speech-language pathology and audiology programs', *Contemporary Issues in Communication Science and Disorders*, vol. 42, pp. 122–137. https://doi.org/10.1044/cicsd_42_S_122

Grol, R & Grimshaw, J 2003, 'From best evidence to best practice: Effective implementation of change in patient care', *The Lancet*, vol. 362, no. 9391, pp. 1225–1230.

Hayes, D 2012, 'Infant diagnostic evaluation using tele-audiology', *Hearing Review*, vol. 19, no. 10, pp. 30–31.

Hughes, ML, Sevier, JD & Choi, S 2018, 'Techniques for remotely programming children with cochlear implants using pediatric audiological methods via telepractice', *American Journal of Audiology*, vol. 27, no. 3s, pp. 385–390. https://doi.org/10.1044/2018_AJA-IMIA3-18-0002

Hussein, SY, Swanepoel, DW, Mahomed, F & Biagio de Jager, L 2018, 'Community-based hearing screening for young children using an mHealth service-delivery model', *Global Health Action*, vol. 11, no. 1, a1467077. https://doi.org/10.1080/16549716.2018.1467077

Kanji, A & Khoza-Shangase, K 2019, 'Early detection of hearing impairment in high-risk neonates: Let's talk about the high-risk registry in the South African context', *South African Journal of Child Health*, vol. 13, no. 2, pp. 53–55. https://doi.org/10.7196/SAJCH.2019.v13i2.1675

Keeton, C 2010, 'Bridging the gap in South Africa', *Bulletin of the World Health Organization*, vol. 88, no. 11, pp. 803–804. https://doi.org/10.2471/BLT.10.021110

Khan, NB, Joseph, L & Adhikari, M 2018, 'The hearing screening experiences and practices of primary health care nurses: Indications for referral-based on high-risk factors and community views about hearing loss', *African Journal of Primary Health Care and Family Medicine*, vol. 10, no. 1, pp. 1–11. https://doi.org/10.4102/phcfm.v10i1.1848

Khoza-Shangase, K 2010, 'Is there a need for ototoxicity monitoring in patients with HIV/AIDS?', *African Journal of Pharmacy and Pharmacology*, vol. 4, no. 9, pp. 574–579.

Khoza-Shangase, K 2013, 'Ototoxicity in tuberculosis treatment in South Africa: Views from healthcare workers involved in the management of TB', *African Journal of Pharmacy and Pharmacology*, vol. 7, no. 30, pp. 2141–2145. https://doi.org/10.5897/AJPP12.722

Khoza-Shangase, K 2017, 'Risk versus benefit: who assesses this in the management of patients on ototoxic drugs?', *Journal of Pharmacy and BioAllied Sciences*, vol. 9, no. 3, pp. 171–177. https://doi.org/10.4103/jpbs.JPBS_17_17

Khoza-Shangase, K 2019, 'Early hearing detection and intervention in South Africa: Exploring factors compromising service delivery as expressed by caregivers', *International Journal of Pediatric Otorhinolaryngology*, vol. 118, pp. 73–78.

Khoza-Shangase, K 2020a, 'Pharmaco-audiology vigilance in the treatment of adult patients with HIV/AIDS: Ototoxicity monitoring protocol recommendation', *Infectious Disorders-Drug Targets (Formerly Current Drug Targets-Infectious Disorders)*, vol. 20, no. 1, pp. 33–42. https://doi.org/10.2174/1871526518666181016102102

Khoza-Shangase, K 2020b, *HPCSA news bulletin*, viewed 10 December 2020, <https://www.hpcsa.co.za/Uploads/SLH/Newsletter/SLH_newsletter_2020.pdf>.

Khoza-Shangase, K 2022, 'In pursuit of increasing the application of tele-audiology in South Africa: COVID-19 puts on the alert for patient site facilitator training', *South African Journal of Communication Disorders*, vol. 69, no. 2, a900. https://doi.org/10.4102/sajcd.v69i2.900

Khoza-Shangase, K, Kanji, A, Petrocchi-Bartal, L & Farr, K 2017, 'Infant hearing screening from a developing country context: Status from two South African provinces', *South African Journal of Child Health*, vol. 11, no. 4, pp. 159–163. https://doi.org/1010.7196/sajch.2017.v11i4.1267

Khoza-Shangase, K & Mophosho, M 2018, 'Language and culture in speech-language and hearing professions in South Africa: The dangers of a single story', *South African Journal of Communication Disorders*, vol. 65, no. 1, pp. 1–7. https://doi.org/10.4102/sajcd.v65i1.594

Khoza-Shangase, K & Mophosho, M 2021, 'Language and culture in speech-language and hearing professions in South Africa: Re-imagining practice', *South African Journal of Communication Disorders*, vol. 68, no. 1, a793. https://doi.org/10.4102/sajcd.v68i1.793

Khoza-Shangase, K & Moroe, N 2020, 'South African hearing conservation programmes in the context of tele-audiology: A scoping review', *South African Journal of Communication Disorders*, vol. 67, no. 2, a670. https://doi.org/10.4102/sajcd.v67i2.670

Khoza-Shangase, K, Moroe, N & Neille, J 2021a, 'Speech-language pathology and audiology in South Africa: Clinical training and service in the era of COVID-19', *International Journal of Telerehabilitation*, vol. 13, no. 1, n.p. https://doi.org/10.5195/ijt.2021.6376

Khoza-Shangase, K, Sebothoma, B & Moroe, NF 2021b, 'Teleaudiology as part of efforts to enhance inclusivity and equality through ICT in South African schools: Some considerations', eds. M Maguvhe, RS Mphahlele & S Moonsamy, *Empowering students and maximising inclusiveness and equality through ICT*, Brill Sense, Boston, pp. 223–243.

Khoza-Shangase, K & Stirk, M 2016, 'Audiological testing for ototoxicity monitoring in adults with tuberculosis in state hospitals in Gauteng, South Africa', *Southern African Journal of Infectious Diseases*, vol. 31, no. 2, pp. 44–49. https://doi.org/10.1080/23120053.2016.1128143

Krumm, M & Syms, M.J 2011, 'Teleaudiology', *Otolaryngologic Clinics of North America*, vol. 44, no. 6, pp. 1297–1304. https://doi.org/10.1016/j.otc.2011.08.006

Krumm, M & Vento, BA 2013, 'Applications in teleaudiology', in S Kumar & E Cohn, *Telerehabilitation: Health informatics*, Springer, London, pp. 125–138. https://doi.org/10.1007/978-1-4471-4198-3_9

Krupinski, E 2015, 'Innovations and possibilities in connected health', *Journal of American Academy of Audiology*, vol. 26, no. 9, pp. 761–767. https://doi.org/10.3766/jaaa.14047

Lehmann, U, Van Damme, W, Barten, F & Sanders, D 2009, 'Task shifting: The answer to the human resources crisis in Africa?', *Human Resources for Health*, vol. 7, no. 1, pp. 1–4. https://doi.org/10.1186/1478-4491-7-49

Magidson, JF, Gouse, H, Psaros, C, Remmert, JE, O'Cleirigh, C & Safren, SA 2017, 'Task shifting and delivery of behavioral medicine interventions in resource-poor global settings: HIV/AIDS treatment in sub-Saharan Africa', in A-M Vranceanu, JA Greer & SA Safren, *The Massachusetts General Hospital handbook of behavioral medicine*, Humana Press, Cham, pp. 297–320.

Mahlathi, P & Dlamini, J 2015, *Minimum data sets for human resources for health and the surgical workforce in South Africa's health system: A rapid analysis of stock and migration*, viewed n.d., <https://www.who.int/workforcealliance/031616south_africa_case_studiesweb.pdf>

Mhlanga, D & Garidzirai, R 2020, 'The influence of racial differences in the demand for healthcare in South Africa: A case of public healthcare', *International Journal of Environmental Research and Public Health*, vol. 17, no. 14, p. 5043. https://doi.org/10.3390/ijerph17145043

Mulwafu, W, Ensink, R, Kuper, H & Fagan, J 2017, 'Survey of ENT services in sub-Saharan Africa: Little progress between 2009 and 2015', *Global Health Action*, vol. 10, no. 1, a1289736. https://doi.org/10.1080/16549716.2017.1289736

Mulwafu, W, Kuper, H & Ensink, RJH 2016, 'Prevalence and causes of hearing impairment in Africa', *Tropical Medicine & International Health*, vol. 21, no. 2, pp. 158–165. https://doi.org/10.1111/tmi.12640

Mundeva, H, Snyder, J, Ngilangwa, DP & Kaida, A 2018, 'Ethics of task shifting in the health workforce: Exploring the role of community health workers in HIV service delivery in low-and middle-income countries', *BMC Medical Ethics*, vol. 19, no. 1, pp. 1–11. https://doi.org/10.1186/s12910-018-0312-3

Naidoo, S 2012, 'The South African National Health Insurance: A revolution in health care delivery', *Journal of Public Health*, vol. 34, no. 1, pp. 149–150. https://doi.org/10.1093/pubmed/fds008

National Academies of Sciences Engineering and Medicine 2016, *Hearing health care for adults: Priorities for improving access and affordability*, viewed 05 February 2020, <https://www.nap.edu/catalog/23446/hearing-health-care-for-adults-priorities-for-improving-access-and>

National Department of Health 2012, *eHealth strategy for South Africa (2012–2016)*, Department of Health, Pretoria.

National Department of Health 2019, *National digital health strategy for South Africa (2019–2024)*, viewed 05 February 2020, <https://drive.google.com/file/d/1BZd1srARhDyaeajzpVThlF2bNE1J6f5J/view>

National Health Insurance Bill 2019, *National Health Insurance Bill*, viewed 13 December 2019, <https://www.gov.za/sites/default/files/gcis_document/201908/national-health-insurance-bill-b-11-2019.pdf>

Naudé, A & Bornman, J 2021, 'Ethical considerations and tele-audiology in early hearing detection and intervention', eds. K Khoza-Shangase & A Kanji, *Early detection and intervention in audiology*, Wits University Press, Johannesburg, p. 243.

Ntlhakana, L, Kanji, A & Khoza-Shangase, K 2015, 'The use of hearing protection devices in South Africa: Exploring the current status in gold and non-ferrous mines', *Occupational Health Southern Africa*, vol. 21, no. 2, pp. 10–15.

Nyasulu, J & Pandya, H 2020, 'The effects of coronavirus disease 2019 pandemic on the South African health system: A call to maintain essential health services', *African Journal of Primary Health Care and Family Medicine*, vol. 12, no. 1, a2480. https://doi.org/10.4102/phcfm.v12i1.2480

O'Donovan, J, Verkerk, M, Winters, N, Chadha, S & Bhutta, MF 2019, 'The role of community health workers in addressing the global burden of ear disease and hearing loss: A systematic scoping review of the literature', *BMJ Global Health*, vol. 4, no. 2, a001141. https://doi.org/10.1136/bmjgh-2018-001141

Olusanya, BO, Neumann, KJ & Saunders, JE 2014, 'The global burden of disabling hearing impairment: A call to action', *Bulletin World Health Organization*, vol. 92, no. 5, pp. 367–373. https://doi.org/10.2471/BLT.13.128728

Olusanya, BO, Okolo, AA & Adeosun, AA 2004, 'Predictors of hearing loss in school entrants in a developing country', *Journal of Postgraduate Medicine*, vol. 50, no. 3, p. 173.

Oosthuizen, M & Ehlers, VJ 2007, 'Factors that may influence South African nurses' decision to emigrate', *Health Gesonheid*, vol. 12, no. 12, pp. 14–26. https://doi.org/10.4102/hsag.v12i2.246

Pillay, M, Tiwari, R, Kathard, H & Chikte, U 2020, 'Sustainable workforce: South African audiologists and speech therapists', *Human Resource for Health*, vol. 18, no. 47, pp. 1–13. https://doi.org/10.1186/s12960-020-00488-6

Potgieter, JM, Swanepoel, DW & Smits, C 2018, 'Evaluating a smartphone digits-in-noise test as part of the audiometric test battery', *South African Journal of Communication Disorders*, vol. 65, no. 1, a574. https://doi.org/10.4102/sajcd.v65i1.574

Ramkumar, V, John, KR, Selvakumar, K, Vanaja, CS, Nagarajan, R & Hall, JW 2018, 'Cost and outcome of a community-based paediatric hearing screening programme in rural India with application of tele-audiology for follow-up diagnostic hearing assessment', *International Journal of Audiology*, vol. 57, no. 6, pp. 407–414. https://doi.org/10.1080/14992027.2018.1442592

Sandström, J, Swanepoel, DW, Laurent, C, Umefjord, G & Lundberg, T 2020, 'Accuracy and reliability of smartphone self-test audiometry in community clinics in low-income settings: A comparative study', *Annals of Otology, Rhinology & Laryngology*, vol. 129, no. 6, pp. 578–584. https://doi.org/10.1177/0003489420902162

Saunders, GH & Griest, SE 2009, 'Hearing loss in veterans and the need for hearing loss prevention programs', *Noise Health*, vol. 11, no. 42, pp. 14–21. https://doi.org/10.4103/1463-1741.45308

Schweitzer, C, Mortz, M & Vaughan, N 1999, 'Perhaps not by prescription, but by perception', *High Performance Hearing Solutions*, vol. 3, pp. 58–62.

Sebothoma, B 2020, 'Middle ear pathologies in adults within the mining industry: A systematic review', *South African Journal of Communication Disorders*, vol. 67, no. 2, pp. 1–5. https://doi.org/10.4102/sajcd.v67i2.679

Sebothoma, B, Khoza-Shangase, K, Masege, D & Mol, D 2021, 'The use of tele practice in assessment of middle ear function in adults living with HIV during the COVID-19 pandemic', *Indian Journal of Otolaryngology and Head & Neck Surgery*, n.v., pp. 1–8. https://doi.org/10.1007/s12070-021-02836-x

Siegfried, N, Wilkinson, T & Hofman, K 2017, 'Where from and where to for health technology assessment in South Africa? A legal and policy landscape analysis', *South African Health Review*, vol. 2017, no. 1, pp. 42–48.

State of the Nation Address (SONA) 2020, *President Cyril Ramaphosa: 2020 State of the Nation Address*, viewed 25 February 2020, <https://www.gov.za/speeches/president-cyril-ramaphosa-2020-state-nation-address-13-feb-2020-0000>

Statistics South Africa (StatsSA) 2018, *General Household Survey*, pp. 56–58, viewed 30 May 2019, <https://www.moonstone.co.za/upmedia/uploads/library/Moonstone%20Library/MS%20Industry%20News/General_Household_Survey_Telecommunications.pdf>

Statistics South Africa (StatsSA) 2019, *Mid-year population estimates: 2019*, viewed 25 February 2020, <https://www.statssa.gov.za/publications/P0302/P03022019.pdf>

Steuerwald, W, Windmill, I, Scott, M, Evans, T & Kramer, K 2018, 'Stories from the webcams: Cincinnati children's hospital medical center audiology telehealth and pediatric auditory device services', *American Journal of Audiology*, vol. 27, no. 3S, pp. 391–402.

Suen, JJ, Bhatnagar, K, Emmett, SD, Marrone, N, Kleindienst Robler, S, Swanepoel, W, Wong, A & Nieman, CL 2019, 'Hearing care across the life course provided in the community', *Bulletin of the World Health Organization*, vol. 97, no. 10, pp. 681–690. https://doi.org/10.2471/BLT.18.227371

Swanepoel, DW, Clark, JL, Koekemoer, D, Hall, JW, Krumm, M & Ferrari, DV 2010, 'Telehealth in audiology: The need and potential to reach underserved communities', *International Journal of Audiology*, vol. 49, no. 3, pp. 195–202. https://doi.org/10.3109/14992020903470783

Swanepoel, DW, Myburgh, HC, Howe, DM, Mahomed, F & Eikelboom, RH 2014, 'Smartphone hearing screening with integrated quality control and data management', *International Journal of Audiology*, vol. 53, no. 12, pp. 841–849.

The Lancet Editorial 2016, 'Hearing loss: An important global health concern', *The Lancet*, vol. 387, no. 10036, p. 2351. https://doi.org/10.1016/S0140-6736(16)30777-2

Tshifularo, M, Govender, L & Monama, G 2013, 'Otolaryngological, head and neck manifestations in HIV-infected patients seen at Steve Biko Academic Hospital in Pretoria, South Africa', *South African Medical Journal*, vol. 103, no. 7, pp. 464–466. https://doi.org/10.7196/SAMJ.6786

Tshule, MMN 1994, 'The diploma in community speech and hearing therapy: Students and staff experiences', viewed 25 July 2021, <https://hdl.handle.net/10539/27355>

Van Wyk, T, Mahomed-Asmail, F & Swanepoel, DW 2019, 'Supporting hearing health in vulnerable populations through community care workers using mHealth technologies', *International Journal of Audiology*, vol. 58, no. 11, pp. 790–797. https://doi.org/10.1080/14992027.2019.1649478

Wallace, P 2020, *The price SA will pay for being downgraded to junk: What the loss of the last investment-grade rating means to the country*, viewed 15 March 2021, <https://www.businesslive.co.za/bd/economy/2020-03-31-the-price-sa-will-pay-for-being-downgraded-to-junk/>

Wasserman, H 2020, *South Africa is 'Junk' – Here's what that means to you*, viewed 15 March 2021, <https://www.businessinsider.co.za/south-africa-is-junk-heres-what-that-means-to-you-2020-3>

Wonkam Tingang, E, Noubiap, JJ, Fokouo, JVF, Oluwole, OG, Nguefack, S, Chimusa, ER & Wonkam, A 2020, 'Hearing impairment overview in Africa: The case of Cameroon', *Genes*, vol. 11, no. 2, a233. https://doi.org/10.3390/genes11020233

World Health Organization (WHO) 2008, *Task shifting: Rational redistribution of tasks among health workforce teams: Global recommendations and guidelines*, World Health Organization, Geneva.

World Health Organization (WHO) 2015, *Hearing loss due to recreational exposure to loud sounds: A review*, World Health Organization, Geneva.

World Health Organization (WHO) 2017, *Global health workforce shortage to reach 12.9 million in coming decades*, World Health Organization, Geneva.

World Health Organization (WHO) 2018, *Prevention of blindness and deafness*, World Health Organization, Geneva.

Chapter 3

Adedayo, O & Olawale, O 2014, 'Fighting hearing loss in children – A clarion call', *World Journal of Medical Sciences*, vol. 11 no. 1, pp. 14–21. https://doi.org/10.5829/idosi.wjms.2014.11.1.81172

Adedeji, TO, Tobih, JE, Sogebi, OA & Daniel, AD 2015, 'Management challenges of congenital & early onset childhood hearing loss in a sub-Saharan African country', *The International Journal of Pediatric Otorhinolaryngology*, vol. 79, no. 10, pp. 1625–1629. https://doi.org/10.1016/j.ijporl.2015.06.003

Al-Rowaily, MA, Al-Fayez, AI, Al-Jomiey, MS, Al-Badr, AM & Abolfotouh, MA 2012, 'Hearing impairments among Saudi preschool children', *International Journal of Pediatric Otorhinolaryngology*, vol. 76, no. 11, pp. 1674–1677. https://doi.org/10.1016/j.ijporl.2012.08.004

American Medical Association (AMA) 2014, *Proceedings of the 2014 Annual Meeting of the House of Delegates*, viewed 10 February 2017, <https://www.ama-assn.org/house-delegates/annual-meeting/proceedings-2014-annual-meeting-house-delegates>

American Medical Association (AMA) 2014, *Proceedings of the 2016 Annual Meeting of the House of Delegates*, viewed 10 February 2017, <https://www.ama-assn.org/house-delegates/annual-meeting/proceedings-2016-annual-meeting-house-delegates>

American Medical Association (AMA) 2016, *Coverage of and payment for telemedicine*, Report No. CMS Report7-A-14, viewed 15 April 2019, <https://www.americantelemed.org>

Bess, FH & Tharpe, AM 2008, 'Case history data on unilaterally hearing-impaired children', *Ear and Hearing*, vol. 7, no. 1, pp. 14–19. https://doi.org/10.1097/00003446-198602000-00004

Biehl, J & Petryna, A (eds.) 2013, *When people come first: critical studies in global health*, Princeton University Press, Princeton, NJ.

Bigna, JJ & Noubiap, JJ 2019, 'The rising burden of non-communicable diseases in sub-Saharan Africa', *The Lancet Global Health*, vol. 7, no. 10, pp. e1295–e1296. https://doi.org/10.1016/S2214-109X(19)30370-5

Birkeland, AC & Lesperance, MM 2016, 'Clinical challenges in diagnosing the genetics etiology of hearing loss', in B Vona & T Haaf, *Genetic of deafness*, Karger, Paris, pp. 40–55.

Botasso, M, Sanches, SGG, Bento, RF & Samelli, AG 2015, 'Teleaudiometry as a screening method in school children', *Clinics*, vol. 70, pp. 283–288. https://doi.org/10.6061/clinics/2015(04)11

Bradford, NK, Caffery, LJ & Smith, AC 2015, 'Awareness, experiences and perceptions of telehealth in a rural Queensland community', *BMC Health Services Research*, vol. 15, no. 1, pp. 1–10. https://doi.org/10.1186/s12913-015-1094-7

Brennan-Jones, CG, Eikelboom, RH & Swanepoel, DW 2017, 'Diagnosis of hearing loss using automated audiometry in an asynchronous telehealth model: A pilot accuracy study', *Journal of Telemedicine and Telecare*, vol. 23, no. 2, pp. 256–262. https://doi.org/10.1177/1357633X16641552

Bush, ML, Kaufman, MR & McNulty, BN 2017, 'Disparities in access to pediatric hearing healthcare', *Current Opinion in Otolaryngology & Head and Neck Surgery*, vol. 25, no. 5, pp. 359–364. https://doi.org/10.1097/MOO.0000000000000388

Butler, I 2012, 'Identification and management of childhood hearing loss', *CME: Your SA Journal of CPD*, vol. 30, no. 9, pp. 314–317.

Cason, J & Cohn, ER 2014, 'Telepractice: An overview and best practices', *Perspectives on Augmentative and Alternative Communication*, vol. 23, no. 1, pp. 4–17. https://doi.org/10.1044/aac23.1.4

Centre for Development and Enterprise 2011, *Informing South African Policy: Reforming Healthcare in South Africa*, viewed 20 April 2019, <http://www.cde.org.za/wp-content/uploads/2012/12/REFORMING%20HEALTHCARE%20IN%20SA%20full%20report.pdf>

Ching, TY, Dillon, H, Button, L, Seeto, M, Van Buynder, P, Marnane, V, Cupples, L & Leigh, G 2017, 'Age at intervention for permanent hearing loss and 5-year language outcomes', *Pediatrics*, vol. 140, no. 3, a20164274. https://doi.org/10.1542/peds.2016-4274

Chukwudozie, A 2015, 'Inequalities in health: The role of health insurance in Nigeria', *Journal of Public Health in Africa*, vol. 6, no. 1, a512. https://doi.org/10.4081/jphia.2015.512

Chu, YC, Cheng, YF, Lai, YH, Tsao, Y, Tu, TY, Young, ST, Chen, T-S, Chung, Y-F, Mai, F & Liao, W-H 2019, 'A mobile phone-based approach for hearing screening of school-age children: Cross-sectional validation study', *JMIR mHealth and uHealth*, vol. 7, no. 4, a12033. https://doi.org/10.2196/12033

Deen-Swarray, M 2016, 'Toward digital inclusion: Understanding the literacy effect on adoption and use of mobile phones and the internet in Africa', *Information Technologies & International Development*, vol. 12, no. 2, pp. 29–45.

Desalew, A, Feto Gelano, T, Semahegn, A, Geda, B & Ali, T 2020, 'Childhood hearing impairment and its associated factors in sub-Saharan Africa in the 21st century: A systematic review and meta-analysis', *SAGE Open Medicine*, vol. 8, a2050312120919240. https://doi.org/10.1177/2050312120919240

Edirippulige, S, Armfield, NR & Smith, AC 2012, 'A qualitative study of the careers and professional practices of graduates from an e-health postgraduate programme', *Journal of Telemedicine and Telecare*, vol. 18, no. 8, pp. 455–459. https://doi.org/10.1258/jtt.2012.gth107

Ehnfors, M & Grobe, SJ 2004, 'Nursing curriculum and continuing education: Future directions', *International Journal of Medical Informatics*, vol. 73, no. 7–8, pp. 591–598. https://doi.org/10.1016/j.ijmedinf.2004.04.005

Ferrari, DV & Bernardez-Braga, GRA 2009, 'Remote probe microphone measurement to verify hearing aid performance', *Journal of Telemedicine and Telecare*, vol. 15, no. 3, pp. 122–124. https://doi.org/10.1258/jtt.2009.003005

Frenk, J, Chen, L, Bhutta, ZA, Cohen, J, Crisp, N, Evans, T, Fineberg, H, Garcia, P, Ke, Y, Kelley, P, Kistnasamy, B, Meleis, A, Naylor, D, Pablos-Mendez, A, Reddy, S, Scrimshaw, S, Sepulveda, J, Serwadda, D & Zurayk, H 2010, 'Health professionals for a new century: Transforming education to strengthen health systems in an interdependent world', *The Lancet*, vol. 376, no. 9756, pp. 1923–1958. https://doi.org/10.1016/S0140-6736(10)61854-5

Fulcher, AN, Purcell, A, Baker, E & Munro, N 2015, 'Factors influencing speech and language outcomes of children with early identified severe/profound hearing loss: Clinician-identified facilitators and barriers', *International Journal of Speech-Language Pathology*, vol. 17, no. 3, pp. 325–333. https://doi.org/10.3109/17549507.2015.1032351

George, C, Whitehouse, D & Duquenouy, P 2013, *eHealth: Legal, ethical and governance challenges*, Springer, Berlin.

Global Burden of Disease Study 2013 Collaborators 2015, 'Global, regional, and national incidence, prevalence, and years lived with disability for 301 acute and chronic diseases and injuries in 188 countries, 1990–2013: A systematic analysis for the Global Burden of Disease Study 2013', *The Lancet*, vol. 386, no. 9995, pp. 743–800. https://doi.org/10.1016/S0140-6736(15)60692-4

Govender, S, Latiff, N, Asmal, N, Ramsaroop, S & Mbele, T 2015, 'Evaluating the outcomes of a hearing screening service for grade one learners in urban areas at Durban, South Africa', *Journal of Public Health in Africa*, vol. 6, no. 1, p. 529. https://doi.org/10.4081/jphia.2015.529

Govender, SM & Mars, M 2017, 'The use of telehealth services to facilitate audiological management for children: A scoping review and content analysis', *Journal of Telemedicine and Telecare*, vol. 23, no. 3, pp. 392–401. https://doi.org/10.1177/1357633X16645728

Govender, SM & Mars, M 2018a, 'Assessing the efficacy of asynchronous telehealth-based hearing screening and diagnostic services using automated audiometry in a rural South African school', *South African Journal of Communication Disorders*, vol. 65, no. 1, pp. 1–9. https://doi.org/10.4102/sajcd.v65i1.582

Govender, SM & Mars, M 2018b, 'The perspectives of South African academics within the disciplines of health sciences regarding telehealth and its potential inclusion in student training', *African Journal of Health Professions Education*, vol. 10, no. 1, pp. 38–43. https://doi.org/10.7196/AJHPE.2018.v10i1.957

Havenga, E, Swanepoel, DW, Le Roux, T & Schmid, B 2017, 'Tele-intervention for children with hearing loss: A comparative pilot study', *Journal of Telemedicine and Telecare*, vol. 23, no. 1, pp. 116–125. https://doi.org/10.1177/1357633X15617886

Health Professions Council of South Africa (HPCSA) 2014, *The general ethical guidelines for good practice in telemedicine*, Human Rights, Ethics and Professional Practice Committee, August, viewed 25 November 2019, https://www.hpcsa.co.za/Uploads/Professional_Practice/Conduct%20%26%20Ethics/Booklet%2010%20Telemedicine%20September%20%202016.pdf

Health Professions Council of South Africa (HPCSA) 2019, *Minimum standards for the hearing screening in schools*, Professional Board for Speech, Language and Hearing Professions, October, viewed 10 December 2020, <https://www.hpcsa.co.za/Uploads/SLH/Minimum%20Standards%20for%20the%20Hearing%20Screening%20in%20Schools.pdf>

Hughes, ML, Goehring, JL, Baudhuin, JL & Diaz, GR 2012, 'The use of telehealth for research and clinical measures in cochlear implant recipients: A validation study', *Journal of Speech, Language and Hearing Research*, vol. 55, pp. 1112–1127. https://doi.org/10.1044/1092-4388(2011/11-0237)

Ilinca, S, Di Giorgio, L, Salari, P & Chuma, J 2019, 'Socio-economic inequality and inequity in use of health care services in Kenya: Evidence from the fourth Kenya household health expenditure and utilization survey', *International Journal for Equity in Health*, vol. 18, no. 1, pp. 1–13. https://doi.org/10.1186/s12939-019-1106-z

Jack, C, Hlombe, Y & Mars, M 2014, 'Language, cultural brokerage and informed consent – Will technological terms impede telemedicine use?', *South African Journal of Bioethics and Law*, vol. 7, no. 1, pp. 14–18. https://doi.org/10.7196/sajbl.291

Janardhana, N, Muralidhar, D, Naidu, DM & Raghevendra, G 2015, 'Discrimination against differently abled children among rural communities in India: Need for action', *Journal of Natural Science, Biology, and Medicine*, vol. 6, no. 1, p. 7. https://doi.org/10.4103/0976-9668.149070

Jobson, M 2015, *Structure of the health system in South Africa*, Khulumani Support Group, Johannesburg.

Kam, ACS, Li, LKC, Yeung, KNK, Wu, W, Huang, Z, Wu, H & Tong, MCF 2014, 'Automated hearing screening for preschool children', *Journal of Medical Screening*, vol. 21, no. 2, pp. 71–75. https://doi.org/10.1177/0969141314528322

Karr, S 2012, 'Getting to know telepractice', *The ASHA Leader*, vol. 17, no. 12, p. 30. https://doi.org/10.1044/leader.SCM.17122012.30

Khoza-Shangase, K 2021, 'Continuity of care at school for the hearing-impaired child', eds. K Khoza-Shangase & A Kanji, *Early detection and intervention in audiology: An African perspective*, Wits University Press, Johannesburg, p. 155. https://doi.org/10.18772/22021026567

Khoza-Shangase, K & Kanji, A 2021, 'Best practice in South Africa for early hearing detection and intervention', eds. K Khoza-Shangase & A Kanji, *Early detection and intervention in audiology: an African perspective*, Wits University Press, Johannesburg, p. 264. https://doi.org/10.18772/22021026567

Khoza-Shangase, K & Kassner, L 2013, 'Automated screening audiometry in the digital age: Exploring uhear™ and its use in a resource-stricken developing country', *International Journal of Technology Assessment in Health Care*, vol. 29, no. 1, pp. 42–47. https://doi.org/10.1017/S0266462312000761

Khoza-Shangase, K & Masondo, N 2020, 'What are the current audiological practices for ototoxicity assessment and management in the South African healthcare context?', *International Journal of Environmental Research and Public Health*, vol. 17, no. 7, p. 2613. https://doi.org/10.3390/ijerph17072613

Khoza-Shangase, K & Masondo, N 2021, 'In pursuit of preventive audiology in South Africa: Scoping the context for ototoxicity assessment and management', *Journal of Pharmacy & Bioallied Sciences*, vol. 13, no. 1, p. 46. https://doi.org/10.4103/jpbs.JPBS_334_19

Khoza-Shangase, K & Mophosho, M 2018, 'Language and culture in speech-language and hearing professions in South Africa: The dangers of a single story', *South African Journal of Communication Disorders*, vol. 65, no. 1, pp. 1–7. https://doi.org/10.4102/sajcd.v65i1.594

Khoza-Shangase, K, Sebothoma, B & Moroe, NF 2021, 'Teleaudiology as part of efforts to enhance inclusivity and equality through ICT in South African schools: Some considerations', eds. M Maguvhe, RS Mphahlele & S Moonsamy, *Empowering students and maximising inclusiveness and equality through ICT*, Brill Sense, Boston, pp. 223–243.

Kisling, LA & Das, MJ 2021, *Prevention strategies,* StatPearls Publishing, January, viewed 03 November 2022, <https://www.ncbi.nlm.nih.gov/books/NBK537222/>

Kredo, T, Abrams, A, Young, T, Louw, Q, Volmink, J & Daniels, K 2017, 'Primary care clinical practice guidelines in South Africa: Qualitative study exploring perspectives of national stakeholders', *BMC Health Services Research*, vol. 17, no. 1, pp. 1–12. https://doi.org/10.1186/s12913-017-2546-z

Krumm, M 2007, 'Audiology telemedicine', *Journal of Telemedicine and Telecare*, vol. 13, no. 5, pp. 224–229. https://doi.org/10.1258/135763307781458912

Krupinski, EA & Bernard, J 2014, 'Standards and guidelines in telemedicine and telehealth', *Healthcare*, vol. 2 no. 1, pp. 74–93. https://doi.org/10.3390/healthcare2010074

Kuzovkov, V, Yanov, Y, Levin, S, Bovo, R, Rosignoli, M, Eskilsson, G & Willbas, S 2014, 'Remote programming of MED-EL cochlear implants: Users' and professionals' evaluation of the remote programming experience', *Acta Oto-laryngologica*, vol. 134, no. 7, pp. 709–716. https://doi.org/10.3109/00016489.2014.892212

Lancaster, P, Krumm, M, Ribera, J & Klich, R 2008, 'Remote hearing screenings via telehealth in a rural elementary school', *American Journal of Audiology*, vol. 17, no. 2, pp. 114–122. https://doi.org/10.1044/1059-0889(2008/07-0008)

Maclennan-Smith, F, Swanepoel, D & Hall, JW III 2013, 'Validity of diagnostic pure-tone audiometry without a sound-treated environment', *International Journal of Audiology*, vol. 52, pp. 66–73. https://doi.org/10.3109/14992027.2012.736692

Macrotrends 2020, *Sub-Saharan Africa rural population 1960–2020*, viewed 05 February 2021, <https://www.macrotrends.net/countries/SSF/sub-saharan-africa-/rural-population>

Mahomed-Asmail, F, Eikelboom, RH, Myburgh, HC & Hall, J III 2016a, 'Clinical validity of hearscreen™ smartphone hearing screening for school children', *Ear and Hearing*, vol. 37, no. 1, pp. 11–17. https://doi.org/10.1097/AUD.0000000000000223

Mahomed-Asmail, F, Swanepoel, DW & Eikelboom, RH 2016b, 'Referral criteria for school-based hearing screening in South Africa: Considerations for resource-limited contexts', *Health SA Gesondheid: Journal of Interdisciplinary Health Sciences*, vol. 21, no. 1, pp. 96–102. https://doi.org/10.1016/j.hsag.2015.11.003

Mahomed, F, Swanepoel, DW, Eikelboom, RH & Soer, M 2013, 'Validity of automated threshold audiometry: A systematic review and meta-analysis', *Ear and Hearing: The Official Journal of the American Auditory Society*, vol. 34, no. 6, pp. 745–752. https://doi.org/10.1097/01.aud.0000436255.53747.a4

Mahomed, F, Swanepoel, W & Ayieko, J 2014, *School-age hearing screening: Open access guide to audiology and hearing aids for otolaryngologists*, viewed 10 March 2019, <https://vula.uct.ac.za/access/content/group/27b5cb1b-1b65-4280-9437>

Maluleke, NP, Chiwutsi, R & Khoza-Shangase, K 2021, 'Family-centred early hearing detection and intervention', eds. K Khoza-Shangase & A Kanji, *Early detection and intervention in audiology: An African perspective*, Wits University Press, Johannesburg, p. 196. https://doi.org/10.18772/22021026567

Maphumulo, WT & Bhengu, BR 2019, 'Challenges of quality improvement in the healthcare of South Africa post-apartheid: A critical review', *Curationis*, vol. 42, no. 1, a1901. https://doi.org/10.4102/curationis.v42i1.1901

Margolis, RH, Glasberg, BR, Creeke, S & Moore, BC 2010, 'AMTAS®: Automated method for testing auditory sensitivity: Validation studies', *International Journal of Audiology*, vol. 49, no. 3, pp. 185–194. https://doi.org/10.3109/14992020903092608

Matter, RA & Eide, AH 2018, 'Access to assistive technology in two Southern African countries', *BMC Health Services Research*, vol. 18, p. 792. https://doi.org/10.1186/s12913-018-3605-9

Mayosi, BM & Benatar, SR 2014, 'Health and health care in South Africa-20 years after Mandela', *New England Journal of Medicine*, vol. 371, no. 14, pp. 1344–1353. https://doi.org/10.1056/NEJMsr1405012

Mburu, G & George, G 2017, 'Determining the efficacy of national strategies aimed at addressing the challenges facing health personnel working in rural areas in KwaZulu-Natal, South Africa', *African Journal of Primary Health Care and Family Medicine*, vol. 9, p. 1355. https://doi.org/10.4102/phcfm.v9i1.1355

McLaren, Z, Ardington, C & Leibbrandt, M 2013, *Distance as a barrier to healthcare access in South Africa*, A South African Labour and Development Research Unit (SALDRU) Working Paper (97), SALDRU, University of Cape Town, Cape Town.

Medhanyie, AA, Little, A, Yebyo, H, Spigt, M, Tadesse, K, Blanco, R & Dinant, GJ 2015, 'Health workers' experiences, barriers, preferences and motivating factors in using mHealth forms in Ethiopia', *Human Resources for Health*, vol 13, no. 1, pp. 1–10. https://doi.org/10.1186/1478-4491-13-2

Merugumala, SV, Pothula, V & Cooper, M 2017, 'Barriers to timely diagnosis and treatment for children with hearing impairment in a southern Indian city: A qualitative study of parents and clinic staff', *International Journal of Audiology*, vol. 56, no. 10, pp. 733–739. https://doi.org/10.1080/14992027.2017.1340678

Muwaniki, C & Muvirimi, P 2017, 'Realigning vocational skills for employment and self employment of hearing-impaired youths: The case of Masvingo-Peri Urban', *Journal of Education and Vocational Research*, vol. 8, no. 3, pp. 29–36. https://doi.org/10.22610/jevr.v8i3.1990

Monica, SD, Ramkumar, V, Krumm, M, Raman, N, Nagarajan, R & Venkatesh, L 2017, 'School entry level tele-hearing screening in a town in South India – Lessons learnt', *International Journal of Pediatric Otorhinolaryngology*, vol. 92, pp. 130–135. https://doi.org/10.1016/j.ijporl.2016.11.021

Mpofu, J & Chimhenga, S 2013, 'Challenges faced by hearing impaired pupils in learning: A case study of King George VI Memorial School', *Journal of Research & Method in Education*, vol. 2, no. 1, pp. 69–74.

Mulwafu, W, Kuper, H & Ensink, RJH 2016, 'Systematic review prevalence and causes of hearing impairment in Africa', *Tropical Medicine and International Health*, vol. 21, no. 2, pp. 158–165. https://doi.org/10.1111/tmi.12640

Nada, E, Khater, A & Saeed, A 2014, 'Value of early intervention for hearing impairment on language and speech acquisition', *The Egyptian Journal of Otolaryngology*, vol. 30, no. 3, pp. 237–242. https://doi.org/10.4103/1012-5574.138483

Naipal, S & Rampersad, N 2018, 'A review of visual impairment', *African Vision and Eye Health*, vol. 77, no. 1, pp. 1–4. https://doi.org/10.4102/aveh.v77i1.393

Naudé, A & Bornman, J 2021, 'Early hearing detection and intervention in the context of tele-audiology: Ethical considerations', eds. K Khoza-Shangase & A Kanji, *Early detection and intervention in audiology: An African perspective*, Wits University Press, Johannesburg, pp. 243–263. https://doi.org/10.18772/22021026567

Newton, V 2013, 'Benefits of an early identification and diagnosis of permanent bilateral hearing loss', *Hearing, Balance and Communication*, vol. 11, no. 3, pp. 91–99. https://doi.org/10.3109/21695717.2013.820512

Peer, S & Fagan, JJ 2015, 'Hearing loss in the developing world: Evaluating the iPhone mobile device as a screening tool', *South African Medical Journal*, vol. 105, no. 1, pp. 35–39. https://doi.org/10.7196/samj.8338

Punch, R, Hyde, M & Creed, PA 2004, 'Issues in the school-to-work transition of hard of hearing adolescents', *American Annals of the Deaf*, vol. 149, no. 1, pp. 28–38. https://doi.org/10.1353/aad.2004.0015

Ramkumar, V, Nagarajan, R, Kumaravelu, S & Hall, JW 2014, 'Providing tele ABR in rural India', *Perspectives on Telepractice*, vol. 4, no. 1, pp. 30–36. https://doi.org/10.1044/teles4.1.30

Ramos, A, Rodríguez, C, Martinez-Beneyto, P, Perez, D, Gault, A, Falcon, JC & Boyle, P 2009, 'Use of telemedicine in the remote programming of cochlear implants', *Acta Oto-laryngologica*, vol. 129, no. 5, pp. 533–540. https://doi.org/10.1080/00016480802294369

Rawlings, BW 1994, 'Postsecondary education: Its impact and outcomes', eds. TE Allen, KH Lam, BW Rawlings, DE Rose & AN Schildroth, *Young deaf adults and the transition from high school to postsecondary careers*, Galludet University, Washington DC, pp. 7–16.

Roberton, T, Carter, ED, Chou, VB, Stegmuller, AR, Jackson, BD, Tam, Y, Sawadogo-Lewis, T & Walker, N 2020, 'Early estimates of the indirect effects of the COVID-19 pandemic on maternal and child mortality in low-income and middle-income countries: A modelling study', *The Lancet Global Health*, vol. 8, no. 7, pp. 901–908. https://doi.org/10.1016/S2214-109X(20)30229-1

Roelen, K, Delap, E, Jones, C & Chettri, HK 2017, 'Improving child wellbeing and care in sub-Saharan Africa: The role of social protection', *Children and Youth Services Review*, vol. 73, pp. 309–318.

Rourke, R, Bromwich, M & Chan, D 2014, 'iPad audiometry in Canada's North: A portable and cost-effective method for hearing screening', *Otolaryngology – Head and Neck Surgery*, vol. 151, suppl. 1, a237. https://doi.org/10.1177/0194599814541627a237

Schwarz, F, Ward, J & Willcock, S 2014, 'e-Health readiness in outback communities: An exploratory study', *Rural Remote Health*, vol. 14, a2871. https://doi.org/10.22605/RRH2871

Scott Kruse, C, Karem, P, Shifflett, K, Vegi, L, Ravi, K & Brooks, M 2018, 'Evaluating barriers to adopting telemedicine worldwide: A systematic review', *Journal of Telemedicine and Telecare*, vol. 24, no. 1, pp. 4–12. https://doi.org/10.1177/1357633X16674087

Scott, RE & Mars, M 2015, 'Telehealth in the developing world: Current status and future prospects', *Smart Homecare Technology and TeleHealth*, vol. 2015, no. 3, pp. 25–37. https://doi.org/10.2147/SHTT.S75184

Skarzyński, PH, Świerniak, W, Piłka, A, Skarżynska, MB, Włodarczyk, AW, Kholmatov, D, Makhamadiev, A & Hatzopoulos, S 2016, 'A hearing screening program for children in primary schools in Tajikistan: A telemedicine model', *Medical Science Monitor: International Medical Journal of Experimental and Clinical Research*, vol. 22, p. 2424. https://doi.org/10.12659/msm.895967

South Africa 1997, 'White paper on an Integrated National Disability Strategy', viewed 20 February 2018, <https://www.gov.za/sites/default/files/gcis_document/201409/disability2.pdf>

South African National Department of Health 2012, *South Africa eHealth Strategy*, viewed 18 March 2019, <http://www.health-e.org.za/wp-content/uploads/2014/08/South-Africa-eHealth-Strategy-2012-2017.2012.pdf>

South African National Department of Health 2019, *The National Health Insurance Bill*, viewed 26 March 2020, <http://www.health.gov.za/nhi/>

South African Department of Basic Education and Department of Health 2012, *Integrated School Health Policy (ISHP)*, October, viewed 10 December 2018, <https://www.health-e.org.za/wpcontent/uploads/2013/10/Integrated_School_Health_Policy.pdf>

South African Department of Education White Paper on Special Needs Education: Building an Inclusive Education and Training System 2001, 'White Paper 6', viewed 10 December 2019, <https://wcedonline.westerncape.gov.za/Specialised-ed/documents/WP6.pdf>

Standards and Guidelines for Quality Assurance in the European Higher Education Area (ESG) 2015, *Brussels*, viewed 15 November 2019, <https://www.enqa.eu/wp-content/uploads/2015/11/ESG_2015.pdf>

Stevenson, J, Kreppner, J, Pimperton, H, Worsfold, S & Kennedy, C 2015, 'Emotional and behavioural difficulties in children and adolescents with hearing impairment: A systematic review and meta-analysis', *European Child & Adolescent Psychiatry*, vol. 24, no. 5, pp. 477–496. https://doi.org/10.1007/s00787-015-0697-1

Swanepoel, DW, Maclennan-Smith, F & Hall, JW 2013, 'Diagnostic pure-tone audiometry in schools: Mobile testing without a sound-treated environment', *Journal of the American Academy of Audiology*, vol. 24, no. 10, pp. 992–1000. https://doi.org/10.3766/jaaa.24.10.10

Swanepoel, DW, Mngemane, S, Molemong, S, Mkwanazi, H & Tutshini, S 2010b, 'Hearing assessment – Reliability, accuracy, and efficiency of automated audiometry', *Telemedicine and e-Health*, vol. 16, no. 5, pp. 557–563. https://doi.org/10.1089/tmj.2009.0143

Swanepoel, DW, Olusanya, BO & Mars, M 2010, 'Hearing health-care delivery in sub-Saharan Africa – A role for tele-audiology', *Journal of Telemedicine and Telecare*, vol. 16, no. 2, pp. 53–56. https://doi.org/10.1258/jtt.2009.009003.

Tharpe, AM 2008, 'Unilateral and mild bilateral hearing loss in children: Past and current perspectives', *Trends in Amplification*, vol. 12, no. 1, pp. 7–15. https://doi.org/10.1177/1084713807304668

The African Report on Children with Disabilities 2014, *The African report on children with disabilities: Promising starts and persisting challenges*, viewed 20 December 2019, <www.africanchildforum.org>

Theunissen, SC, Rieffe, C, Netten, AP, Briaire, JJ, Soede, W, Schoones, JW & Frijns, JHM 2014, 'Psychopathology and its risk and protective factors in hearing-impaired children and adolescents: A systematic review', *JAMA Pediatrics*, vol. 168, no. 2, pp. 170–177. https://doi.org/10.1001/jamapediatrics.2013.3974

The World Bank 2017, *The World Bank in South Africa*, viewed 20 December 2019, <http://www.worldbank.org/en/country/southafrica/overview>

Tian, H, Lu, C, Yang, J, Banger, K, Huntzinger, DN, Schwalm, CR, Michalak, AM, Cook, R, Ciais, P, Hayes, D, Huang, M, Ito, A, Jain, AK, Lei, H, Mao, J, Pan, S, Post, WM, Peng, S, Poulter, B, Ren, W, Ricciuto, D, Schaefer, K, Shi, X, Tao, B, Wang, W, Wei, Y, Yang, Q, Zhang, B & Zeng, N 2015, 'WHO global estimates on prevalence of hearing loss', *Global Biogeochemistry Cycles*, vol. 29, no. 6, pp. 775–792.

Townsend, BA & Scott, RE 2019, 'The development of ethical guidelines for telemedicine in South Africa', *South African Journal of Bioethics and Law*, vol. 12, no. 1, pp. 19–26.

United Nations (UN) 2015, *Transforming our world: The 2030 agenda for sustainable development*, viewed 17 November 2019, <https://sustainabledevelopment.un.org/content/documents/21252030%20Agenda%20for%20Sustain>

United Nations (UN) 2017, *Income inequality trends in sub-Saharan Africa divergence, determinants and consequences*, viewed 17 November 2019, <africa.undp.org>

UNESCO Institute for Statistics 2015, *Information and Communication Technology (ICT) in Education in sub-Saharan Africa: A comparative analysis of basic e-readiness in schools*, viewed 17 November 2019, <http://uis.unesco.org/sites/default/files/documents/information-and-communication-technology-ict-in-education-in-sub-saharan-africa-2015-en.pdf>

United Nations Department of Economic and Social Affairs, Population Division 2017, *World population prospects: The 2017 revision*, viewed 17 November 2019, <https://www.un.org/development/desa/publications/world-population-prospects-the-2017-revision.html>

Warner-Czyz, AD, Loy, BA, Evans, C, Wetsel, A & Tobey, EA 2015, 'Self-esteem in children and adolescents with hearing loss', *Trends in Hearing*, vol. 19, a2331216515572615. https://doi.org/10.1177/2331216515572615

Western Cape Government 1998, *Employment Equity Act, No 55 of 1998*, viewed 03 July 2018, <https://www.westerncape.gov.za/legislation/employment-equity-act-55-1998>

Wilson, BS, Tucci, DL, Merson, MH & O'Donoghue, GM 2017, 'Global hearing health care: New findings and perspectives', *The Lancet*, vol. 390, no. 10111, pp. 2503–2515. https://doi.org/10.1016/S0140-6736(17)31073-5

Wimer, C, Fox, L, Garfinkel, I, Kaushal, N & Waldfogel, J 2016, 'Progress on poverty? New estimates of historical trends using an anchored supplemental poverty measure', *Demography*, vol. 53, no. 4, pp. 1207–1218. https://doi.org/10.1007/s13524-016-0485-7

World Health Organization (WHO) 2001, *International classification of functioning, disability and health (ICF)*, World Health Organization, Geneva.

World Health Organization (WHO) 2013, *eHealth and WHO*, World Health Organization, Geneva.

World Health Organization (WHO) 2017, *Deafness and hearing loss*, World Health Organization, Geneva.

World Health Organization (WHO) 2019, *Statistics overview 2019: Monitoring health for the SDGs, Sustainable Development Goals*, World Health Organization, Geneva.

World Health Organization (WHO) 2020, *Child health: Fact sheet*, World Health Organization, Geneva.

World Medical Association (WMA) 2009, *WMA statement on the ethics of telemedicine*, viewed 13 January 2017, <http://www.wma.net/en/30publications/10policies/t3/>

Yousuf Hussein, S, Swanepoel, DW, Mahomed, F & Biagio De Jager, L 2018, 'Community-based hearing screening for young children using an mHealth service-delivery model', *Global Health Action*,vol. 11, no. 1, a1467077. https://doi.org/10.1080/16549716.2018.1467077

Chapter 4

Asmail, FM, Swanepoel, DW & Eikelboom, RH 2016, 'Referral criteria for school-based hearing screening in South Africa: Considerations for resource-limited contexts', *Health SA Gesondheid*, vol. 21, no. 1, pp. 96–102. https://doi.org/10.4102/hsag.v21i0.939

Assegaai, T & Schneider, H 2019, 'National guidance and district-level practices in the supervision of community health workers in South Africa: A qualitative study', *Human Resources for Health*, vol. 17, no. 1, p. 25. https://doi.org/10.1186/s12960-019-0360-x

Billard, I 2014, 'The hearing and otitis program: A model of community based ear and hearing care services for Inuit of Nunavik', *Revue canadienne d'orthophonie et d'audiologie*, vol. 38, no. 2, n.p.

Burger, R & Christian, C 2018, 'Access to health care in post-Apartheid South Africa: Availability, affordability, acceptability', *Health Economics, Policy and Law*, vol. 15, no. 1, pp. 1–13. https://doi.org/10.1017/S1744133118000300

Burnett, RJ, Dlamini, NR, Meyer, JC, Fernandes, L, Motloung, BR, Ndlovu, TH, Simango, HA, Kibuuka, DK, Dochez, C, Montwedi, DN, Nkwinika, VV & Mphahlele, MJ 2019, 'Progress towards obtaining valid vaccination coverage data in South Africa', *South African Journal of Science*, vol. 115, no. 5/6, pp. 1–4. https://doi.org/10.17159/sajs.2019/6060

Chadha, S, Kamenov, K & Cieza, A 2019, 'Health system requirements for hearing care services', *Bulletin of the World Health Organization*, vol. 97, a647. https://doi.org/10.2471/BLT.19.243683

Chan, S, Hixon, B, Adkins, M, Au, D, Shinn, JB & Bush, ML 2018, 'Rurality and determinants of hearing healthcare in adult hearing aid recipients', *Laryngoscope*, vol. 127, no. 10, pp. 2362–2367. https://doi.org/10.1002/lary.26490

Coco, L, Champlin, CA & Eikelboom, RH 2006, 'Community-based intervention determines tele-audiology site candidacy', *American Journal of Audiology*, vol. 25, no. 3 suppl. pp. 264–267. https://doi.org/10.1044/2016_AJA-16-0002

Collins Dictionary 2020, *Access*, viewed 30 November 2020, <https://www.collinsdictionary.com/dictionary/english/access>

Davis, A, McMahon, CM, Pichora-Fuller, KM, Russ, S, Lin, F, Olusanya, BO, Chadha, S & Tremblay, KL 2016, 'Aging and hearing health: The life-course approach', *Gerontologist*, vol. 56, pp. 256–267. https://doi.org/10.1093/geront/gnw033

Davis, S 2019, 'The what, why and when of childhood vaccination in South Africa – 2019', *Professional Nursing Today*, vol. 23, no. 2, pp. 27–29.

Day, C, Gray, A & Ndlovu, N 2018, 'Health and related indicators 2018', eds. LC Rispel & A Padarath, *South African health review 2018*, Health Systems Trust, Durban, pp. 139–250.

De Kock, T, Swanepoel, D & Hall, JW 2016, 'Newborn hearing screening at a community-based obstetric unit: Screening and diagnostic outcomes', *International Journal of Pediatric Otorhinolaryngology*, vol. 84, pp. 124–131. https://doi.org/10.1016/j.ijporl.2016.02.031

Department of Health 2006, *Health on community service by health professionals*, viewed 28 November 2019, <https://www.gov.za/health-community-service-health-professionals>

Department of Health 2014, *Vaccinator's manual: Expanded programme on immunisation in South Africa (EPI-SA)*, viewed 13 March 2019, <http://www.health.gov.za/index.php/shortcodes/2015-03-29-10-42-47/2015-04-30-08-29-27/immunization/category/165-immunisation?download=503:vaccinators-manual-final>

Department of Health 2017, *White paper on National Health Insurance for South Africa: Towards universal health coverage*, viewed 13 March 2019, <http://www.health.gov.za/index.php/nhi-documents?download=2257:white-paper-nhi-2017>

Departments of Health and Basic Education 2012, *Integrated school health policy 2012*, viewed 13 March 2019, <https://serve.mg.co.za/content/documents/2017/06/14/integratedschoolhealthpolicydbeanddoh.pdf>

Dhai, A & Mahomed, S 2018, 'Healthcare in crisis: A shameful disrespect of our constitution', *South African Journal of Bioethics and Law*, vol. 11, no. 1, pp. 8–10. https://doi.org/10.7196/SAJBL.2018.v11i1.00649

Duncan, M, Sherry, K & Watson, R 2011, 'Disability and rurality', ed. T Lorenzo, *Intentions, pillars and players. Disability catalyst Africa Series 1*, Disability Innovations Africa, Cape Town, pp. 29–36.

Eagar, D, Rensburg, R & Versteeg-Mojanaga, M 2013, *Defining rural – What do we mean by rurality? How rural is your facility?*, Rural Health Advocacy Project, viewed 27 March 2017, <http://rhap.org.za/our-projects/defining-rural/>

Edusei, J & Amoah, PA 2014, 'Appreciating the complexities in accessing health care among urban poor: The case of street children in Kumasi Metropolitan Area, Ghana', *Developing Country Studies*, vol. 4, no. 8, pp. 69–89.

Erasmus, D, Ranchod, S, Abraham, M, Bloch, J, Carvounes, A & Dreyer, K 2016, *Challenges and opportunities for health finance in South Africa: A supply and regulatory perspective*, viewed 27 March 2017, <https://www.mm3admin.co.za/documents/docmanager/f447b607-3c8f-4eb7-8da4-11bca747079f/00104931.pdf>

Fridrichs, N, Swanepoel, D & Hall, JW 2012, 'Efficacy of a community-based infant hearing screening program utilizing existing clinic personnel in Western Cape, South Africa', *International Journal of Pediatric Otorhinolaryngology*, vol. 76, no. 4, pp. 552–559. https://doi.org/10.1016/j.ijporl.2012.01.015

Glenister, KM, Bourke, L, Bolitho, L, Wright, S, Roberts, S, Kemp, W, Rhode, L, Bhat, R, Tremper, S, Magliano, DJ, Morgan, M, Marino, R, Adam, W & Simmons, D 2018, 'Longitudinal study of health, disease and access to care in Rural Victoria: The Crossroads-II Study: methods', *BMC Public Health*, vol. 18, p. 670. https://doi.org/10.1186/s12889-018-5511-9

Goulios, H & Patuzzi, RB 2008, 'Audiology education and practice from an international perspective', *International Journal of Audiology*, vol. 47, no. 10, pp. 647–664. https://doi.org/10.1080/14992020802203322

Halfon, N & Hochstein, M 2002, 'Life course health development: An integrated framework for developing health, policy, and research', *Milbank Quarterly*, vol. 80, no. 3, pp. 433–479. https://doi.org/10.1111/1468-0009.00019

Halfon, N, Larson, K, Lu, M, Tullis, E & Russ, S 2014, 'Life course health development: Past, present and future', *Maternal and Child Health Journal*, vol. 18, pp. 344–365. https://doi.org/10.1007/s10995-013-1346-2

Health Professions Council of South Africa (HPCSA) 2017, *A guideline for planning STA services at all levels of health care*, viewed 30 November 2019, <https://www.hpcsa.co.za/Uploads/SLH/Policy%20and%20Guidelines/guideline_planning_STA_services_at_all_levels_health%20care.pdf>

Health Professions Council of South Africa (HPCSA) 2018a, *Minimum standards for hearing screening in schools*, viewed 30 November 2019, <https://www.hpcsa.co.za/Uploads/SLH/Minimum%20Standards%20for%20the%20Hearing%20Screening%20in%20Schools.pdf>

Health Professions Council of South Africa (HPCSA) 2018b, *Guidelines for early hearing detection and intervention (EHDI)*, viewed 30 November 2019, <https://www.hpcsa.co.za/Uploads/SLH/Guidelines%20for%20Early_Hearing_Detection_and_Intervention_(EHDI)_2018.pdf>

Health Professions Council of South Africa (HPCSA) 2019, *Guidelines for speech, language and hearing practice in a culturally and linguistically diverse South Africa*, viewed 10 February 2020, <https://www.hpcsa.co.za/Uploads/SLH/Guidelines%20for%20practice%20in%20a%20culturally%20and%20linguistically%20divers---.pdf>

Janse van Rensburg, Z 2020, 'Levels of health literacy and English comprehension in patients presenting to South African primary healthcare facilities', *African Journal of Primary Health Care and Family Medicine*, vol. 12, no. 1, a2047. https://doi.org/10.4102/phcfm.v12i1.2047

Jayakody, DMP, Friedland, PL, Martins, RN & Sohrabi, HR 2018, 'Impact of aging on the auditory system and related cognitive functions: A narrative review', *Frontiers in Neuroscience*, vol. 12, p. 125. https://doi.org/10.3389/fnins.2018.00125

Jennings, G 2015, *Public transport interventions and transport justice in South Africa: A literature and policy review*, viewed 20 November 2019, <https://www.researchgate.net/publication/309673621>

Joubert, K & Botha, D 2019, 'Contributing factors to high prevalence of hearing impairment in the Elias Motsoaledi Local Municipal Area, South Africa: A rural perspective', *South African Journal of Communication Disorders*, vol. 66, no. 1, a611. https://doi.org/10.4102/sajcd.v66i1.611

Joubert, K & Githinji, E 2014, 'Quality and readability of information pamphlets on hearing and paediatric hearing loss in the Gauteng province, South Africa', *International Journal of Pediatric Otorhinolaryngology*, vol. 78, no. 2, pp. 354–358. https://doi.org/10.1016/j.ijporl.2013.12.018

Joubert, K, Sebothoma, B & Kgare, KS 2017, 'Public awareness of audiology, hearing and hearing health in the Limpopo province, South Africa', *South African Journal of Communication Disorders*, vol. 64, no. 1, a557. https://doi.org/10.4102/sajcd.v64i1.557

Kanji, A 2018, 'Early hearing detection and intervention: Reflections from the South African context', *South African Journal of Communication Disorders*, vol. 65, no. 1, a581. https://doi.org/10.4102/sajcd.v65i1.581

Kgare, KS 2018, *Effectiveness of a clinic-based newborn hearing screening programme in rural South Africa: Parental perspectives*, viewed 10 March 2019, <http://wiredspace.wits.ac.za/jspui/handle/10539/27380>

Khan, NB, Joseph, L & Adhikari, M 2018, 'The hearing screening experiences and practices of primary health care nurses: Indications for referral based on high-risk factors and community views about hearing loss', *African Journal of Primary Health Care and Family Medicine*, vol. 10, no. 1, a1848. https://doi.org/10.4102/phcfm.v10i1.1848

Khoza-Shangase, K, Kanji, A, Petrocchi-Bartal, L & Farr, K 2017, 'Infant hearing screening in a developing-country context: Status in two South African provinces', *South African Journal of Child Health*, vol. 11, no. 4, pp. 159–163.

Levesque, JF, Harris, MF & Russell, G 2013, 'Patient-centred access to health care: Conceptualising access at the interface of health systems and populations', *International Journal for Equity in Health*, vol. 12, no. 1, n.p. https://doi.org/10.1186/1475-9276-12-18

Liu, C, Wang, A, Huang, Y, Zhang, Y, Ding, H, Wu, J, Du, L, Yang, J, Mai, F, Zeng, Y, Liu, L, Zhao, X, Zhang, C & Yin, A 2019, 'Development of a community-based hearing loss prevention and control service model in Guangdong, China', *BMC Public Health*, vol. 19, p. 1601. https://doi.org/10.1186/s12889-019-7910-y

Lubetzky, AV 2020, 'Balance, falls, and hearing Loss: Is it time for a paradigm shift?', *JAMA Otolaryngology – Head & Neck Surgery*, vol. 146, no. 6, pp. 355–356. https://doi.org/10.1001/jamaoto.2020.0415

Malakoane, B, Heunis, JC, Chikobvu, P, Kigozi, NG & Kruger, WH 2020, 'Public health system challenges in the Free State, South Africa: A situation appraisal to inform health system strengthening', *BMC Health Service Research*, vol. 20, p. 58. https://doi.org/10.1186/s12913-019-4862-y

Maphumulo, WT & Bhengu, BR 2019, 'Challenges of quality improvement in the healthcare of South Africa post-apartheid: A critical review', *Curationis*, vol. 42, no. 1, a1901. https://doi.org/10.4102/curationis.v42i1.1901

Marimwe, C & Dowse, R 2019, 'Health literacy test for limited literacy populations (HELT-LL): validation in South Africa', *Cogent Medicine*, vol. 6, no. 1, p. 1. https://doi.org/10.1080/2331205X.2019.1650417

McIntyre, D & Ataguba, J 2017, *Access to quality health care in South Africa: Is the health sector contributing to addressing the inequality challenge?*, viewed 20 November 2019, <https://www.parliament.gov.za/.../Diagnostic_Report_on_Access_to_Quality_Healthcare.pdf>

McLaren, ZM, Ardington, C & Leibbrandt, M 2014, 'Distance decay and persistent health care disparities in South Africa', *BMC Health Services Research*, vol. 14, a541. https://doi.org/10.1186/s12913-014-0541-1

Moonsamy, S, Mupawose, A, Seedat, J, Mophosho, M & Pillay, D 2017, 'Speech-language pathology and audiology in South Africa: Reflections on transformation in professional training and practice since the end of apartheid', *Perspectives of the ASHA Special Interest Groups*, vol. 2, no. 17, pp. 30–41. https://doi.org/10.1044/persp2.SIG17.30

Mthimkhulu, N 2017, 'Southern African solutions to public transport challenges', *36th Southern African Transport conference (SATC 2017)*, Pretoria, South Africa, July 10–13, 2017, n.p.

Mulwafu, W, Ensink, R, Kuper, H & Fagan, J 2017, 'Survey of ENT services in sub-Saharan Africa: Little progress between 2009 and 2015', *Global Health Action*, vol. 10, no. 1, a1289736. https://doi.org/10.1080/16549716.2017.1289736

Mulwafu, W, Kuper, H & Ensink, RJH 2016, 'Prevalence and causes of hearing impairment in Africa', *Tropical Medicine and International Health*, vol. 21, no. 2, pp. 158–165. https://doi.org/10.1111/tmi.12640

Ned, L, Cloete, L & Mji, G 2017, 'The experiences and challenges faced by rehabilitation community service therapists within the South African primary healthcare health system', *African Journal of Disability*, vol. 6, a311. https://doi.org/10.4102/ajod.v6i0.311

Nicol, A, Knowlton, LM, Schuurman, N, Matzopoulos, R, Zargaran, E, Cinnamon, J, Fawcett, V, Taulu, T & Hameed, SM 2014, 'Trauma surveillance in Cape Town, South Africa: An analysis of 9236 consecutive trauma center admissions', *JAMA Otolaryngology – Head & Neck Surgery*, vol. 49, no. 6, pp. 549–556. https://doi.org/10.1001/jamasurg.2013.5267

Nielsen-Bohlman, L, Panzer, A & Kindig, D (eds.) 2004, *Health literacy: A prescription to end confusion*, National Academies Press, Washington DC.

Nxumalo, N, Goudge, J & Liz Thomas, L 2013, 'Outreach services to improve access to health care in South Africa: Lessons from three community health worker programmes', *Global Health Action*, vol. 6, no. 1, a19283. https://doi.org/10.3402/gha.v6i0.19283

O'Donovan, J, Verkerk, M, Winters, N, Chadna, S & Bhutta, MF 2019, 'The role of community health workers in addressing global burden of ear disease and hearing loss: A systematic scoping review of literature', *BMJ Global Health*, vol. 4, no. 2, a001141. https://doi.org/10.1136/bmjgh-2018-001141

Olaniran, A, Smith, H, Unkels, R, Bar-Zeev, S & Van Den Broek, N 2017, 'Who is a community health worker? A systematic review of definitions', *Global Health Action*, vol. 10, no. 1, a1272223. https://doi.org/10.1080/16549716.2017.1272223

Olusanya, BO, Neumann, KJ & Saunders, JE 2014, 'The global burden of disabling hearing impairment: A call to action', *Bulletin of the World Health Organization*, vol. 92, pp. 367–373. https://doi.org/10.2471/BLT.13.128728

Penchansky, R & Thomas, WJ 1981, 'The concept of access: definition and relationship to consumer satisfaction', *Medical Care*, vol. 19, no. 2, pp. 127–140. https://doi.org/10.1097/00005650-198102000-00001

Peters, DH, Garg, A, Bloom, G, Walker, DG, Brieger, WR & Rahman, HM 2008, 'Poverty and access to healthcare in developing countries', *Annals of the New York Academy of Sciences*, vol. 1136, no. 1, pp. 161–171. https://doi.org/10.1196/annals.1425.011

Pillay, M, Tiwari, R, Kathard, H & Chikte, U 2020, 'Sustainable workforce: South African audiologists and speech therapists', *Human Resources for Health*, vol. 18, no. 1, pp. 1–13. https://doi.org/10.1186/s12960-020-00488-6

Plaks, N, Khoza-Shangase, K & Joubert, K 2014, 'Hearing loss in the South African closed head injured population: Two to five years post onset', *Journal of Pharmaceutical and Biomedical Sciences (JPBMS)*, vol. 4, no. 10, pp. 839–851.

Protheroe, J, Nutbeam, D & Rowlands, G 2009, 'Health literacy: A necessity for increasing participation in health care', *British Journal of General Practice*, vol. 59, no. 567, pp. 721–723. https://doi.org/10.3399/bjgp09X472584

Ramkumar, V, John, KR, Selvakumar, K, Vanaja, CS, Nagarajan, R & Hall, JW 2018, 'Cost and outcome of a community-based paediatric hearing screening programme in rural India with application of tele-audiology for follow up diagnostic hearing assessment', *International Journal of Audiology*, vol. 57, no. 6, pp. 407–414. https://doi.org/10.1080/14992027.2018.1442592

Ramma, L & Sebothoma, B 2016, 'The prevalence of hearing impairment within the Cape Town Metropolitan Area', *South African Journal of Communication Disorders*, vol. 63, no. 1, a105. https://doi.org/10.4102/sajcd.v63i1.105

Ratanji-Vanmala, H, Swanepoel, DW & Laplante-Lévesque, A 2020, 'Patient uptake, experience, and satisfaction using web-based and face-to-face hearing health services: Process evaluation study', *Journal of Medical Internet Research*, vol. 2, no. 3, a15875. https://doi.org/10.2196/15875

Rispel, LC, Blaauw, D, Ditlopo, P & White, J 2018, 'Human resources for health and universal health coverage: Progress, complexities and contestations', eds. LC Rispel & A Padarath, *South African health review 2018*, Health Systems Trust, Durban, pp. 23–32.

Rosenhall, U & Sundh, V 2006, 'Age-related hearing loss and blood pressure', *Noise and Health*, vol. 8, no. 31, pp. 88–94. https://doi.org/10.4103/1463-1741.33539

Saprii, L, Richards, E, Kokho, P & Theobald, S 2015, 'Community health workers in rural India: Analysing the opportunities and challenges accredited social health activists (ASHAs) face in realising their multiple roles', *Human Resources in Health*, vol. 13, p. 95. https://doi.org/10.1186/s12960-015-0094-3

Solanki, T 2012, *The prevalence of hearing loss in adults presenting with cardiovascular disease*, viewed 10 April 2019, <http://hdl.handle.net/10539/11572>

Sooful, P, Van Dijk, C & Avenant, C 2009, 'The maintenance and utilization of government fitted hearing aids', *Central European Journal of Medicine*, vol. 4, no. 1, pp. 110–118. https://doi.org/10.2478/s11536-009-0014-9

South African National Department of Health 2011, *Human resources for health South Africa: HRH strategy for the health sector: 2012/13–2016/17*, viewed 10 April 2019, <https://www.gov.za/sites/default/files/gcis_document/201409/hrhstrategy0.pdf>

Statistics South Africa 2012, *Census 2011: Prevalence of disability in South Africa*, viewed 15 November 2019, <http://www.statssa.gov.za/>

Statistics South Africa 2017, *General household survey 2016*, viewed 15 November 2019, <https://www.statssa.gov.za/publications/P0318/P03182016.pdf>

Statistics South Africa 2019, *Inequality trends in South Africa: A multidimensional diagnostic of inequality*, viewed 10 February 2020, <http://www.statssa.gov.za/publications/Report-03-10-19/Report-03-10-192017.pdf>

Swanepoel, DW 2006, 'Audiology in South Africa', *International Journal of Audiology*, vol. 45, no. 5, pp. 262–266. https://doi.org/10.1080/14992020500485650

Taylor, B, Van Waart, J, Ranchod, S & Taylor, A 2018, 'Medicolegal storm threatening maternal and child healthcare services', *South African Medical Journal*, vol. 108, no. 3, pp. 149–150. https://doi.org/10.7196/SAMJ.2018.v108i3.13139

Teixeira, L & Joubert, K 2014, 'Availability of audiological equipment and protocols for paediatric assessment and hearing aid fitting in Gauteng, South Africa', *South African Journal of Communication Disorders*, vol. 61, no. 1, pp. 354–358. https://doi.org/10.4102/sajcd.v61i1.58

Theunissen, M & Swanepoel, D 2008, 'Early hearing detection and intervention services in the public health sector in South Africa', *International Journal of Audiology*, vol. 47, no. Suppl 1, pp. 23–29. https://doi.org/10.1080/14992020802294032

Uys, IC & Hugo, R 1997, 'Speech-language pathology and audiology: Transformation in teaching, research and service delivery', *Health SA Gesondheid*, vol. 2, no. 2, a327. https://doi.org/10.4102/hsag.v2i2.327

Van Wyk, T, Mahomed-Asmail, F & Swanepoel, DW 2019, 'Supporting hearing health in vulnerable populations through community care workers using m-Health technologies', *International Journal of Audiology*, vol. 58, no. 11, pp. 790–797. https://doi.org/10.1080/14992027.2019.1649478

Visagie, S, Eide, AH, Mannan, H, Schneider, M, Swartz, L, Mji, G, Munthali, A, Khogali, M, Van Rooy, G, Hem, K-G & MacLachlan, M 2017, 'A description of assistive technology sources, services and outcomes of use in a number of African settings', *Disability and Rehabilitation: Assistive Technology*, vol. 12, no. 7, pp. 705–712. https://doi.org/10.1080/17483107.2016.1244293

Watermeyer, J & Barratt, J 2013, '"I live in a bubble": Speech-language therapy and audiology students' expectations and experiences of a rural community work practicum', *Rural and Remote Health*, vol. 13, a2131. https://doi.org/10.22605/RRH2131

Wilson, BS, Tucci, DL, Merson, MH & O'Donoghue, GM 2017, 'Global hearing health care: New findings and perspectives', *Lancet*, vol. 390, no. 10111, pp. 2503–2515. https://doi.org/10.1016/S0140-6736(17)31073-5

World Bank 2019, *Rural population*, viewed 10 January 2020, <https://data.worldbank.org/indicator/SP.RUR.TOTL?view=chart>

World Health Organization (WHO) 1978, *Declaration of Alma-Ata*, World Health Organization, Geneva.

World Health Organization (WHO) 2006, *Primary ear and hearing care training resources*, viewed 10 January 2020, <https://www.who.int/pbd/deafness/activities/hearing_care/trainer.pdf?ua=1>

World Health Organization (WHO) 2007, *Everybody's business: Strengthening health systems to improve health outcomes: WHO's framework for action*, WHO Press, Geneva.

World Health Organization (WHO) 2008, *Task shifting: Rational redistribution of tasks among health workforce teams: Global recommendations and guidelines*, World Health Organization, Geneva.

World Health Organization (WHO) 2017a, *Global costs of unaddressed hearing loss and cost-effectiveness of interventions: An executive summary*, World Health Organization, Geneva.

World Health Organization (WHO) 2017b, *World Health assembly resolution on hearing, 2017*, World Health Organization, Geneva.

World Health Organization (WHO) 2018, *Addressing the rising prevalence of hearing loss*, World Health Organization, Geneva.

World Health Organization (WHO) 2019, *Deafness and hearing loss*, World Health Organization, Geneva.

World Health Organization (WHO) 2020a, *Universal health coverage*, viewed n.d., <https://www.who.int/healthsystems/universal_health_coverage/en/>

World Health Organization (WHO) 2020b, *Deafness and hearing loss*, World Health Organization, Geneva.

World Health Organization (WHO) 2020c, *National health policies, strategies and plans: Situation analysis and priority setting*, World Health Organization, Geneva.

Chapter 5

Aithal, S, Kei, J, Aithal, V, Manuel, A, Myers, J, Driscoll, C & Khan, A 2017, 'Normative study of wideband acoustic immittance measures in newborn infants', *Journal of Speech, Language, and Hearing Research*, vol. 60, no. 5, pp. 1417–1426. https://doi.org/10.1044/2016_JSLHR-H-16-0237

Anderson, S, Parbery-Clark, A, White-Schwoch, T, Drehobl, S & Kraus, N 2013, 'Effects of hearing loss on the subcortical representation of speech cues', *The Journal of the Acoustical Society of America*, vol. 133, no. 5, pp. 3030–3038. https://doi.org/10.1121/1.4799804

Avnstorp, MB, Homøe, P, Bjerregaard, P & Jensen, RG 2016, 'Chronic suppurative otitis media, middle ear pathology and corresponding hearing loss in a cohort of Greenlandic children', *International Journal of Pediatric Otorhinolaryngology*, vol. 83, pp. 148–153. https://doi.org/10.1016/j.ijporl.2016.01.017

Balbani, AP & Montovani, JC 2003, 'Impact of otitis media on language acquisition in children', *Jornal de Pediatria*, vol. 79, no. 5, pp. 391–396.

Barron, P, Pillay, Y, Fernandes, A, Sebidi, J & Allen, R 2016, 'The MomConnect mHealth initiative in South Africa: Early impact on the supply side of MCH services', *Journal of Public Health Policy*, vol. 37, no. 2, pp. 201–212. https://doi.org/10.1057/s41271-016-0015-2

Benatar, S & Gill, S 2021, 'Universal access to healthcare: The case of South Africa in the comparative global context of the late Anthropocene era', *International Journal of Health Policy and Management*, vol. 10, no. 2, pp. 49–54. https://doi.org/10.34172/IJHPM.2020.28

Bezuidenhout, KJ, Khoza-Shangase, K, De Maayer, T & Strehlau, R 2018, 'Universal newborn hearing screening in public health care in South Africa: Challenges to implementation', *South African Journal of Child Health*, vol. 12, no. 4, pp. 159–163. https://doi.org/10.7196/SAJCH.2018.v12i4.1522

Biagio, L, Swanepoel, DW, Adeyemo, A, Hall, JW & Vinck, B 2013, 'Asynchronous video-otoscopy with a telehealth facilitator', *Telemedicine and e-Health*, vol. 19, no. 4, pp. 252–258. https://doi.org/10.1089/tmj.2012.0161

Biagio, L, Swanepoel, DW, Laurent, C & Lundberg, T 2014, 'Paediatric otitis media at a primary healthcare clinic in South Africa', *South African Medical Journal*, vol. 104, no. 6, pp. 431–435. https://doi.org/10.7196/SAMJ.7534

Chang, YS, Ryu, G, Kim, K & Cho, YS 2019, 'Normative wideband absorbance measures in healthy neonates in Korea: A preliminary study', *International Journal of Pediatric Otorhinolaryngology*, vol. 117, pp. 6–11. https://doi.org/10.1016/j.ijporl.2018.11.012

Choi, SY, Cho, YS, Lee, NJ, Lee, J, Chung, WH & Hong, SH 2012, 'Factors associated with quality of life after ear surgery in patients with chronic otitis media', *Archives of Otolaryngology – Head & Neck Surgery*, vol. 138, no. 9, pp. 840–845. https://doi.org/10.1001/archoto.2012.1800

Dobbie, F, Purves, R, McKell, J, Dougall, N, Campbell, R, White, J, Amos, A, Moore, L & Bauld, L 2019, 'Implementation of a peer-led school based smoking prevention programme: A mixed methods process evaluation', *BMC Public Health*, vol. 19, no. 1, pp. 1–9. https://doi.org/10.1186/s12889-019-7112-7

Emanuel, DC, Henson, OEC & Knapp, RR 2012, 'Survey of audiological immittance practice', *American Journal of Audiology*, vol. 21, no. 1, pp. 60–70. https://doi.org/10.1044/1059-0889(2012/11-0037)

English, R, Peer, N, Honikman, S, Tugendhaft, A & Hofman, KJ 2017, '"First 1000 days" health interventions in low-and middle-income countries: Alignment of South African policies with high-quality evidence', *Global Health Action*, vol. 10, no. 1, a1340396. https://doi.org/10.1080/16549716.2017.1340396

Erkkola-Anttinen, N, Tähtinen, PA, Laine, MK & Ruohola, A 2014, 'Parental role in the diagnostics of otitis media: Can parents be taught to use tympanometry reliably?', *International Journal of Pediatric Otorhinolaryngology*, vol. 78, no. 7, pp. 1036–1039. https://doi.org/10.1016/j.ijporl.2014.03.035

Fagan, J & Jacobs, M 2009, 'Survey of ENT services in Africa: Need for a comprehensive intervention', *Global Health Action*, vol. 2, no. 1, a1932. https://doi.org/10.3402/gha.v2i0.1932

Fick, C 2017, 'Twenty years of IMCI implementation in South Africa: Accelerating impact for the next decade', *South African Health Review*, vol. 2017, no. 1, pp. 207–204.

Frantz, JM 2015, 'A peer-led approach to promoting health education in schools: The views of peers', *South African Journal of Education*, vol. 35, no. 1, pp. 1–7. https://doi.org/10.15700/201503070006

Ghasemi, V, Simbar, M, Rashidi Fakari, F & Kiani, Z 2019, 'The effect of peer education on health promotion of Iranian adolescents: A systematic review', *International Journal of Pediatrics*, vol. 7, no. 3, pp. 9139–9157. https://doi.org/10.22038/IJP.2018.36143.3153

Ghebreyesus, TA 2017, 'All roads lead to universal health coverage', *The Lancet Global Health*, vol. 5, no. 9, pp. 839–840. https://doi.org/10.1016/S2214-109X(17)30295-4

Govender, CD, Pillay, M, Paken, J & Sewram, V 2020, 'Perspectives and practices of ototoxicity monitoring', *South African Journal of Communication Disorders*, vol. 67, no. 1, a685. https://doi.org/10.4102/sajcd.v67i1.685

Govender, NG, Maistry, N, Soomar, N & Paken, J 2014, 'Hearing loss within a marriage: Perceptions of the spouse with normal hearing', *South African Family Practice*, vol. 56, no. 1, pp. 50–56. https://doi.org/10.1080/20786204.2014.10844583

Haapala, S, Niemitalo-Haapola, E, Raappana, A, Kujala, T, Suominen, K, Kujala, T & Jansson-Verkasalo, E 2014, 'Effects of recurrent acute otitis media on cortical speech-sound processing in 2-year old children', *Ear and Hearing: The Official Journal of the American Auditory Society*, vol. 35, no. 3, pp. 75–83. https://doi.org/10.1097/AUD.0000000000000002

Health Professional Council of South Africa (HPCSA) 2011, *Regulations defining the scope of the profession of Audiology*, viewed n.d., <https://www.gov.za/sites/default/files/gcis_document/201409/34632rg9594gon803.pdf>

Health Professional Council of South Africa (HPCSA) 2018, *Minimum standards for the hearing screening in schools*, viewed 20 February 2019, <https://www.hpcsa.co.za/Uploads/SLH/Minimum%20Standards%20for%20the%20Hearing%20Screening%20in%20Schools.pdf>

Hsieh, VC 2020, 'Putting resiliency of a health system to the test: COVID-19 in Taiwan', *Journal of the Formosan Medical Association = Taiwan yi zhi*, vol. 119, no. 4, pp. 884–885. https://doi.org/10.1016/j.jfma.2020.03.002

Hunter, LL & Sanford, CA 2015, 'Tympanometry and wideband acoustic immittance', eds. J Katz, M Chasin, K English, LJ Hood & KL Tillery, *Handbook of clinical audiology*, 7th edn, Wolters Kluver, Philadelphia.

Ibekwe, TS & Nwaorgu, OGB 2011, 'Classification and management challenges of otitis media in a resource-poor country', *Nigerian Journal of Clinical Practice*, vol. 14, no. 3, pp. 262–269. https://doi.org/10.4103/1119-3077.86764

Jaffer, S 2016, 'Wideband acoustic immittance: Instrument, ethnicity, and gender specific normative data', PhD dissertation, University of British Columbia.

Joubert, K & Botha, D 2019, 'Contributing factors to high prevalence of hearing impairment in the Elias Motsoaledi Local Municipal area, South Africa: A rural perspective', *South African Journal of Communication Disorders*, vol. 66, no. 1, a611. https://doi.org/10.4102/sajcd.v66i1.611

Joubert, K, Sebothoma, B & Kgare, KS 2017, 'Public awareness of audiology, hearing and hearing health in the Limpopo province, South Africa', *South African Journal of Communication Disorders*, vol. 64, no. 1, a557. https://doi.org/10.4102/sajcd.v64i1.557

Kaf, WA 2011, 'Wideband energy reflectance findings in presence of normal tympanogram in children with Down's syndrome', *International Journal of Pediatric Otorhinolaryngology*, vol. 75, no. 2, pp. 219–226. https://doi.org/10.1016/j.ijporl.2010.11.004

Kanji, A & Khoza-Shangase, K 2018, 'Objective hearing screening measures: An exploration of a suitable combination for risk-based newborn hearing screening', *Journal of the American Academy of Audiology*, vol. 29, no. 6, pp. 495–502. https://doi.org/10.3766/jaaa.16155

Kanji, A & Khoza-Shangase, K 2021, 'A paradigm shift in early hearing detection and intervention in South Africa', eds. K Khoza-Shangase & A Kanji, *Early detection and intervention in audiology: An African perspective*, Wits University Press, Johannesburg, p. 1. https://doi.org/10.18772/22021026567

Keefe, DH, Sanford, CA, Ellison, JC, Fitzpatrick, DF & Gorga, MP 2012, 'Wideband aural acoustic absorbance predicts conductive hearing loss in children', *International Journal of Audiology*, vol. 51, no. 12, pp. 880–891. https://doi.org/10.3109/14992027.2012.721936

Khan, NB, Thaver, S & Govender, SM 2017, 'Self-ear cleaning practices and the associated risk of ear injuries and ear-related symptoms in a group of university students', *Journal of Public Health in Africa*, vol. 8, no. 2, a555. https://doi.org/10.4081/jphia.2017.555

Khoza, K & Ross, E 2002, 'Auditory function in a group of adults infected with HIV/AIDS in Gauteng, South Africa', *South African Journal of Communication Disorders*, vol. 49, no. 1, pp. 17–27. https://doi.org/10.4102/sajcd.v49i1.214

Khoza-Shangase, K 2010, 'HIV/AIDS and auditory function in adults: The need for intensified research in the developing world', *African Journal of AIDS Research*, vol. 9, no. 1, pp. 1–9. https://doi.org/10.2989/16085906.2010.484531

Khoza-Shangase, K 2017, 'Risk versus benefit: Who assesses this in the management of patients on ototoxic drugs?', *Journal of Pharmacy & Bioallied Sciences*, vol. 9, no. 3, pp. 171–177. https://doi.org/10.4103/jpbs.JPBS_17_17

Khoza-Shangase, K 2019, 'Best/next practice in speech-language and hearing professions: Being responsible and responsive to context', *HPCSA Bulletin*, viewed 10 December 2019, <https://www.hpcsa.co.za/Uploads/SLH/Newsletter/SLH_newsletter_2020.pdf>

Khoza-Shangase, K 2020a, 'Burden of disease: A scoping review of HIV/AIDS and TB in occupational noise-induced hearing loss', *South African Journal of Communication Disorders*, vol. 67, no. 2, a669. https://doi.org/10.4102/sajcd.v67i2.669

Khoza-Shangase, K 2020b, 'Pharmaco-audiology vigilance in the treatment of adult patients with HIV/AIDS: Ototoxicity monitoring protocol recommendation', *Infectious Disorders-Drug Targets (Formerly Current Drug Targets-Infectious Disorders)*, vol. 20, no. 1, pp. 33–42. https://doi.org/10.2174/1871526518666181016102102

Khoza-Shangase, K 2021a, 'Continuity of care at school for the hearing-impaired child', eds. K Khoza-Shangase & A Kanji, *Early detection and intervention in audiology: An African perspective*, Wits University Press, Johannesburg, p. 155. https://doi.org/10.18772/22021026567

Khoza-Shangase, K 2021b, 'Confronting realities to early hearing detection in South Africa', eds. K Khoza-Shangase & A Kanji, *Early detection and intervention in audiology: An African perspective*, Wits University Press, Johannesburg, pp. 66–68. https://doi.org/10.18772/22021026567

Khoza-Shangase, K & Anastasiou, J 2020, 'An exploration of recorded otological manifestations in South African children with HIV/AIDS: A pilot study', *International Journal of Pediatric Otorhinolaryngology*, vol. 133, a109960. https://doi.org/10.1016/j.ijporl.2020.109960

Khoza-Shangase, K & Harbinson, S 2015, 'Evaluation of universal newborn hearing screening in South African primary care', *African Journal of Primary Health Care and Family Medicine*, vol. 7, no. 1, pp. 1–12. https://doi.org/10.4102/phcfm.v7i1.769

Khoza-Shangase, K & Kanji, A 2021, 'Best practice in South Africa for early hearing detection and intervention', eds. K Khoza-Shangase & A Kanji, *Early detection and intervention in audiology: An African perspective*, Wits University Press, Johannesburg, p. 264. https://doi.org/10.18772/22021026567

Khoza-Shangase, K & Masondo, N 2020, 'What are the current audiological practices for ototoxicity assessment and management in the South African healthcare context?', *International Journal of Environmental Research and Public Health*, vol. 17, no. 7, a2613. https://doi.org/10.3390/ijerph17072613

Khoza-Shangase, K & Mophosho, M 2021, 'Language and culture in speech-language and hearing professions in South Africa: Re-imagining practice', *South African Journal of Communication Disorders*, vol. 68, no. 1, a793. https://doi.org/10.4102/sajcd.v68i1.793

Khoza-Shangase, K & Moroe, N 2020, 'South African hearing conservation programmes in the context of tele-audiology: A scoping review', *South African Journal of Communication Disorders*, vol. 67, no. 2, a670. https://doi.org/10.4102/sajcd.v67i2.670

Khoza-Shangase, K, Moroe, N & Neille, J 2021a, 'Speech-language pathology and audiology in South Africa: Clinical training and service in the era of COVID-19', *International Journal of Telerehabilitation*, vol. 13, no. 1, a6376. https://doi.org/10.5195/ijt.2021.6376

Khoza-Shangase, K, Sebothoma, B & Moroe, NF 2021b, 'Teleaudiology as part of efforts to enhance inclusivity and equality through ICT in South African schools: Some considerations', eds. M Maguvhe, RS Mphahlele & S Moonsamy, *Empowering students and maximising inclusiveness and equality through ICT*, Brill Sense, Boston, pp. 223–243.

Khoza-Shangase, K & Riva, R 2021, 'Hearing function in adults with rheumatoid arthritis: A scoping review for preventive audiology planning', *Indian Journal of Otolaryngology and Head & Neck Surgery*, n.v., pp. 1–12. https://doi.org/10.1007/s12070-021-02747-x

Khoza-Shangase, K & Turnbull, T 2009, 'Hearing screening in a group of paediatric patients attending an HIV/AIDS clinic: A pilot study', *African Journal of Infectious Diseases*, vol. 3, no. 2, pp. 57–68. https://doi.org/10.4314/ajid.v3i2.55082

King, MS, Mhlanga, RE & De Pinho, H 2006, 'The context of maternal and child health: Maternal, child and women's health', *South African Health Review*, vol. 2006, no. 1, pp. 107–126.

Kolo, ES, Salisu, AD, Yaro, AM & Nwaorgu, OGB 2012, 'Sensorineural hearing loss in patients with chronic suppurative otitis media', *Indian Journal of Otolaryngology and Head & Neck Surgery*, vol. 64, no. 1, pp. 59–62. https://doi.org/10.1007/s12070-011-0251-5

Kreisman, BM, Smart, JL & John, AB 2015, 'Diagnostic audiology', eds. J Katz, M Chasin, K English, LJ Hood & KL Tillery, *Handbook of clinical audiology*, Wolters Kluwer, Philadelphia, pp. 119–134.

Krupinski, EA 2015, 'Innovations and possibilities in connected health', *Journal of the American Academy of Audiology*, vol. 26, no. 9, pp. 761–767. https://doi.org/10.3766/jaaa.14047

Le Roux, IM, Rotheram-Borus, MJ, Stein, J & Tomlinson, M 2014, 'The impact of paraprofessional home visitors on infants' growth and health at 18 months', *Vulnerable Children and Youth Studies*, vol. 9, no. 4, pp. 291–304. https://doi.org/10.1080/17450128.2014.940413

Lundberg, T, De Jager, LB, Swanepoel, DW & Laurent, C 2017, 'Diagnostic accuracy of a general practitioner with video-otoscopy collected by a health care facilitator compared to traditional otoscopy', *International Journal of Pediatric Otorhinolaryngology*, vol. 99, pp. 49–53. https://doi.org/10.1016/j.ijporl.2017.04.045

MacDonald, L & Green, WB 2001, 'A survey of Canadian audiological practices: Immittance measures', *Journal of Speech-Language Pathology and Audiology*, vol. 25, no. 4, pp. 212–220.

Mahomed-Asmail, F, Swanepoel, DW & Eikelboom, RH 2016, 'Hearing loss in urban South African school children (grade 1 to 3)', *International Journal of Pediatric Otorhinolaryngology*, vol. 84, pp. 27–31. https://doi.org/10.1016/j.ijporl.2016.02.021

Margolis, RH, Saly, GL & Keefe, DH 1999, 'Wideband reflectance tympanometry in normal adults', *The Journal of the Acoustical Society of America*, vol. 106, no. 1, pp. 265–280. https://doi.org/10.1121/1.427055

Martin, FN & Clark, JG 2019, *Introduction to audiology*, 13th edn, Pearson Education Limited, Hoboken, NJ.

Mayosi, BM & Benatar, SR 2014, 'Health and health care in South Africa – 20 years after Mandela', *New England Journal of Medicine*, vol. 371, no. 14, pp. 1344–1353. https://doi.org/10.1056/NEJMsr1405012

Mellanby, AR, Rees, JB & Tripp, JH 2000, 'Peer-led and adult-led school health education: A critical review of available comparative research', *Health Education Research*, vol. 15, no. 5, pp. 533–545. https://doi.org/10.1093/her/15.5.533

Merchant, GR, Al-Salim, S, Tempero, RM, Fitzpatrick, D & Neely, ST 2021, 'Improving the differential diagnosis of otitis media with effusion using wideband acoustic immittance', *Ear and Hearing: The Official Journal of the American Auditory Society*, vol. 42, no. 5, pp. 1183–1194. https://doi.org/10.1097/AUD.0000000000001037

Moroe, NF 2020, 'Occupational noise-induced hearing loss in South African large-scale mines: Exploring hearing conservation programmes as complex interventions embedded in a realist approach', *International Journal of Occupational Safety and Ergonomics*, vol. 26, no. 4, pp. 753–761. https://doi.org/10.1080/10803548.2018.1498183

Moroe, N & Khoza-Shangase, K 2018, 'Management of occupational noise induced hearing loss in the mining sector in South Africa: Where are the audiologists?', *Journal of Occupational Health*, vol. 60, no. 5, pp. 376–382. https://doi.org/10.1539/joh.2018-0020-OA

Mosam, A, Goldstein, S, Erzse, A, Tugendhaft, A & Hofman, K 2020, 'Building trust during COVID 19: Value-driven and ethical priority-setting', *South African Medical Journal*, vol. 110, no. 6, pp. 443–444. https://doi.org/10.7196/SAMJ.2020.v110i6.14893

Mottiar, S & Lodge, T 2018, 'The role of community health workers in supporting South Africa's HIV/AIDS treatment programme', *African Journal of AIDS Research*, vol. 17, no. 1, pp. 54–61. https://doi.org/10.2989/16085906.2017.1402793

Mulwafu, W, Ensink, R, Kuper, H & Fagan, J 2017b, 'Survey of ENT services in sub-Saharan Africa: Little progress between 2009 and 2015', *Global Health Action*, vol. 10, no. 1, a1289736. https://doi.org/10.1080/16549716.2017.1289736

Mulwafu, W, Kuper, H & Ensink, RJH 2017a, 'Prevalence and causes of hearing impairment in Africa', *Tropical Medicine and International Health*, vol. 21, no. 2, pp. 158–165. https://doi.org/10.1111/tmi.12640

Myers, J, Kei, J, Aithal, S, Aithal, V, Driscoll, C, Khan, A, Manuel, A, Joseph, A & Malicka, AN 2018, 'Development of a diagnostic prediction model for conductive conditions in neonates using wideband acoustic immittance', *Ear and Hearing: The Official Journal of the American Auditory Society*, vol. 39, no. 6, pp. 1116–1135. https://doi.org/10.1097/AUD.0000000000000565

O'Donovan, J, Verkerk, M, Winters, N, Chadha, S & Bhutta, MF 2019, 'The role of community health workers in addressing the global burden of ear disease and hearing loss: A systematic scoping review of the literature', *BMJ Global Health*, vol. 4, no. 2, a001141. https://doi.org/10.1136/bmjgh-2018-001141

Ohannessian, R, Duong, TA & Odone, A 2020, 'Global telemedicine implementation and integration within health systems to fight the COVID-19 pandemic: A call to action', *JMIR Public Health and Surveillance*, vol. 6, no. 2, a18810. https://doi.org/10.2196/18810

Okeyo, I, Lehmann, U & Schneider, H 2021, 'Policy adoption and the implementation woes of the intersectoral first 1000 days of childhood initiative, in the Western Cape province of South Africa', *International Journal of Health Policy and Management*, vol. 10, no. 7, pp. 364–375. https://doi.org/10.34172/IJHPM.2020.173

Olajide, TG, Olajuyin, OA, Eletta, AP, Agboola, SM, Busari, AO & Adebara, I 2019, 'Self-ear cleaning: Prevalence and profile among school children in Ekiti, Nigeria', *Journal of Biosciences and Medicines*, vol. 7, no. 4, pp. 25–32. https://doi.org/10.4236/jbm.2019.74003

Olusanya, BO, Okolo, AA & Adeosun, AA 2004, 'Predictors of hearing loss in school entrants in a developing country', *Journal of Postgraduate Medicine*, vol. 50, no. 3, pp. 173–179.

Park, J, Cheng, JT, Ferguson, D, Maguluri, G, Chang, EW, Clancy, C, Lee, DJ & Iftimia, N 2016, 'Investigation of middle ear anatomy and function with combined video otoscopy-phase sensitive OCT', *Biomedical Optics Express*, vol. 7, no. 2, pp. 238–250. https://doi.org/10.1364/BOE.7.000238

Passchier, RV 2017, 'Exploring the barriers to implementing national health insurance in South Africa: The people's perspective', *South African Medical Journal*, vol. 107, no. 10, pp. 836–838. https://doi.org/10.7196/SAMJ.2017.v107i10.12726

Peter, VZ, Paken, J & Joseph, L 2020, 'An audiological profile of a cohort of school-aged children with HIV and AIDS attending an antiretroviral clinic in South Africa', *South African Journal of Communication Disorders*, vol. 67, no. 1, pp. 1–9. https://doi.org/10.4102/sajcd.v67i1.651

Petrocchi-Bartal, L & Khoza-Shangase, K 2014, 'Hearing screening procedures and protocols in use at immunisation clinics in South Africa', *South African Journal of Communication Disorders*, vol. 61, no. 1, a66. https://doi.org/10.4102/sajcd.v61i1.66

Phanguphangu, MC 2017, 'Otoscopic examinations reveal high prevalence of outer and middle ear pathologies in paediatrics in Limpopo, South Africa', *International Journal of Audiology*, vol. 56, no. 4, pp. 215–218. https://doi.org/10.1080/14992027.2016.1244868

Pillay, M, Tiwari, R, Kathard, H & Chikte, U 2020, 'Sustainable workforce: South African audiologists and speech therapists', *Human Resources for Health*, vol. 18, no. 1, pp. 1–13. https://doi.org/10.1186/s12960-020-00488-6

Polat, Z, Baş, B, Hayır, D, Bulut, F & Ataş, A 2015, 'Wideband tympanometry normative data for Turkish young adult population', *Journal of International Advanced Otology*, vol. 11, no. 2, pp. 157–162. https://doi.org/10.5152/iao.2015.809

Ramma, L & Sebothoma, B 2016, 'The prevalence of hearing impairment within the Cape Town Metropolitan area', *South African Journal of Communication Disorders*, vol. 63, no. 1, a105. https://doi.org/10.4102/sajcd.v63i1.105

Ramma, L & Sebothoma, B 2017, 'Exploring factors associated with a higher likelihood of seeking audiology services by individuals with hearing loss', *JSM Communication Disorders*, vol. 1, no. 1, p. 1001.

Ranchod, S, Adams, C, Burger, R, Carvounes, A, Dreyer, K, Smith, A, Stewart, J & Biljon, CV 2017, 'South Africa's hospital sector: Old divisions and new developments', eds. A Padarath & P Barron, *South African health review 2017*, Health Systems Trust, Durban, pp. 101–110.

Reid, S 2020, 'Coronavirus pandemic holds lessons for South Africa's universal health care plans', *The Conversation*, viewed 10 July 2021, <https://theconversation.com/coronavirus-pandemic-holds-lessons-for-south-africas-universal-health-care-plans-137443>

Rushbrooke, E & Houston, KT 2013, *Telepractice in audiology*, Plural Publishing, San Diego.

Sandström, J, Swanepoel, D, Laurent, C, Umefjord, G & Lundberg, T 2020, 'Accuracy and reliability of smartphone self-test audiometry in community clinics in low income settings: A comparative study', *Annals of Otology, Rhinology & Laryngology*, vol. 129, no. 6, pp. 578–584. https://doi.org/10.1177/0003489420902162

Sanjar, FA, Queiroz, BEUP & Miziara, ID 2011, 'Otolaryngologic manifestations in HIV disease: Clinical aspects and treatment', *Brazilian Journal of Otorhinolaryngology*, vol. 77, pp. 391–400. https://doi.org/10.1590/S1808-86942011000300020

Schneider, H, Besada, D, Sanders, D, Daviaud, E & Rohde, S 2018, *Ward-based primary health care outreach teams in South Africa: Developments, challenges and future direction*, viewed 05 December 2019, <https://www.hst.org.za/publications/South%20African%20Health%20Reviews/SAHR%202018.pdf>

Sebothoma, B 2020, 'Middle ear pathologies in adults within the mining industry: A systematic review', *South African Journal of Communication Disorders*, vol. 67, no. 2, pp. 1–5.

Sebothoma, B & Khoza-Shangase, K 2018, 'A comparison between video otoscopy and standard tympanometry findings in adults living with human immunodeficiency virus (HIV) in South Africa', *South African Journal of Communication Disorders*, vol. 65, no. 1, a591. https://doi.org/10.4102/sajcd.v65i1.591

Sebothoma, B & Khoza-Shangase, K 2020, 'Middle ear pathologies in adults living with human immunodeficiency virus: A systematic review', *Annals of Otology, Rhinology & Laryngology*, vol. 129, no. 8, pp. 821–828. https://doi.org/10.1177/0003489420909847

Sebothoma, B & Khoza-Shangase, K 2021, 'Acoustic immittance measures and middle ear assessment: Current practice by South African Audiologists', *South African Journal of Communication Disorders*, vol. 68, no. 1, a818. https://doi.org/10.4102/sajcd.v68i1.818

Sebothoma, B & Khoza-Shangase, K in press, 'Wideband absorbance measure in adults living with and without human immunodeficiency virus', *Journal of Otolaryngology - Head and Neck Surgery* n.v., n.p.

Sebothoma, B, Khoza-Shangase, K, Mol, D & Masege, D 2021, 'The sensitivity and specificity of wideband absorbance measure in identifying pathologic middle ears in adults living with HIV', *South African Journal of Communication Disorders*, vol. 68, no. 1, a820. https://doi.org/10.4102/sajcd.v68i1.820

Shahnaz, N, Bork, K, Polka, L, Longridge, N, Bell, D & Westerberg, BD 2009, 'Energy reflectance and tympanometry in normal and otosclerotic ears', *Ear and Hearing: The Official Journal of the American Auditory Society*, vol. 30, no. 2, pp. 219–233. https://doi.org/10.1097/AUD.0b013e3181976a14

Shahnaz, N, Feeney, MP & Schairer, KS 2013, 'Wideband acoustic immittance normative data: Ethnicity, gender, aging, and instrumentation', *Ear and Hearing: The Official Journal of the American Auditory Society*, vol. 34, pp. 27–35. https://doi.org/10.1097/AUD.0b013e31829d5328

Shapiro, J & Galowitz, P 2016, 'Peer support for clinicians: A programmatic approach', *Academic Medicine*, vol. 91, no. 9, pp. 1200–1204. https://doi.org/10.1097/ACM.0000000000001297

Sharma, N, Jaiswal, AA, Banerjee, PK & Garg, AK 2015, 'Complications of chronic suppurative otitis media and their management: A single institution 12 years' experience', *Indian Journal of Otolaryngology and Head & Neck Surgery*, vol. 67, no. 4, pp. 353–360. https://doi.org/10.1007/s12070-015-0836-5

Statistics South Africa 2019, *Mid-year population estimates*, viewed 07 February 2020, <http://www.statssa.gov.za/publications/P0302/P03022019.pdf#:~:text=For%202019%2C%20Statistics%20South%20Africa%20%28Stats%20SA%29%20estimates,the%20South%20African%20population%2C%20with%20approximately%2015%2C2%20million>

Stock, S, Miranda, C, Evas, S, Plessis, S, Ridley, J, Yeh, S & Chanoine, J-P 2007, 'Healthy buddies: A novel, peer-led health promotion program for the prevention of obesity and eating disorders in children in elementary school', *Pediatrics*, vol. 120, no. 4, pp. 1059–1068. https://doi.org/10.1542/peds.2006-3003

Swanepoel, DW 2006, 'Audiology in South Africa: Audiología en Sudáfrica', *International Journal of Audiology*, vol. 45, no. 5, pp. 262–266. https://doi.org/10.1080/14992020500485650

Swanepoel, DW 2015, 'Tele-audiology', eds. J Katz, M Chasin, K English, L Hood & KL Tillery, *Handbook of clinical audiology*, 7th edn, Wolters Kluver Health, Philadelphia, pp. 539–560.

Swanepoel, DW 2020, 'eHealth technologies enable more accessible hearing care', *Seminars in Hearing*, vol. 41, no. 2, pp. 133–140. https://doi.org/10.1055/s-0040-1708510

Swanepoel, DW & Hall, JW 2010, 'A systematic review of telehealth applications in audiology', *Telemedicine and e-Health*, vol. 16, no. 2, pp. 181–200. https://doi.org/10.1089/tmj.2009.0111

Swanepoel, DW, Myburgh, HC, Howe, DM, Mahomed, F & Eikelboom, RH 2014, 'Smartphone hearing screening with integrated quality control and data management', *International Journal of Audiology*, vol. 53, no. 12, pp. 841–849.

Taipale, A, Pelkonen, T, Taipale, M, Roine, I, Bernardino, L, Peltola, H & Pitkaranta, A 2011, 'Otorhinolaryngological findings and hearing in HIV-positive and HIV-negative children in a developing country', *European Archives of Oto-rhino-laryngology*, vol. 268, no. 10, pp. 1527–1532. https://doi.org/10.1007/s00405-011-1579-x

Thobejane, GSV & Ntuli-Ngcobo, B 2014, 'The prevalence and types of auditory pathologies in patients presenting with HIV/AIDS at Dr George Mukhari Academic Hospital, Ga-Rankuwa, South Africa', Doctoral dissertation, Sefako Makgatho Health Sciences University.

Torre, III P, Cook, A, Elliott, H, Dawood, G & Laughton, B 2016, 'Middle ear function in human immunodeficiency virus (HIV)-infected South African children', *Journal of Paediatric Care Insight*, vol. 1, no. 1, pp. 13–17. https://doi.org/10.24218/jpci.2016.04

UNAIDS 2014, *UNAIDS sets 90-90-90 target for 2020 to end AIDS by 2030*, viewed 19 October 2018, <http://i-base.info/htb/27174>

UNAIDS 2019, *UNAIDS DATA 2019*, viewed 10 March 2020, <https://www.unaids.org/sites/default/files/media_asset/2019-UNAIDS-data_en.pdf>

Van der Westhuizen, Y, Swanepoel, DW, Heinze, B & Hofmeyr, LM 2013, 'Auditory and otological manifestations in adults with HIV/AIDS', *International Journal of Audiology*, vol. 52, pp. 37–43. https://doi.org/10.3109/14992027.2012.721935

Van Wyk, T, Mahomed-Asmail, F & Swanepoel, DW 2019, 'Supporting hearing health in vulnerable populations through community care workers using mHealth technologies', *International Journal of Audiology*, vol. 58, no. 11, pp. 790–797. https://doi.org/10.1080/14992027.2019.1649478

Vouloumanou, EK, Karageorgopoulos, DE, Kazantzi, MS, Kapaskelis, AM & Falagas, ME 2009, 'Antibiotics versus placebo or watchful waiting for acute otitis media: A meta-analysis of randomized controlled trials', *Journal of Antimicrobial Chemotherapy*, vol. 64, no. 1, pp. 16–24. https://doi.org/10.1093/jac/dkp166

World Health Organization (WHO) 2013, *Multi-country assessment of national capacity to provide hearing care*, WHO Document Production Services, Geneva.

World Health Organization (WHO) 2017, *Tracking universal health coverage: 2017 global monitoring report*, World Health Organization & World Bank, Geneva.

World Health Organization (WHO) 2018, *Addressing the rising prevalence of hearing loss*, World Health Organization, Geneva.

World Health Organization (WHO) 2020, *Basic ear and hearing care resource*, World Health Organization, Geneva.

Chapter 6

Adams, S, Ehrlich, R, Quail, Z, Jeebhay, MF & Ismail, N 2012, 'Occupational health challenges facing the Department of Health: Protecting employees against tuberculosis and caring for former mineworkers with occupational health disease', *South African Health Review*, vol. 2012, no. 1, pp. 67–82.

American Speech-Language-Hearing Association (ASHA) 1994, 'Audiologic management of individuals receiving cochleotoxic therapy (Guidelines)', *ASHA*, vol. 36, no. Suppl 12, pp. 11–19.

American Speech-Language-Hearing Association (ASHA) 2015, 'Audiology information series: Ototoxic medications', viewed 10 December 2018, <https://www.asha.org/uploadedFiles/AIS-Ototoxic-Medications.pdf>

AngloGold Ashanti 2012, *Country fact sheet South Africa*, viewed 27 October 2019, <http://www.aga-reports.com/12/>

Baguley, DM & Prayuenyong, P 2020, 'Looking beyond the audiogram in ototoxicity associated with platinum-based chemotherapy', *Cancer Chemotherapy and Pharmacology*, vol. 85, no. 2, pp. 245–250. https://doi.org/10.1007/s00280-019-04012-z

Bankaitis, AE & Schountz, T 1998, 'HIV-related ototoxicity', *Seminars in Hearing*, vol. 19, no. 2, pp. 155–163. https://doi.org/10.1055/s-0028-1082965

Bardien, J, Schaaf, H, Fagan, JJ & Petersen, L 2009, 'Aminoglycoside-induced hearing loss: South Africans at risk', *South African Medical Journal*, vol. 99, no. 6, pp. 440–441.

Benatar, S & Gill, S 2021, 'Universal access to healthcare: The case of South Africa in the comparative global context of the late Anthropocene era', *International Journal of Health Policy and Management*, vol. 10, no. 2, p. 49. https://doi.org/10.34172/IJHPM.2020.28

Bess, FH & Humes, LE 1990, *Audiology: The fundamentals*, Williams & Wilkins, Philadelphia.

Bisht, M & Bist, SS 2011, 'Ototoxicity: The hidden menace', *Indian Journal of Otolaryngology and Head & Neck Surgery*, vol. 63, no. 3, pp. 255–259.

Bistline, KL 2018, *Does the inclusion of the cost and burden of adverse drug reactions associated with drug-resistant TB treatment affect the incremental cost-effectiveness of new treatment regimens? A case study from the introduction of bedaquiline in South Africa National TB Programme*, viewed 10 February 2019, <https://open.uct.ac.za/handle/11427/28441>

Blaschke, TF, Nies, AS & Mamelok, RD 1995, 'Principles of therapeutics', eds. AG Gilman, LS Goodman & TW Rall, *Goodman and Gilman's the pharmacological basis of therapeutics*, 7th edn, MacGraw-Hill, New York, pp. 49–65.

Boettcher, FA, Henderson, D, Gratton, MA, Danielson, RW & Byrne, CD 1987, 'Synergistic interactions of noise and other ototraumatic agents', *Ear and Hearing: The Official Journal of the American Auditory Society*, vol. 8, no. 4, pp. 192–212. https://doi.org/10.1097/00003446-198708000-00003

Bogdanov, G, Bogdanov, I, Kazandjieva, J & Tsankov, N 2021, 'Cutaneous adverse effects of the available COVID-19 vaccines', *Clinics in Dermatology*, vol. 39, no. 3, pp. 523–531. https://doi.org/10.1016/j.clindermatol.2021.04.001

Burgoyne, RW & Tan, DH 2008, 'Prolongation and quality of life for HIV-infected adults treated with highly active antiretroviral therapy (HAART): A balancing act', *Journal of Antimicrobial Chemotherapy*, vol. 61, no. 3, pp. 469–473. https://doi.org/10.1093/jac/dkm499

Campbell, CKM 2004, 'Audiologic monitoring for ototoxicity', eds. PS Roland & JA Rutka, *Ototoxicity*, BC Decker Inc., Hamilton, pp. 153–160.

Campbell, KC 2018, 'Ototoxicity', eds. RS Ackley, TN Decker & CJ Limb, *An essential guide to hearing and balance disorders*, Psychology Press, London, pp. 117–138.

Cassidy, C, Dever, D, Stanbery, L, Edelman, G, Dworkin, L & Nemunaitis, J 2020, 'FDA efficiency for approval process of COVID-19 therapeutics', *Infectious Agents and Cancer*, vol. 15, no. 1, pp. 1–13. https://doi.org/10.1186/s13027-020-00338-z

Colopy, MW, Damaraju, CV, He, W, Jiang, Q, Levitan, BS, Ruan, S & Yuan, Z 2015, 'Benefit-risk evaluation and decision making: Some practical insights', *Therapeutic Innovation & Regulatory Science*, vol. 49, no. 3, pp. 425–433. https://doi.org/10.1177/2168479014565469

Conradie, F, Meintjes, G, Hughes, J, Maartens, G, Ferreira, H, Siwendu, S, Master, I & Ndjeka, N 2014, 'Clinical access program for bedaquiline for the treatment of drug-resistant tuberculosis', *South African Medical Journal*, vol. 104, no. 3, pp. 164–166. https://doi.org/10.7196/SAMJ.7263

Coovadia, H, Jewkes, R, Barron, P, Sanders, D & McIntyre, D 2009, 'The health and health system of South Africa: Historical roots of current public health challenges', *The Lancet*, vol. 374, no. 9692, pp. 817–834. https://doi.org/10.1016/S0140-6736(09)60951-X

Coplan, PM, Noel, RA, Levitan, BS, Ferguson, J & Mussen, F 2011, 'Development of a framework for enhancing the transparency, reproducibility and communication of the benefit-risk balance of medicines', *Clinical Pharmacology & Therapeutics*, vol. 89, no. 2, pp. 312–315. https://doi.org/10.1038/clpt.2010.291

Council for International Organizations of Medical Sciences (CIOMS) 1998, *Benefit-risk balance for marketed drugs: Evaluating safety signals: Report of CIOMS working group IV*, viewed 29 September 2010, <http://www.cioms.ch/publications/g4-benefit-risk.pdf>

Danckers, M, Lesko, MB, Adamson, R & Leibert, E 2014, 'Compassionate use of bedaquiline in the treatment of pulmonary XDR-TB', *The International Journal of Tuberculosis and Lung Disease*, vol. 18, no. 12, pp. 1522–1525. https://doi.org/10.5588/ijtld.14.0338

Davies, NECG 2013, 'Fixed-dose combination for adults accessing antiretroviral therapy: Advice document', *Southern African Journal of HIV Medicine*, vol. 14, no. 1, pp. 41–43. https://doi.org/10.4102/sajhivmed.v14i1.104

Duggal, P & Sarkar, M 2007, 'Audiologic monitoring of multi-drug resistant tuberculosis patients on aminoglycoside treatment with long term follow-up', *BMC Ear, Nose and Throat Disorders*, vol. 7, no. 1, pp. 1–7. https://doi.org/10.1186/1472-6815-7-5

Duong, D 2021, 'What's important to know about the new COVID-19 variants?', *CAMJ*, vol. 193, no. 4, pp. e141–e142. https://doi.org/10.1503/cmaj.1095915

Eichler, HG, Pignatti, F, Flamion, B, Leufkens, H & Breckenridge, A 2008, 'Balancing early market access to new drugs with the need for benefit/risk data: A mounting dilemma', *Nature Reviews Drug Discovery*, vol. 7, no. 10, pp. 818–826. https://doi.org/10.1038/nrd2664

Fairall, LR, Bachmann, MO, Louwagie, GM, Van Vuuren, C, Chikobvu, P, Steyn, D, Staniland, GH, Timmerman, V, Msimanga, M, Seebregts, CJ, Boulle, A, Nhiwatiwa, R, Bateman, ED, Zwarenstein, MF & Chapman, RD 2008, 'Effectiveness of antiretroviral treatment in a South African program: A cohort study', *Archives of Internal Medicine*, vol. 168, no. 1, pp. 86–93. https://doi.org/10.1001/archinternmed.2007.10

Floyd, K, Glaziou, P, Raviglione, M & Zumla, A 2018, 'The global tuberculosis epidemic – Progress in patient care. Prevention and control efforts in year three of the "end TB era"', *Lancet Respiratory Medicine*, vol. 6, no. 4, pp. 299–314. https://doi.org/10.1016/S2213-2600(18)30057-2

Freeman, M n.d., *Should non-communicable conditions of high burden but low mortality be prioritised in South Africa?*, viewed 13 February 2021, https://www.health.gov.za/2014-08-11-13-19-27?download=89:commission-presentation-should-non-communicable-conditionsof-high-burden-but-low-mortality-be-prioritised-in-south-africa-melvyn-freeman

Ganesan, P, Schmiedge, J, Manchaiah, V, Swapna, S, Dhandayutham, S & Kothandaraman, PP 2018, 'Ototoxicity: A challenge in diagnosis and treatment', *Journal of Audiology & Otology*, vol. 22, no. 2, pp. 59–68. https://doi.org/10.7874/jao.2017.00360

García, CC, Sánchez, EA, Huerta, DH & Gómez-Arnau, J 2020, 'COVID-19 treatment-induced neuropsychiatric adverse effects', *General Hospital Psychiatry*, vol. 67, p. 163. https://doi.org/10.1016/j.genhosppsych.2020.06.001

Govender, CD, Pillay, M, Paken, J & Sewram, V 2020, 'Perspectives and practices of ototoxicity monitoring', *South African Journal of Communication Disorders*, vol. 67, no. 1, a685. https://doi.org/10.4102/sajcd.v67i1.685

Govender, M & Paken, J 2015, 'Practices employed by audiologists in the management of adult patients with multidrug-resistant tuberculosis in South Africa', *South African Family Practice*, vol. 57, no. 6, pp. 363–372. https://doi.org/10.1080/20786190.2015.1085222

Guastalla, JP & Dieras, V 2003, 'The taxanes: Toxicity and quality of life considerations in advanced ovarian cancer', *British Journal of Cancer*, vol. 89, no. 3, pp. 16–22. https://doi.org/10.1038/sj.bjc.6601496

Guglielmetti, L, Hewison, C, Avaliani, Z, Hughes, J, Kiria, N, Lomtadze, N, Ndjeka, N, Setkina, S, Shabangu, A, Sikhondze, W, Skrahina, A, Veziris, N & Furin, J 2017, 'Examples of bedaquiline introduction for the management of multidrug-resistant tuberculosis in five countries', *The International Journal of Tuberculosis and Lung Disease*, vol. 21, no. 2, pp. 167–174. https://doi.org/10.5588/ijtld.16.0493

Guo, JJ, Pandey, S, Doyle, J, Bian, B, Lis, Y & Raisch, DW 2010, 'A review of quantitative risk-benefit methodologies for assessing drug safety and efficacy – Report of the ISPOR risk-benefit management working group', *Value in Health*, vol. 13, no. 5, pp. 657–666. https://doi.org/10.1111/j.1524-4733.2010.00725.x

Hall, JW 2000, *Handbook of otoacoustic emissions*, Singular Publishing Group, San Diego.

Harris, T, Peer, S & Fagan, JJ 2012, 'Audiological monitoring for ototoxic tuberculosis, human immunodeficiency virus and cancer therapies in a developing world setting', *The Journal of Laryngology & Otology*, vol. 126, no. 6, pp. 548–551. https://doi.org/10.1017/S0022215112000357

Health Professions' Council of South Africa (HPCSA) 2018, *Audiological management of patients on treatment that includes ototoxic medication: Guidelines*, viewed 10 January 2019, <https://www.hpcsa.co.za/Uploads/SLH/Guidelines%20for%20Audiological%20Management%20of%20Patients%20on%20Treatment%20that%20includes%20Ototoxic%20Medications.pdf>

Higashi, K, Medic, G, Littlewood, KJ, Diez, T, Granström, O & De Hert, M 2013, 'Medication adherence in schizophrenia: Factors influencing adherence and consequences of nonadherence, a systematic literature review', *Therapeutic Advances in Psychopharmacology*, vol. 3, no. 4, pp. 200–218. https://doi.org/10.1177/2045125312474019

Hofman, K & Madhi, S 2020, 'The unanticipated costs of COVID-19 to South Africa's quadruple disease burden', *South African Medical Journal*, vol. 110, no. 8, pp. 698–699. https://doi.org/10.7196/SAMJ.2020.v110i8.15125

Hollander, C, Joubert, K & Schellack, N 2020, 'An ototoxicity grading system within a mobile app (OtoCalc) for a resource-limited setting to guide grading and management of drug-induced hearing loss in patients with drug-resistant tuberculosis: Prospective, cross-sectional case series', *JMIR mHealth and uHealth*, vol. 8, no. 1, a14036. https://doi.org/10.2196/14036

Hong, H, Dowdy, DW, Dooley, KE, Francis, HW, Budhathoki, C, Han, HR & Farley, JE 2020, 'Aminoglycoside-induced hearing loss among patients being treated for drug-resistant tuberculosis in South Africa: A prediction model', *Clinical Infectious Diseases*, vol. 70, no. 5, pp. 917–924. https://doi.org/10.1093/cid/ciz289

Institute for Health Metrics and Evaluation (IHME) 2018, *Findings from the global burden of disease study in 2017*, viewed 15 February 2020, <https://www.healthdata.org/sites/default/files/files/policy_report/2019/GBD_2017_Booklet.pdf>

Juhaeri, J 2019, 'Benefit-risk evaluation: The past, present and future', *Therapeutic Advances in Drug Safety*, vol. 10. https://doi.org/10.1177/2042098619871180

Kallail, KJ, Downs, DW & Scherz, JW 2008, 'Communication disorders in individuals with HIV/AIDS', *Kansas Journal of Medicine*, vol. 1, no. 3, pp. 62–69. https://doi.org/10.17161/kjm.v1i3.11273

Khoza-Shangase, K 2010a, 'Is there a need for ototoxicity monitoring in patients with HIV/AIDS?', *African Journal of Pharmacy and Pharmacology*, vol. 4, no. 9, pp. 574–579.

Khoza-Shangase, K 2010b, 'HIV/AIDS and auditory function in adults: The need for intensified research in the developing world', *African Journal of AIDS Research*, vol. 9, no. 1, pp. 1–9. https://doi.org/10.2989/16085906.2010.484531

Khoza-Shangase, K 2011, 'Highly active antiretroviral therapy: Does it sound toxic?', *Journal of Pharmacy and Bioallied Sciences*, vol. 3, no. 1, p. 142. https://doi.org/10.4103/0975-7406.76494

Khoza-Shangase, K 2013, 'Ototoxicity in tuberculosis treatment in South Africa: Views from healthcare workers involved in the management of TB', *African Journal of Pharmacy & Pharmacology*, vol. 7, no. 30, pp. 2141–2145. https://doi.org/10.5897/AJPP12.722

Khoza-Shangase, K 2014, 'Pharmaco-audiology vigilance and highly active antiretroviral therapy (HAART) in South Africa: Ototoxicity monitoring pursued', *Journal of AIDS Clinical Research in Sexually Transmitted Diseases*, vol. 1, no. 1, pp. 1–10. https://doi.org/10.24966/ACRS-7370/100001

Khoza-Shangase, K 2017, 'Risk versus benefit: Who assesses this in the management of patients on ototoxic drugs?', *Journal of Pharmacy & Bioallied Sciences*, vol. 9, no. 3, pp. 171–177. https://doi.org/10.4103/jpbs.JPBS_17_17

Khoza-Shangase, K 2018, 'Vestibular function in a group of adults with HIV/AIDS on HAART', *African Journal of Infectious Diseases*, vol. 12, no. 1, pp. 7–14. https://doi.org/10.21010/ajid.v12i1.2

Khoza-Shangase, K 2020a, 'Pharmaco-audiology vigilance in the treatment of patients with HIV/AIDS: Ototoxicity monitoring protocol recommendation', *Infectious Disorders – Drug Targets*, vol. 20, no. 1, pp. 33–42. https://doi.org/10.2174/1871526518666181016102102

Khoza-Shangase, K 2020b, 'Burden of disease: A scoping review of HIV/AIDS and TB in occupational noise-induced hearing loss', *South African Journal of Communication Disorders*, vol. 67, no. 2, a669. https://doi.org/10.4102/sajcd.v67i2.669

Khoza-Shangase, K 2020c, 'Hearing function of gold miners with and without a history of tuberculosis treatment: A retrospective data review', *Brazilian Journal of Otorhinolaryngology*, vol. 86, no. 3, pp. 294–299. https://doi.org/10.1016/j.bjorl.2018.12.003

Khoza-Shangase, K & Jina, K 2013, 'Ototoxicity monitoring in general medical practice: Exploring perceptions and practices of general practitioners about drug-induced auditory symptoms', *Innovations in Pharmaceuticals and Pharmacotherapy*, vol. 1, no. 3, pp. 250–259.

Khoza-Shangase, K, Lecheko, L & Ntlhakana, L 2020, 'The impact of medical interventions for reducing ototoxicity during treatment for multi-drug resistant tuberculosis', *Acta Otorrinolaringológica Española*, vol. 71, no. 6, pp. 349–357. https://doi.org/10.1016/j.otorri.2019.12.003

Khoza-Shangase, K & Masondo, N 2020, 'What are the current audiological practices for ototoxicity assessment and management in the South African healthcare context?', *International Journal of Environmental Research and Public Health*, vol. 17, no. 7, a2613. https://doi.org/10.3390/ijerph17072613

Khoza-Shangase, K & Masondo, N 2021, 'In pursuit of preventive audiology in South Africa: Scoping the context for ototoxicity assessment and management', *Journal of Pharmacy & Bioallied Sciences*, vol. 13, no. 1, p. 46. https://doi.org/10.4103/jpbs.JPBS_334_19

Khoza-Shangase, K & Mophosho, M 2018, 'Language and culture in speech-language and hearing professions in South Africa: The dangers of a single story', *South African Journal of Communication Disorders*, vol. 65, no. 1, a594. https://doi.org/10.4102/sajcd.v65i1.594

Khoza-Shangase, K & Mophosho, M 2021, 'Language and culture in speech-language and hearing professions in South Africa: Re-imagining practice', *South African Journal of Communication Disorders*, vol. 68, no. 1, a793. https://doi.org/10.4102/sajcd.v68i1.793

Khoza-Shangase, K & Moroe, N 2020, 'South African hearing conservation programmes in the context of tele-audiology: A scoping review', *South African Journal of Communication Disorders*, vol. 67, no. 2, a670. https://doi.org/10.4102/sajcd.v67i2.670

Khoza-Shangase, K, Moroe, N & Neille, J 2021, 'Speech-language pathology and audiology in South Africa: Clinical training and service in the era of COVID-19', *International Journal of Telerehabilitation*, vol. 13, no. 1, pp. 1–31. https://doi.org/10.5195/ijt.2021.6376

Khoza-Shangase, K & Prodromos, M 2021, 'Impact of drug-resistant tuberculosis treatment on hearing function in South African adults: Bedaquiline versus kanamycin', *South African Journal of Communication Disorders*, vol. 68, no. 1, a784. https://doi.org/10.4102/sajcd.v68i1.784

Khoza-Shangase, K & Stirk, M 2016, 'Audiological testing for ototoxicity monitoring in adults with tuberculosis in state hospitals in Gauteng, South Africa', *Southern African Journal of Infectious Diseases*, vol. 31, no. 2, pp. 44–49. https://doi.org/10.1080/23120053.2016.1128143

Khoza-Shangase, K & Van Rie, KJ 2017, 'Pathological vestibular symptoms presenting in a group of adults with HIV/AIDS in Johannesburg, South Africa', *Southern African Journal of Infectious Diseases*, vol. 32, no. 2, a53. https://doi.org/10.4102/sajid.v32i2.53

Konrad-Martin, D, Reavis, KM, McMillan, G, Helt, WJ & Dille, M 2014, 'Proposed comprehensive ototoxicity monitoring program for VA healthcare (COMP-VA)', *Journal of Rehabilitation Research and Development*, vol. 51, no. 1, pp. 81–100. https://doi.org/10.1682/JRRD.2013.04.0092

Kros, CJ & Steyger, PS 2019, 'Aminoglycoside-and cisplatin-induced ototoxicity: Mechanisms and otoprotective strategies', *Cold Spring Harbor Perspectives in Medicine*, vol. 9, no. 11, a033548. https://doi.org/10.1101/cshperspect.a033548

Kürzinger, ML, Douarin, L, Uzun, I, El-Haddad, C, Hurst, W, Juhaeri, J & Tcherny-Lessenot, S 2020, 'Structured benefit-risk evaluation for medicinal products: Review of quantitative benefit-risk assessment findings in the literature', *Therapeutic Advances in Drug Safety*, vol. 11. https://doi.org/10.1177/2042098620976951

Landier, W 2016, 'Ototoxicity and cancer therapy', *Cancer*, vol. 122, no. 11, pp. 1647–1658. https://doi.org/10.1002/cncr.29779

Le Prell, CG, Ojano-Dirain, C, Rudnick, EW, Nelson, MA, DeRemer, SJ, Prieskorn, DM and Miller JM 2014, 'Assessment of nutrient supplement to reduce gentamicin-induced ototoxicity', *Journal of the Association for Research in Otolaryngology*, vol. 15, no. 3, pp. 375–393. https://doi.org/10.1007/s10162-014-0448-x

Li, H & Steyger, P 2009, 'Synergistic ototoxicity due to noise exposure and aminoglycoside antibiotics', *Noise & Health*, vol. 11, no. 42, p. 26. https://doi.org/10.4103/1463-1741.45310

Lonsbury-Martin, BL & Martin, GK 2001, 'Evoked otoacoustic emissions as objective screeners for ototoxicity', *Seminars in Hearing*, vol. 22, no. 4, pp. 377–392. https://doi.org/10.1055/s-2001-19111

Manchaiah, V, Beukes, EW, Granberg, S, Durisala, N, Baguley, DM, Allen, PM & Andersson, G 2018, 'Problems and life effects experienced by tinnitus research study volunteers: An exploratory study using the ICF classification', *Journal of the American Academy of Audiology*, vol. 29, no. 10, pp. 936–947. https://doi.org/10.3766/jaaa.17094

Maphumulo, WT & Bhengu, BR 2019, 'Challenges of quality improvement in the healthcare of South Africa post-apartheid: A critical review', *Curationis*, vol. 42, no. 1, a1901. https://doi.org/10.4102/curationis.v42i1.1901

Mayosi, BM, Flisher, AJ, Lalloo, UG, Sitas, F, Tollman, SM & Bradshaw, D 2009, 'The burden of non-communicable diseases in South Africa', *The lancet*, vol. 374, no. 9693, pp. 934–947.

Mayosi, BM, Lawn, JE, Van Niekerk, A, Bradshaw, D, Karim, SSA, Coovadia, HM & Lancet South Africa Team 2012, 'Health in South Africa: Changes and challenges since 2009', *The Lancet*, vol. 380, no. 9858, pp. 2029–2043. https://doi.org/10.1016/S0140-6736(12)61814-5

McKenna, L 2018, *The price of Bedaquiline*, Treatment Action Group, viewed 30 January 2019, <http://www.treatmentactiongroup.org/sites/default/files/realitycheckbedaquiline101618.pdf>

Moodley, S, Störbeck, C, Gama, N, Moodley, S, Moodley, S & Störbeck, C 2021, 'Ototoxicity: A review of South African studies', *South African Family Practice*, vol. 63, no. 1, a5187. https://doi.org/10.4102/safp.v63i1.5187

Moore, TJ, Cohen, MR & Furberg, CD 2007, 'Serious adverse drug events reported to the food and drug administration, 1998–2005', *Archives of Internal Medicine*, vol. 167, no. 16, pp. 1752–1759. https://doi.org/10.1001/archinte.167.16.1752

Morata, TC 2007, 'Promoting hearing health and the combined risk of noise-induced hearing loss and ototoxicity', *Audiological Medicine*, vol. 5, no. 1, pp. 33–40. https://doi.org/10.1080/16513860601159018

Mustafa, MWM 2020, 'Audiological profile of asymptomatic COVID-19 PCR-positive cases', *American Journal of Otolaryngology*, vol. 41, no. 3, p. 102483. https://doi.org/10.1016/j.amjoto.2020.102483

Nachega, JB, Hislop, M, Dowdy, DW, Lo, M, Omer, SB, Regensberg, L, Chaisson, RE & Maartens, G 2006, 'Adherence to highly active antiretroviral therapy assessed by pharmacy claims predicts survival in HIV-infected South African adults', *JAIDS Journal of Acquired Immune Deficiency Syndromes*, vol. 43, no. 1, pp. 78–84. https://doi.org/10.1097/qai.0b013e3181743955

Nebeker, JR, Barach, P & Samore, MH 2004, 'Clarifying adverse drug events: A clinician's guide to terminology, documentation, and reporting', *Annals of Internal Medicine*, vol. 140, no. 10, pp. 795–801. https://doi.org/10.7326/0003-4819-140-10-200405180-00009

Ntlhakana, L, Khoza-Shangase, K & Nelson, G 2020, 'Occupational noise-induced hearing loss in platinum miners: What do the data tell us?', *Occupational Health Southern Africa*, vol. 26, no. 1, pp. 8–14. https://doi.org/10.17159/2411-9717/1318/2021

Nunes, MC, Von Gottberg, A, De Gouveia, L, Cohen, C, Moore, DP, Klugman, KP & Madhi, SA 2011, 'The impact of antiretroviral treatment on the burden of invasive pneumococcal disease in South African children: A time series analysis', *AIDS*, vol. 25, no. 4, pp. 453–462. https://doi.org/10.1097/QAD.0b013e328341b7f1

Paken, J, Govender, CD, Pillay, M, Ayele, BT & Sewram, V 2021, 'Feasibility and first results of a prospective cohort study to investigate cisplatin-associated ototoxicity amongst cancer patients in South Africa', *BMC Cancer*, vol. 21, no. 1, pp. 1–11. https://doi.org/10.1186/s12885-021-08567-0

Perez, RB 2015, 'A review of ototoxic medications: Implications for professionals working with consumers with hearing loss', *JADARA*, vol. 49, no. 2, pp. 57–65.

Pillay, M, Tiwari, R, Kathard, H & Chikte, U 2020, 'Sustainable workforce: South African audiologists and speech therapists', *Human Resources for Health*, vol. 18, no. 1, pp. 1–13. https://doi.org/10.1186/s12960-020-00488-6

Pillay-Van Wyk, V, Msemburi, W, Laubscher, R, Dorrington, RE, Groenewald, P, Glass, T, Nojilana, B, Joubert, JD, Matzopoulos, R, Prinsloo, M, Nannan, N, Gwebushe, N, Vos, T, Somdyala, N, Sithole, N, Neethling, I, Nicol, E, Rossouw, A & Bradshaw, D 2016, 'Mortality trends and differentials in South Africa from 1997 to 2012: Second national burden of disease study', *The Lancet Global Health*, vol. 4, no. 9, pp. 642–653. https://doi.org/10.1016/S2214-109X(16)30113-9

Ramma, L, Schellack, N & Heinze, B 2019, 'Prevention of treatment-induced ototoxicity: An update for clinicians', *South African Medical Journal*, vol. 109, no. 3, pp. 145–149. https://doi.org/10.7196/SAMJ.2019.v109i3.013903

Reddy, M & Swanepoel, B 2006, *Cutting the cost of HIV/AIDS*, viewed n.d., <http://www.deloitte.com/assets/DcomSouthAfrica/Local%20Assets/Documents/HIVAIDS_Deloitte.pdf>

Rohde, J, Cousens, S, Chopra, M, Tangcharoensathien, V, Black, R, Bhutta, ZA & Lawn, JE 2008, '30 years after Alma-Ata: Has primary health care worked in countries?', *The Lancet*, vol. 372, no. 9642, pp. 950–961. https://doi.org/10.1016/S0140-6736(08)61405-1

Rome, BN & Avorn, J 2020, 'Drug evaluation during the Covid-19 pandemic', *New England Journal of Medicine*, vol. 382, no. 24, pp. 2282–2284. https://doi.org/10.1056/NEJMp2009457

Rybak, LP & Ramkumar, V 2007, 'Ototoxicity', *Kidney international*, vol. 72, no. 8, pp. 931–935.

Scheffler, RM, Mahoney, CB, Fulton, BD, Dal Poz, MR & Preker, AS 2009, 'Estimates of health care professional shortages in sub-Saharan Africa by 2015: Critical shortages of health workers are projected in 2015 throughout sub-Saharan Africa, and the projected cost to eliminate them approaches $20 billion', *Health Affairs*, vol. 28, no. Suppl 1, pp. 849–862. https://doi.org/10.1377/hlthaff.28.5.w849

Schellack, N, Wium, AM, Ehlert, K, Van Aswegen, Y & Gous, A 2015, 'Establishing a pharmacotherapy induced ototoxicity programme within a service-learning approach', *South African Journal of Communication Disorders*, vol. 62, no. 1, a96. https://doi.org/10.4102/sajcd.v62i1.96

Sebothoma, B, Khoza-Shangase, K, Mol, D & Masege, D 2021, 'The sensitivity and specificity of wideband absorbance measure in identifying pathologic middle ears in adults living with HIV', *South African Journal of Communication Disorders*, vol. 68, no. 1, a820. https://doi.org/10.4102/sajcd.v68i1.820

Sheth, S, Mukherjea, D, Rybak, LP & Ramkumar, V 2017, 'Mechanisms of cisplatin-induced ototoxicity and otoprotection', *Frontiers in Cellular Neuroscience*, vol. 11, a338. https://doi.org/10.3389/fncel.2017.00338

Siemieniuk, RA, Bartoszko, JJ, Ge, L, Zeraatkar, D, Izcovich, A, Kum, E, Pardo-Hernandez, H, Rochwerg, B, Lamontagne, F, Han, MA, Liu, Q, Agarwal, A, Agoritsas, T, Alexander, P, Chu, D, Couban, R, Darzi, A, Devji, T, Fang, B, Fang, C, Flottorp, SA, Foroutan, F, Heels-Ansdell, D, Honarmand, K, Hou, L, Hou, X, Ibrahim, Q, Loeb, M, Marcucci, M, Mcleod, S, Motaghi, S, Murthy, S, Mustafa, R, Neary, JD, Qasim, A, Rada, G, Riaz, IB, Sadeghirad, B, Sekercioglu, N, Sheng, L, Switzer, C, Tendal, B, Thabane, L, Tomlinson, G, Turner, T, Vandvik, PO, Vernooji, R, Viteri-Garcia, A, Wang, Y, Yao, L, Ye, Z, Guyatt, GH & Brignardello-Peterson, R 2020, 'Drug treatments for covid-19: Living systematic review and network meta-analysis', *BMJ*, vol. 370, a2980. https://doi.org/10.1136/bmj.m2980

Singh, K 2017, 'Over 100 TB patients go deaf because of negligence', *News24*, viewed 30 August 2018, <https://www.news24.com/SouthAfrica/News/over-100-tb-patients-go-deaf-because-of-negligence-da-20170906>

Stevenson, LJ, Biagio-De Jager, L, Graham, MA & Swanepoel, DW 2021, 'Community-based ototoxicity monitoring for drug-resistant tuberculosis in South Africa: An evaluation study',

International Journal of Environmental Research and Public Health, vol. 18, no. 21, a11342. https://doi.org/10.3390/ijerph182111342

Stuckler, D, Basu, S, McKee, M & Lurie, M 2011, 'Mining and risk of tuberculosis in sub-Saharan Africa', *American Journal of Public Health*, vol. 101, no. 3, pp. 524–530. https://doi.org/10.2105/AJPH.2009.175646

Stuckler, D, Steele, S, Lurie, M & Basu, S 2013, 'Introduction: "Dying for gold": The effects of mineral mining on HIV, tuberculosis, silicosis, and occupational diseases in southern Africa', *International Journal of Health Services*, vol. 43, no. 4, pp. 639–649. https://doi.org/10.2190/HS.43.4.c

Sun, DQ, Ward, BK, Semenov, YR, Carey, JP & Della Santina, CC 2014, 'Bilateral vestibular deficiency: Quality of life and economic implications', *JAMA Otolaryngology – Head & Neck Surgery*, vol. 140, no. 6, pp. 527–534. https://doi.org/10.1001/jamaoto.2014.490

Swanepoel, DW 2006, 'Audiology in South Africa: Audiología en Sudáfrica', *International Journal of Audiology*, vol. 45, no. 5, pp. 262–266. https://doi.org/10.1080/14992020500485650

Thomson, K & Nachlis, H 2020, 'Emergency use authorizations during the COVID-19 pandemic: Lessons from hydroxychloroquine for vaccine authorization and approval', *JAMA Otolaryngology – Head & Neck Surgery*, vol. 324, no. 13, pp. 1282–1283. https://doi.org/10.1001/jama.2020.16253

Tsintis, P & La Mache, E 2004, 'CIOMS and ICH initiatives in pharmacovigilance and risk management', *Drug Safety*, vol. 27, no. 8, pp. 509–517. https://doi.org/10.2165/00002018-200427080-00004

UNAIDS 2014, *UNAIDS sets 90-90-90 target for 2020 to end AIDS by 2030*, viewed 30 August 2019, <http://i-base.info/htb/27174>

UNAIDS 2020, *Country factsheets: South Africa, 2019*, viewed 13 January 2020, <https://www.unaids.org/en/regionscountries/countries/southafrica>

Valente, M, Hosford-Dunn, H & Roeser, RJ 2008, *Audiology: Treatment*, 2nd edn, Thieme, New York.

Wissink, TF, Moes, C, Beisel, KW & Fritzsch, B 2006, 'Neurotrophins and hearing dysfunction: Comparing models to stop nerve fiber loss', *Drug Discovery Today: Disease Models*, vol. 3, no. 4, pp. 391–396. https://doi.org/10.1016/j.ddmod.2006.10.011

World Health Organization (WHO) 2014a, *Companion handbook to the WHO guidelines for the programmatic management of drug-resistant tuberculosis*, World Health Organization, Geneva.

World Health Organization (WHO) 2014b, *Global tuberculosis report*, World Health Organization, Geneva.

World Health Organization (WHO) 2017, *Multi-drug resistant tuberculosis (MDR TB)*, World Health Organization, Geneva.

World Health Organization (WHO) 2019, *Fact sheets: Deafness and hearing loss: Estimates*, World Health Organization, Geneva.

World Health Organization (WHO) 2020, *TB and HIV, and other comorbidities*, World Health Organization, Geneva.

Zheng, JL & Gao, WQ 1996, 'Differential damage to auditory neurons and hair cells by ototoxins and neuroprotection by specific neurotrophins in rat cochlear organotypic cultures', *European Journal of Neuroscience*, vol. 8, no. 9, pp. 1897–1905. https://doi.org/10.1111/j.1460-9568.1996.tb01333.x

Chapter 7

Abdalla, FM & Omar, MA 2011, 'The role of the health system in the prevention of hearing loss among children in sub-Saharan Africa', *Sudanese Journal of Paediatrics*, vol. 11, no. 1, pp. 8–19.

Albino, N & Berry, L 2013, 'Early childhood development services in South Africa: What are the next steps?', *South African Child Gauge*, viewed 10 March 2017, <http://hdl.handle.net/11427/3896>

Alvarez, AE 2008, *An evaluation of the Virginia early hearing detection and intervention program*, viewed 10 March 2017, <http://www.infanthearing.org/states/documents/evaluation_tools/Virginia%20VEHDIP_Evaluation_July2008.pdf>

ASHA 2020, *Telepractice*, viewed 08 May 2020, <https://www.asha.org/Practice-Portal/Professional-Issues/Telepractice/>

Aubrey, C 2017, 'Sources of inequality in South African early child development services', *South African Journal of Childhood Education*, vol. 7, no. 1, pp. 1–9. https://doi.org/10.4102/sajce.v7i1.450

Bhardwaj, S, Pattinson, R, Kauchali, S, Dlamini, N, Marshall, C, Van der Merwe, M & Barron, P 2018, 'Implementation of strategies to improve programme effectiveness lead to an improvement in maternal and child health outcomes in South Africa', *South African Medical Journal*, vol. 108, no. 3 Suppl 1, pp. 44–49. https://doi.org/10.7196/SAMJ.2017.v108i3b.12812

Bradshaw, D, Nannan, N, Pillay-van Wyk, V, Laubscher, R, Groenewald, P & Dorrington, RE 2019, 'Burden of disease in South Africa: Protracted transitions driven by social pathologies', *South African Medical Journal*, vol. 109, no. 11, pp. 69–76. https://doi.org/10.7196/SAMJ.2019.v109i11b.14273

Brennan-Jones, C, Eikelboom, R & Swanepoel, D n.d. 'Telehealth for diagnosis of hearing loss', *Open Access Guide to Audiology and Hearing Aids for Otolaryngologists*, viewed 08 May 2020, <http://www.entdev.uct.ac.za/guides/open-access-guide-to-audiology-and-hearing-aids-for-otolaryngologists>

Butler, I 2010, 'Vaccine offers meningitis hope', *Nature*, vol. 468, p. 143. https://doi.org/10.1038/468143a

Chopra, M, Lawn, JE, Sanders, D, Barron, P, Karim, SSA, Bradshaw, D, Jewkes, R, Karim, QA, Flisher, AJ, Mayosi, BM, Tollman, SM, Churchyard, GJ, Coovadia, H & Lancet South Africa Team 2009, 'Achieving the health millennium development goals for South Africa: Challenges and priorities', *The Lancet*, vol. 374, no. 9694, pp. 1023–1031. https://doi.org/10.1016/S0140-6736(09)61122-3

Colella-Santos, MF, Hein, TAD, De Souza, GL, Do Amaral, MIR & Casali, RL 2014, 'Newborn hearing screening and early diagnostic in the NICU', *BioMed Research International*, vol. 2014, pp. 1–11. https://doi.org/10.1155/2014/845308

Crowley, L, Fink, G & Karlan, D 2014, *Increasing vaccination coverage using a mobile phone application in mozambique*, viewed 11 March 2020, <https://www.povertyactionlab.org/evaluation/increasingvaccination-coverage-using-mobile-phone-application-mozambique>

Davis, A 2019, 'The what, why and when of childhood vaccination in South Africa – 2019', *Prof Nurs Today*, vol. 23, no. 2, pp. 27–29.

De Kock, T, Swaepoel, D & Hall III JW 2016, 'Newborn hearing screening at a community-based obstetric unit: Screening and diagnostic outcomes', *International Journal of Pediatric Otorhinolaryngology*, vol. 84, pp. 124–131. https://doi.org/10.1016/j.ijporl.2016.02.031

Department of Education Culture and Employment n.d., *Early childhood development framework and action plan*, viewed 15 April 2020, <https://www.ece.gov.nt.ca/en/services/early-childhood-development/early-childhood-development-framework-and-action-plan>

Department of Health (DoH) 2011, *National health insurance: Policy paper*, viewed 15 April 2020, <http://www.bowman.co.za/FileBrowser/ContentDocuments/NHI.pdf>

Department of Health (DoH) 2015, *National health insurance for South Africa: Towards universal health coverage*, viewed 15 April 2020, <http://www.bhfglobal.com/wp-content/uploads/2015/03/National_Health_Insurance_White_Paper_10Dec2015.pdf>

Department of Health (DoH) 2017, *National health insurance for South Africa: Towards universal health coverage*, viewed 15 April 2020, <https://www.gov.za/sites/default/files/gcis_document/201707/40955gon627.pdf>

Dlamini, NR & Maja, P 2016, 'The expanded programme on immunisation in South Africa: A story yet to be told', *South African Medical Journal*, vol. 106, no. 7, pp. 675–677. https://doi.org/10.7196/SAMJ.2016.v106i7.10956

Dookie, S & Singh, S 2012, 'Primary health services at district level in South Africa: A critique of the primary health care approach', *BMC Family Practice*, vol. 13, pp. 67–70. https://doi.org/10.1186/1471-2296-13-67

Dovlo, D 2020, 'People and their health systems: The right to universal health coverage and the SDGs in Africa', eds. M Kaltenborn, M Krajewski & H Kuhn, *Sustainable development goals and human rights. Interdisciplinary studies in human rights*, Vol. 5, Springer, Cham, pp. 53–71.

Dramowski, A & Whitelaw, A 2017, 'A framework for preventing healthcare-associated infection in neonates and children in South Africa', *South African Medical Journal*, vol. 107, pp. 192–195. https://doi.org/10.7196/SAMJ.2017.v107i3.12035

Ehlert, K & Naudé, AM 2014, 'Infection prevention and control measures currently applied in South African audiology', *South African Journal of Communication Disorders*, vol. 61, no. 1, pp. 1–10. https://doi.org/10.4102/sajcd.v61i1.55

Engelman, D 2014, *The status of neonatal hearing screening in sub-Saharan Africa: A systematic review*, City University of New York, New York.

Feucht, UD 2013, 'Keeping children alive and healthy in South Africa-how do we reach this goal? Perspectives from a paediatrician in a District Clinical Specialist Team', *South African Journal of Child Health*, vol. 7, no. 4, pp. 124–126. https://doi.org/10.7196/sajch.680

Govender, SM & Mars, M 2016, 'The use of telehealth services to facilitate audiological management for children: A scoping review and content analysis', *Journal of Telemedicine and Telecare*, vol. 23, no. 3, pp. 392–401. https://doi.org/10.1177/1357633X16645728

Health Professions Council of South Africa (HPCSA) 2007, *Early hearing detection and intervention programmes in South Africa, position statement year 2007*, viewed 08 May 2020, <http://www.hpsca.co.za/hpcsa/default.aspx?id=137>

Health Professions Council of South Africa (HPCSA) 2018, *Early hearing detection and intervention (EHDI) guidelines*, viewed 02 March 2019, <http://www.hpcsa.co.za/Uploads/editor/UserFiles/downloads/speech/Early_Hearing_Detection_and_Intervention_(EHDI)_2018.pdf>

HIHOPES 2019, *Our vision*, viewed 08 May 2020, <https://www.hihopes.co.za/>

Houston, KT, Behl, D & Mottershead, S 2018, 'Using telepractice to improve outcomes for children who are deaf or hard of hearing & their families', viewed 15 May 2019, <http://www.infanthearing.org/ehdi-ebook/2018_ebook/17%20Chapter17UsingTelepractice2018.pdf>

Institute of Health Economics 2012, *The safety and efficacy/effectiveness of using automated testing devices for universal newborn hearing screening: An update*, viewed 02 February 2019, <http://www.inahta.org/upload/Briefs_12/12026_The_safety_and_efficacy_effectiveness_of_using_automated_testing_devices_for_universal_newborn_hearing_screening.pdf>

Jamoulle, M 2015, 'Quaternary prevention: First, do not harm', *Revista Brasileira de Medicina de Família e Comunidade*, vol. 10, no. 35, pp. 1–3. https://doi.org/10.5712/rbmfc10(35)1064

Joint Committee on Infant Hearing (JCIH) 2007, 'Year 2007 position statement: Principles and guidelines for early hearing detection and intervention programs', *Pediatrics*, vol. 120, no. 4, pp. 898–921. https://doi.org/10.1542/peds.2007-2333

Joint Committee on Infant Hearing (JCIH) 2019, 'Year 2019 position statement: Principles and guidelines for early hearing detection and intervention programs,' *The Journal of Ealy Hearing Detection and Intervention*, vol. 4, no. 2, pp. 1–44.

Joint Committee on Infant Hearing (JCIH), Muse, C, Harrison, J, Yoshinaga-Itano, C, Grimes, A, Brookhouser, PE, Epstein, S, Buchman, C, Mehl, A, Vohr, B, Moeller, MP, Martin, P, Benedict, BS, Scoggins, B, Crace, J, King, M, Sette, A & Martin, B 2013, 'Supplement to the JCIH 2007 position statement: Principles and guidelines for early intervention after confirmation that a child is deaf or hard of hearing', *Pediatrics*, vol. 131, no. 4, pp. 1324–1349. https://doi.org/10.1542/peds.2013-0008

Kanji, A 2016a, 'Early detection of hearing loss: Exploring risk-based hearing screening within a developing country context', Phd thesis, University of the Witwatersrand.

Kanji, A 2016b, 'Early hearing screening in South Africa – Time to get real about context', *South African Journal of Child Health*, vol. 10, no. 4, p. 192. https://doi.org/10.7196/SAJCH.2016.v10i4.1298

Kanji, A & Khoza-Shangase, K 2018, 'Objective hearing screening measures: An exploration of a suitable combination for risk-based newborn hearing screening', *Journal of the American Academy of Audiology*, vol. 29, pp. 495–502. https://doi.org/10.3766/jaaa.16155

Kanji, A & Khoza-Shangase, K 2019, 'Early detection of hearing impairment in high-risk neonates: Let's talk about the high-risk registry in the South African context', *South African Journal of Child Health*, vol. 13, no. 2, pp. 53–55.

Kanji, A, Khoza-Shangase, K & Moroe, N 2018, 'Newborn hearing screening protocols and their outcomes: A systematic review', *International Journal of Pediatric Otorhinolaryngology*, vol. 115, pp. 104–109. https://doi.org/10.1016/j.ijporl.2018.09.026

Keleher, H 2001, 'Why primary health care offers a more comprehensive approach for tackling health inequities than primary care', *Australian Journal of Primary Health*, vol. 7, no. 2, pp. 57–61. https://doi.org/10.1071/PY01035

Khan, N, Charles, C, Naidoo, N, Nokubonga, A, Mkhwanazi, N & Moustache, H 2019, 'Infection prevention and control measures in audiology practice within public healthcare facilities in KwaZulu-Natal province, South Africa', *South African Journal of Communication Disorders*, vol. 66, no. 1, a636. https://doi.org/10.4102/sajcd.v66i1.636

Khoza-Shangase, K & Harbinson, S 2015, 'Evaluation of universal newborn hearing screening in South African primary care', *African Journal of Primary Health Care and Family Medicine*, vol. 7, no. 1, a769. https://doi.org/10.4102/phcfm.v7i1.769

Khoza-Shangase, K, Kanji, A, Petrocchi-Bartal, B & Farr, K 2017, 'Infant hearing screening from a developing country context: Status from two South African Provinces,' *South African Journal of Child Health*, vol. 11, no. 4, pp. 159–163.

KiDS 2019, *South African early childhood review 2019*, viewed 08 May 2020, <http://www.ci.uct.ac.za/sites/default/files/image_tool/images/367/SA-ECR_2019_12_09_2019_online_pages_0.pdf>

Kisling, LA & Das, JM 2019, *Prevention strategies*, StatPearls Publishing LLC, St. Petersburg.

Malakoane, B, Heunis, JC, Chikobvu, P, Kigozi, NG & Kruger, WH 2020, 'Public health system challenges in the Free State, South Africa: A situation appraisal to inform health system strengthening', *BMC Health Service Research*, vol. 20, no. 1, p. 58. https://doi.org/10.1186/s12913-019-4862-y

Maphumulo, WT & Bhengu, BR 2019, 'Challenges of quality improvement in the healthcare of South Africa post-apartheid: A critical review', *Curationis*, vol. 42, no. 1, a1901. https://doi.org/10.4102/curationis.v42i1.1901

Matsoso, MP & Fryatt, R 2013, 'National health insurance: The first 18 months', *South African Medical Journal*, vol. 103, no. 3, pp. 156–158. https://doi.org/10.7196/SAMJ.6601

Mayosi, BM, Lawn, JE, Van Niekerk, A, Bradshaw, D, Abdool Karim, SS & Coovadia, HM 2012a, 'Health in South Africa: Changes and challenges since 2009,' *Lancet*, vol. 380, pp. 2029–2043. https://doi.org/10.1016/S0140-6736(12)61814-5

Mayosi, BM, Lawn, JE, Van Niekerk, A, Bradshaw, D, Abdool Karim, SS & Coovadia, HM 2012b, 'Health in South Africa: Changes and challenges since 2009', *Lancet*, vol. 380, pp. 2029–2043. https://doi.org/10.1016/S0140-6736(12)61814-5

Meinzen-Derr, J, Wiley, S & Choo, DI 2011, 'Impact of early intervention on expressive and receptive language development among young children with permanent hearing loss', *American Annals of the Deaf*, vol. 155, no. 5, pp. 580–591. https://doi.org/10.1353/aad.2011.0010

Monasta, L, Ronfani, L, Marchetti, F, Montico, M, Vecchi Brumatti, L, Bavcar, A, Grasso, D, Barbiero, C & Tamburlini, G 2012, 'Burden of disease caused by otitis media: Systematic review and global estimates', *PLoS One*, vol. 7, no. 4, p. 36226. https://doi.org/10.1371/journal.pone.0036226

Moodley, S & Störbeck, C 2017, 'Data management for early hearing detection and intervention in South Africa', *South African Journal of Information Management*, vol. 19, no. 1, a779. https://doi.org/10.4102/sajim.v19i1.779

Nabhan, M, Elraiyah, T, Brown, DR, Dilling, J, LeBlanc, A, Montori, VM, Morgenthaler, T, Naessens, J, Prokop, L, Roger, V, Swensen, S, Thompson, RL & Murad, MH 2012, 'What is preventable harm in healthcare? A systematic review of definitions', *BMC Health Services Research*, vol. 12, no. 128, pp. 1–8. https://doi.org/10.1186/1472-6963-12-128

Naidoo, S 2012, 'The South African national health insurance: A revolution in health-care delivery!', *Journal of Public Health*, vol. 34, no. 1, pp. 149–150. https://doi.org/10.1093/pubmed/fds008

National Committee for Confidential Enquiries into Maternal Deaths 2008, *Saving mothers 2005-2007: Fourth report on confidential enquiries into maternal deaths in South Africa*, viewed 18 April 2020, <http://www.health.gov.za/index.php/2014-08-15-12-55-04/category/101-2011rp?download=190:saving-mothers-2005-2007-fourth-report-on-confidential-enquiries-intomaternal-deaths-in-south-africa-full-report>

National Department of Health (NDoH) n.d., *mHealth strategy*, viewed 08 May 2020, <https://www.hst.org.za/publications/GCCStars/Resources/mhealth%20strategy%20web_1%20(1).pdf>

Nelson, C & Madiba, S 2020, 'Barriers to the implementation of the ward-based outreach team program in Mpumalanga province: Results from process evaluation', *Journal of Primary Care & Community Health*, vol. 11, pp. 1–13. https://doi.org/10.1177/2150132720975552

Neumann, K, Chadha, S, Tavartkiladze, G, Bu, X & White, KR 2019, 'Newborn and infant hearing screening facing globally growing numbers of people suffering from disabling hearing loss', *International Journal of Neonatal Screening*, vol. 5, no. 7, pp. 1–11. https://doi.org/10.3390/ijns5010007

Ojo, AI 2018, 'mHealth interventions in South Africa: A review', *Sage Open*, vol. 8, no. 1, pp. 1–8. https://doi.org/10.1177/2158244018767223

Olu, O, Muneene, D, Bataringaya, JE, Nahimana, M-R, Ba, H, Turgeon, Y, Karamagi, HC & Dovlo, D 2019, 'How can digital health technologies contribute to sustainable attainment of universal health coverage in Africa? A perspective', *Frontiers in Public Health*, vol. 7, pp. 1–7. https://doi.org/10.3389/fpubh.2019.00341

Olusanya, B 2006, 'Early hearing detection and intervention in developing countries: Current status and prospects', *Volta Review*, vol. 106, no. 3, pp. 381–418. https://doi.org/10.17955/tvr.106.3.m.575

Olusanya, BO 2009, 'Newborns at risk of sensorineural hearing loss in low-income countries', *Archives of Disease in Childhood*, vol. 94, pp. 227–229. https://doi.org/10.1136/adc.2008.144550

Olusanya, BO, Neumann, KJ & Saunders, JE 2014, 'The global burden of disabling hearing impairment: A call to action', *Bulletin of the World Health Organization*, vol. 92, no. 5, pp. 367–373. https://doi.org/10.2471/BLT.13.128728

Olusanya, BO, Swanepoel, DW, Chapchap, MJ, Castillo, S, Habib, H, Mukari, SZ, Martinez, NV, Lin, H-C & McPherson, B 2007, 'Progress towards early detection services for infants with hearing loss in developing countries', *BMC Health Services Research*, vol. 7, no. 1, pp. 1–15. https://doi.org/10.1186/1472-6963-7-14

Pasupathy, S & Kumar, HS 2018, 'Critical appraisal of appropriate method for early detection of hearing impairment in newborns in a Tertiary Care Centre', *International Journal of Contemporary Pediatrics*, vol. 5, no. 6, pp. 2064–2070. https://doi.org/10.18203/2349-3291.ijcp20183843

Patel, B, Engelbrecht, H, McDonald, H, Morris, V & Smythe, W 2016, 'A multifaceted hospital-wide intervention increases hand hygiene compliance', *South African Medical Journal*, vol. 106, no. 4, pp. 335–341. https://doi.org/10.7196/SAMJ.2016.v106i4.10671

Peter, JE, Barron, P & Pillay, Y 2015, 'Using mobile technology to improve maternal, child and youth health and treatment of HIV patients', *South African Medical Journal*, vol. 106, pp. 3–4. https://doi.org/10.7196/SAMJ.2016.v106i1.10209

Peters, A, Otter, J, Moldovan, A, Parneix, P, Voss, A & Pittet, D 2018, 'Keeping hospitals clean and safe without breaking the bank: Summary of the healthcare cleaning forum', *Antimicrobial Resistance and Infection Control*, vol. 7, no. 132, pp. 1–12. https://doi.org/10.1186/s13756-018-0420-3

Pillay-Van Wyk, V, Msemburi, W, Laubscher, R, Dorrington, RE, Groenewald, P, Glass, T, Nojilana, B, Joubert, JD, Matzopoulos, R, Prinsloo, M, Nannan, N, Gwebushe, N, Vos, T, Somdyala, N, Sithole, N, Neethling, I, Nicol, E, Rossouw, A & Bradshaw, D 2016, 'Mortality trends and differentials in South Africa from 1997 to 2012: Second national burden of disease study', *The Lancet Global Health*, vol. 4, no. 9, pp. 642–653. https://doi.org/10.1016/S2214-109X(16)30113-9

Pillay, Y & Motsoaledi, PA 2018, 'Digital health in South Africa: Innovating to improve health', *BMJ Global Health*, vol. 3, no. Suppl 2, a000722. https://doi.org/10.1136/bmjgh-2018-000722

Puoanei, TH, Tsolekilei, LP, Egbujiei, BA, Lewyi, M & Sandersi, D 2017, 'Advancing the agenda on noncommunicable diseases: Prevention and management at community level', *South African Health Review*, vol. 2017, no. 1, pp. 171–179.

Qureishi, A, Lee, Y, Belfield, K, Birchall, JP & Daniel, M 2014, 'Update on otitis media-prevention and treatment', *Infection and Drug Resistance*, vol. 7, pp. 15–24. https://doi.org/10.2147/IDR.S39637

Republic of South Africa (RSA) 2015, *National integrated early childhood development policy*, viewed n.d., <https://unicef.org/southafrica/SAF_resources_integratedecdpolicy.pdf>

Republic of South Africa (RSA) 2019, *National health insurance bill*, viewed 08 May 2020, <https://www.gov.za/sites/default/files/gcis_document/201908/national-health-insurance-bill-b-11-2019.pdf>

Rifkin, E & Bouwer, E 2007, 'Cause and effect vs. risk factors', eds. E Rifkin & E Bouwer, *The illusion of certainty: health benefits and risks*, Springer, Baltimore, MD, pp. 15–31.

SADHS 2016, *South Africa demographic and health survey 2016*, viewed 15 April 2019, <https://dhsprogram.com/pubs/pdf/FR337/FR337.pdf>

Schellack, N, Meyer, JC, Gous, AGS & Winters, C 2011, 'Part II. Health and economic context', *South African Medical Journal*, vol. 101, no. 8, pp. 558–561.

Shekari, E, Nakhshab, M, Valinejad, V, Modarres Zadeh, A & Hosseinpour, A 2017, 'A systematic review of the effectiveness of early intervention and the role of parents in language development of hearing loss children', *Iranian Rehabilitation Journal*, vol. 15, no. 1, pp. 5–14. https://doi.org/10.18869/nrip.irj.15.1.5

Shetty, HN, Koohnoor, V & Rajalakshmi, G 2016, 'Sensitivity and specificity of combined physiological tests in newborn hearing screening', *Journal of Phonetics & Audiology*, vol. 2, no. 2, pp. 1–7. https://doi.org/10.4172/2471-9455.1000119

Sodo, P & Bosman, A 2017, 'Progress of the municipal ward-based primary healthcare outreach teams in Vhembe, Limpopo province', *Southern African Journal of Public Health Incorporating Strengthening Health Systems*, vol. 2, no. 1, pp. 18–22.

South African Government 2018, *Presidential health summit 2018*, viewed 08 May 2020, <https://www.gov.za/sites/default/files/gcis_document/201902/presidential-health-summit-report.pdf>

South African Government 2020a, *Child immunisation*, viewed 08 May 2020, <https://www.gov.za/services/child-care/child-immunisation>

South African Government 2020b, *Health*, viewed 08 May 2020, <https://www.gov.za/about-sa/health>

South African Speech Language and Hearing Association (SASLHA) 2011, *Guidelines infection control: Guidelines for speech-language therapists and audiologists regarding infection control*, viewed 17 June 2018, <http://www.saslha.co.za>

Statistics South Africa 2016, *Education series volume IV: Early childhood development in South Africa, 2016*, viewed 08 May 2020, <http://www.statssa.gov.za/publications/92-01-04/92-01-042016.pdf>

Stevenson, S 2019, *The National Health Act Guide*, viewed 10 March 2020, <http://section27.org.za/wp-content/uploads/2019/07/Stevenson-National-Health-Act-Guide-2019-1.pdf>

Störbeck, C & Young, A 2016, 'The HI HOPES data set of deaf children under the age of 6 in South Africa: Maternal suspicion, age of identification and newborn hearing screening', *BMC Pediatrics*, vol. 16, no. 45, pp. 1–10. https://doi.org/10.1186/s12887-016-0574-1

Swanepoel, D 2010, 'The global epidemic of infant hearing loss-priorities for prevention', in *Sound foundation through early amplification*, Judith Gravel Lecture, Chicago.

Swanepoel, D 2017, 'Screening for hearing loss with mHealth solutions', *ENT and Audiology News*, vol. 26, no. 1, pp. 72–74.

Swanepoel, D, Koekemoer, D & Clark, J 2010, 'Intercontinental hearing assessment – A study in tele-audiology', *Telemedicine and Telecare*, vol. 16, pp. 248–252. https://doi.org/10.1258/jtt.2010.090906

Taipale, A, Pelkonen, T, Taipale, M, Bernardino, L, Peltola, H & Pitkaranta, A 2011, 'Chronic suppurative otitis media in children of Luanda, Angola', *Acta Paediatrica*, vol. 100, no. 8, pp. 84–88. https://doi.org/10.1111/j.1651-2227.2011.02192.x

Tesser, CD 2017, 'Why is quaternary prevention important in prevention?', *Revista de Saude Publica*, vol. 51, no. 116, pp. 1–9.

United Nations (UN) 2018, *Sustainable development goals*, viewed 05 January 2019, <https://www.un.org/sustainabledevelopment/%20sustainable-development-goals/>

Upadhya, I & Datar, J 2014, 'Treatment options in otitis media with effusion', *Indian Journal of Otolaryngology and Head & Neck Surgery*, vol. 66, no. 1, pp. 191–197. https://doi.org/10.1007/s12070-011-0423-3

Van Rensburg, HCJ 2014, 'South Africa's protracted struggle for equal distribution and equitable access – Still not there', *Human Resources for Health*, vol. 12, pp. 1–16. https://doi.org/10.1186/1478-4491-12-26

World Health Organization (WHO) 1995, *WHA48.9 prevention of hearing impairment*, World Health Organization, Geneva.

World Health Organization (WHO) 2006, *Primary ear and hearing care*, World Health Organization, Geneva.

World Health Organization (WHO) 2007, *Task shifting to tackle health worker shortages*, World Health Organization, Geneva.

World Health Organization (WHO) 2013, *Millions of people in the world have hearing loss that can be treated or prevented*, World Health Organization, Geneva.

World Health Organization (WHO) 2016, *Childhood hearing loss: strategies for prevention and care*, World Health Organization, Geneva.

World Health Organization (WHO) 2017, *SDGs and progress towards universal health coverage*, World Health Organization, Geneva.

World Health Organization (WHO) 2018a, *Addressing the rising prevalence of hearing loss*, World Health Organization, Geneva.

World Health Organization (WHO) 2018b, *Country cooperation strategy at a glance*, World Health Organization, Geneva.

World Health Organization (WHO) 2020a, *Deafness and hearing loss*, World Health Organization, Geneva.

World Health Organization (WHO) 2020b, *Deafness prevention: Estimates*, World Health Organization, Geneva.

World Health Organization (WHO) 2020c, *SDG 3: Ensure healthy lives and promote wellbeing for all at all ages*, World Health Organization, Geneva.

World Health Organization (WHO) 2021, *World report on hearing: Executive summary*, World Health Organization, Geneva.

Yang, Y, Liu, YH, Fu, MF, Li, CL, Wang, LY, Wang, Q & Sun, X-B 2015, 'Home-based early intervention on auditory and speech development in Mandarin-speaking deaf infants and toddlers with chronological aged 7–24 months', *Chinese Medical Journal*, vol. 128, no. 16, pp. 2202–2207. https://doi.org/10.4103/0366-6999.162504

Yoshinaga-Itano, C & Mah-Rya, LA 1998, 'Identification of hearing loss after age 18 months is not early enough', *American Annals of the Deaf*, vol. 143, no. 5, pp. 380–387. https://doi.org/10.1353/aad.2012.0151

Young, M 2016, *Private vs. public healthcare in South Africa*, viewed 31 January 2020, <https://scholarworks.wmich.edu/cgi/viewcontent.cgi?article=3752&context=honors_theses>

Chapter 8

Adedeji, TO, Tobih, JE, Sogebi, OA & Daniel, AD 2015, 'Management challenges of congenital & early onset childhood hearing loss in a sub-Saharan African country', *International Journal of Pediatric Otorhinolaryngology*, vol. 79, no. 10, pp. 1625–1629.

Alvarez, AE 2008, *An evaluation of the Virginia early hearing detection and intervention program*, viewed 08 May 2018, <http://www.infanthearing.org/states/documents/evaluation_tools/Virginia%20VEHDIP_Evaluation_July2008.pdf>

Babalola, S & Fatusi, A 2009, 'Determinants of use of maternal health services in Nigeria – looking beyond individual and household factors', *BMC Pregnancy and Childbirth*, vol. 9, no. 43, pp. 1–13. https://doi.org/10.1186/1471-2393-9-43

Balton, S, Uys, K & Alant, E 2019, 'Family-based activity settings of children in a low-income African context', *African Journal of Disability*, vol. 8, a364. https://doi.org/10.4102/ajod.v8i0.364

Behl, DD & Kahn, G 2015, 'Provider perspectives on telepractice for serving families of children who are deaf or hard of hearing', *International Journal of Telerehabilitation*, vol. 7, no. 1, pp. 1–12. https://doi.org/10.5195/IJT.2015.6170

Bezuidenhout, KJ, Khoza-Shangase, K, De Maayer, T & Strehlau, R 2018, 'Universal newborn hearing screening in public health care in South Africa: Challenges to implementation', *South African Journal of Child Health*, vol. 12, no. 4, pp. 159–163. https://doi.org/10.7196/SAJCH.2018.v12i4.1522

Blaiser, KM, Behl, D, Callow-Heusser, C & White, KR 2013, 'Measuring costs and outcomes of tele-intervention when serving families of children who are deaf/hard-of-hearing', *International Journal of Telerehabilitation*, vol. 5, no. 2, pp. 3–10. https://doi.org/10.5195/ijt.2013.6129

Bowe, FW 2004, *Early childhood special education: Birth to eight*, Delmar Centage Learning, Clifton Park, New York.

Cavalcanti, HG & Guerra, RO 2012, 'The role of maternal socioeconomic factors in the commitment to universal newborn hearing screening in the northeastern region of Brazil', *International Journal of Pediatric Otorhinolaryngology*, vol. 76, pp. 1661–1667. https://doi.org/10.1016/j.ijporl.2012.07.041

Ching, TYC, Dillon, H, Leigh, G & Cupples, L 2018a, 'Learning from the longitudinal outcomes of children with hearing impairment (LOCHI) study: Summary of 5-year findings and implications', *International Journal of Audiology*, vol. 57, suppl. 2, pp. 105–111. https://doi.org/10.1080/14992027.2017.1385865

Ching, TYC, Scarinci, N, Marnane, V, Sjahalam-King, J, Button, L & Whitfield, J 2018b, 'Factors influencing parents' decisions about communication choices during early education of their child with hearing loss: A qualitative study', *Deafness & Education International*, vol. 20, no. 3–4, pp. 154–181. https://doi.org/10.1080/14643154.2018.1512393

Conroy, AM, McGarth, N, Van Rooyen, H, Hosegood, V, Johnson, MO, Fritz, K, Marr, A, Ngubane, T & Darbes, LA 2016, 'Power and the association with relationship quality in South African couples: Implications for HIV/AIDS interventions', *Social Science & Medicine*, vol. 153, pp. 1–11. https://doi.org/10.1016/j.socscimed.2016.01.035

Crowe, K, Fordham, L, Mcleod, S & Ching, TYC 2014, '"Part of our world": Influences on caregiver decisions about communication choices for children with hearing loss', *Deafness & Education International*, vol. 16, no. 2, pp. 61–85. https://doi.org/10.1179/1557069X13Y.0000000026

Dalmau, M, Balcells-Balcells, A, Gine, C, Canadas, M, Casa, D, Salat, Y, Farre, V & Calaf, N 2017, 'How to implement the family-centred model in early intervention', *Annals of Psychology*, vol. 3, no. 6, pp. 641–651. https://doi.org/10.6018/analesps.33.3.26341

De Kock, T, Swanepoel, D & Hall III JW 2016, 'Newborn hearing screening at a community-based obstetric unit: Screening and diagnostic outcomes', *International Journal of Pediatric Otorhinolaryngology*, vol. 84, pp. 124–131. https://doi.org/10.1016/j.ijporl.2016.02.031

Department of Health (DoH) 2017, *National Health Insurance for South Africa: Towards universal health coverage*, viewed 08 May 2019, <http://www.health.gov.za/index.php/nhi?download=2257:white-paper-nhi-2017>.

Elpers, J, Lester, C, Shinn, JB & Bush, ML 2016, 'Rural family perspectives and experiences with early infant hearing detection and intervention: A qualitative study', *Journal of Community Health*, vol. 41, no. 2, pp. 226–233. https://doi.org/10.1007/s10900-015-0086-1

Epley, P, Summers, AA & Turnbull, A 2010, 'Characteristics and trends in family-centered conceptualizations', *Journal of Family Social Work*, vol. 13, no. 3, pp. 269–285. https://doi.org/10.1080/10522150903514017

Erbasi, E, Scarinci, N, Hickson, L & Ching, TYC 2018, 'Parental involvement in the care and intervention of children with hearing loss', *International Journal of Audiology*, vol. 57, suppl. 2, pp. 15–26. https://doi.org/10.1080/14992027.2016.1220679

Fitzgibbons, J, Beswick, R & Driscoll, CJ 2021, 'Contextualisation of risk factors for hearing impairment', eds. K Khoza-Shangase & A Kanji, *Early detection and intervention in audiology: An African perspective*, Wits University Press, Johannesburg, pp. 89–116. https://doi.org/10.18772/22021026567

Flood, D & Rohloff, P 2018, 'Indigenous languages and global health: Comment', *The Lancet*, vol. 6, no. 2, pp. 134–135. https://doi.org/10.1016/S2214-109X(17)30493-X

Ganle, JK, Obeng, B, Segbefia, AY, Mwinyuri, V, Yeboah, JY & Baatiema, L 2015, 'How intra-familial decision-making affects women's access to, and use of maternal healthcare services in Ghana: A qualitative study', *Pregnancy and Childbirth*, vol. 15, p. 173. https://doi.org/10.1186/s12884-015-0590-4

Gravel, JS & McCaughey, CC 2004, 'Family-centered audiologic assessment for infants and young children with hearing loss', *Seminars in Hearing*, vol. 25, no. 4, pp. 309–317. https://doi.org/10.1055/s-2004-836133

Graydon, K, Waterworth, C, Miller, H & Gunasekera, H 2019, 'Global burden of hearing impairment and ear disease', *The Journal of Laryngology & Otology*, vol. 133, no. 1, pp. 18–25. https://doi.org/10.1017/S0022215118001275

Guralnick, MJ 1998, 'Effectiveness of early intervention for vulnerable children: A developmental perspective', *American Journal of Mental Retardation*, vol. 102, no. 4, pp. 319–345. https://doi.org/10.1352/0895-8017(1998)102<0319:eoeifv>2.0.co;2

Guralnick, MJ (ed.) 2005, *The developmental systems approach to early intervention*, Brookes Pub. Co., Baltimore.

Harrison, M & Roush, J 1996, 'Age of suspicion, identification, and intervention for infants and young children with hearing loss: A national study', *Journal of the American Audiology Society*, vol. 17, no. 1, pp. 55–62. https://doi.org/10.1097/00003446-199602000-00007

Health Professions Council of South Africa (HPCSA) 2007, *Early hearing detection and intervention programmes in South Africa: Position statement year 2007*, viewed 26 March 2020, <http://www.hpsca.co.za/hpcsa/default.aspx?id=137>

Health Professions Council of South Africa (HPCSA) 2018, *Early hearing detection and intervention (EHDI) guidelines*, viewed 26 March 2020, <http://www.hpcsa.co.za/Uploads/editor/UserFiles/downloads/speech/Early_Hearing_Detection_and_Intervention_(EHDI)_2018.pdf>

Health Professions Council of South Africa (HPCSA) 2019, *Guidelines for practice in a culturally and linguistically diverse South Africa*, viewed 26 March 2020, <https://www.hpcsa.co.za/Uploads/SLH/Guidelines%20for%20practice%20in%20a%20culturally%20and%20linguistically%20divers---.pdf>

Iversen, M, Shimmel, J, Ciacera, S & Prabhakar, M 2003, 'Creating a family-centered approach to early intervention services: Perceptions of parents and professionals', *Pediatric Physical Therapy*, vol. 15, no. 1, pp. 23–31. https://doi.org/10.1097/01.PEP.0000051694.10495.79

Joint Committee on Infant Hearing (JCIH) 2007, 'Year 2007 position statement: Principles and guidelines for early hearing detection and intervention programs', *Pediatrics*, vol. 120, no. 4, pp. 898–921. https://doi.org/10.1542/peds.2007-2333

Kanji, A 2021a, 'Exploring early detection of hearing impairment in sub-Saharan Africa', eds. K Khoza-Shangase & A Kanji, *Early detection and intervention in audiology: An African perspective*, Wits University Press, Johannesburg. https://doi.org/10.18772/22021026567

Kanji, A 2021b, 'Approaches to early detection of hearing impairment in low and middle-income countries', eds. K Khoza-Shangase & A Kanji, *Early detection and intervention in audiology: An African perspective*, Wits University Press, Johannesburg. https://doi.org/10.18772/22021026567

Kanji, A & Khoza-Shangase, K 2018a, 'In pursuit of successful hearing screening: An exploration of factors associated with follow up return rate in a risk-based newborn hearing screening programme', *Iranian Journal of Pediatrics*, vol. 28, no. 4, a56047. https://doi.org/10.5812/ijp.56047

Kanji, A & Khoza-Shangase, K 2018b, 'Objective hearing screening measures: An exploration of a suitable combination for risk-based newborn hearing screening', *Journal of the American Academy of Audiology*, vol. 29, no. 6, pp. 495–502. https://doi.org/10.3766/jaaa.16155

Kanji, A & Khoza-Shangase, K 2019, 'Early detection of hearing impairment in high-risk neonates: Let's talk about the high-risk registry in the South African context', *South African Journal of Child Health*, vol. 13, no. 2, pp. 53–55. https://doi.org/10.7196/SAJCH.2019.v13i2.1675

Kanji, A & Khoza-Shangase, K 2021, 'A paradigm shift in early hearing detection and intervention in South Africa', eds. K Khoza-Shangase & A Kanji, *Early detection and intervention in audiology: An African perspective*, Wits University Press, Johannesburg. https://doi.org/10.18772/22021026567

Kanji, A & Krabbenhoft, K 2018, 'Audiological follow-up in a risk-based newborn hearing screening programme: An exploratory study of the influencing factors', *South African Journal of Communication Disorders*, vol. 65, no. 1, a587. https://doi.org/10.4102/sajcd.v65i1.587

Khoza-Shangase, K 2019, 'Early hearing detection and intervention: Exploring factors compromising service delivery as expressed by caregivers', *International Journal of Pediatric Otorhinolaryngology*, vol. 118, pp. 73–78. https://doi.org/10.1016/j.ijporl.2018.12.021

Khoza-Shangase, K 2021a, 'Confronting realities to early hearing detection in South Africa', eds. K Khoza-Shangase & A Kanji, *Early detection and intervention in audiology: An African perspective*, Wits University Press, Johannesburg. https://doi.org/10.18772/22021026567

Khoza-Shangase, K 2021b, 'Continuity of care at school for the hearing-impaired child', eds. K Khoza-Shangase & A Kanji, *Early detection and intervention in audiologya: An African perspective*, Wits University Press, Johannesburg.

Khoza-Shangase, K & Anastasiou, J 2020, 'An exploration of recorded otological manifestations in South African children with HIV/AIDS: A pilot study', *International Journal of Pediatric Otorhinolaryngology*, vol. 133, a109960. https://doi.org/10.1016/j.ijporl.2020.109960

Khoza-Shangase, K, Barratt, J & Jonosky, J 2010, 'Protocols for early audiology intervention services: Views from early intervention practitioners in a developing country', *South African Journal of Child Health*, vol. 4, no. 4, pp. 100–105. https://doi.org/10.7196/SAJCH.271

Khoza-Shangase, K & Harbinson, S 2015, 'Evaluation of universal newborn hearing screening in South African primary care', *African Journal of Primary Health Care & Family Medicine*, vol. 7, no. 1, pp. 1–12. https://doi.org/10.4102/phcfm.v7i1.769

Khoza-Shangase, K, Kanji, A & Ismail, F 2021a, 'What are the current practices employed by audiologists in early hearing detection and intervention in the South African healthcare context?', *International Journal of Pediatric Otorhinolaryngology*, vol. 141, a110587. https://doi.org/10.1016/j.ijporl.2020.110587

Khoza-Shangase, K & Michal, G 2014, 'Early intervention in audiology: Exploring the current status from a developing country context', *British Journal of Medicine and Medical Research*, vol. 4, no. 11, pp. 2238–2249. https://doi.org/10.9734/BJMMR/2014/7322

Khoza-Shangase, K & Mophosho, M 2018, 'Language and culture in speech-language and hearing professions in South Africa: The dangers of a single story', *South African Journal of Communication Disorders*, vol. 65, no. 1, a594. https://doi.org/10.4102/sajcd.v65i1.594

Khoza-Shangase, K & Mophosho, M 2021, 'Language and culture in speech-language and hearing professions in South Africa: Re-imagining practice', *South African Journal of Communication Disorders*, vol. 68, no. 1, a793. https://doi.org/10.4102/sajcd.v68i1.793

Khoza-Shangase, K & Moroe, N 2020, 'South African hearing conservation programmes in the context of tele-audiology: A scoping review', *South African Journal of Communications Disorders*, vol. 67, no. 2, a670. https://doi.org/10.4102/sajcd.v67i2.670

Khoza-Shangase, K, Moroe, N & Neille, J 2021b, 'Speech-language pathology and audiology in South Africa: Clinical training and service in the era of COVID-19', *International Journal of Telerehabilitation*, vol. 13, no. 1, pp. 1–31. https://doi.org/10.5195/ijt.2021.6376

Khoza-Shangase, K & Rifkind, ER 2010, 'Paediatric meningitis and hearing loss in a developing country: Exploring the current protocols regarding audiological management following meningitis', *African Journal of Infectious Diseases*, vol. 4, no. 2, pp. 51–60. https://doi.org/10.4314/ajid.v4i2.55148

Kiling, IY, Due, C, Gyss, C, Li, DE & Turnbull, D 2019, 'Intervention research addressing environmental risk threatening young children with disabilities in developing countries:

A systematic review', *Disability and Rehabilitation*, vol. 41, no. 17, pp. 1987–2005. https://doi.org/10.1080/09638288.2018.1509142

Kuo, DZ, Houtrow, AJ, Arango, P, Kuhlthau, KA, Simmons, JM & Neff, JM 2012, 'Family-centered care: Current applications and future directions in pediatric health care', *Maternal and Child Health Journal*, vol. 16, no. 2, pp. 297–305. https://doi.org/10.1007/s10995-011-0751-7

Kyarkanaye, T, Dada, S & Samuels, AE 2017, 'Collaboration in early childhood intervention services in Gauteng', *Infants & Young Children*, vol. 30, no. 3, pp. 238–254. https://doi.org/10.1097/IYC.0000000000000095

Lang-Roth, R 2014, 'Hearing impairment and language delay in infants: Diagnostics and genetics', *GMS Current Topics in Otorhinolaryngology, Head and Neck Surgery*, vol. 13, a108. https://doi.org/10.3205/cto000108

Larsen, R, Munoz, K, DesGeorges, J, Nelson, L & Kennedy, S 2012, 'Early hearing detection and intervention: Parent experiences with the diagnostic hearing assessment', *American Journal of Audiology*, vol. 21, no. 1, pp. 91–99. https://doi.org/10.1044/1059-0889(2012/11-0016)

Laugen, NJ 2013, 'Providing information to families in newborn hearing screening follow-up: Professional challenges', *Seminars in Hearing*, vol. 34, no. 1, pp. 11–18. https://doi.org/10.1055/S-0032-1333147

Majid, AHA, Zakaria, MN, Abdullah, NAC, Hamzah, S & Mukari, SZMS 2017, 'Determinants of caregivers' awareness of universal newborn hearing screening in Malaysia', *International Journal of Pediatric Otorhinolaryngology*, vol. 101, pp. 107–111.

Maluleke, NP, Khoza-Shangase, K & Kanji, A 2018, 'Hearing impairment detection and intervention in children from centre-based early intervention programmes', *Journal of Child Health Care*, vol. 23, no. 2, pp. 1–10. https://doi.org/10.1177/1367493518788477

Maluleke, NP, Khoza-Shangase, K & Kanji, A 2019, 'Communication and school readiness abilities of children with hearing impairment in South Africa: A retrospective review of early intervention preschool records', *South African Journal of Communication Disorders*, vol. 66, no. 1, a604. https://doi.org/10.4102/sajcd.v66i1.604

Maluleke, NP, Khoza-Shangase, K & Kanji, A 2021a, 'An integrative review of current practice models and/or process of family-centered early intervention for children who are deaf or hard of hearing', *Family & Community Health*, vol. 44, no. 1, pp. 59–71. https://doi.org/10.1097/FCH.0000000000000276

Maluleke, NP, Chiwutsi, R & Khoza-Shangase, K 2021b, 'Family-centred early hearing detection and intervention', eds. K Khoza-Shangase & A Kanji, *Early detection and intervention in audiology: An African perspective*, Wits University Press, Johannesburg. https://doi.org/10.18772/22021026567

Mehta, K, Hilton, E, Baldwin, M & Watkin, P 2020, 'Parent-to-parent support for the families of deaf children identified by the newborn hearing screen', *Deafness & Education International*, vol. 22, no. 2, pp. 96–112. https://doi.org/10.1080/14643154.2019.1591680

Merugumala, SV, Pothula, V & Cooper, M 2017, 'Barriers to timely diagnosis and treatment for children with hearing impairment in a Southern Indian city: A qualitative study of parents and clinic staff', *International Journal of Audiology*, vol. 56, no. 10, pp. 733–739. https://doi.org/10.1080/14992027.1340678

Moeller, M 2000, 'Early intervention and language development in children who are deaf and hard of hearing', *Pediatrics*, vol. 106, no. 3, a43. https://doi.org/10.1542/peds.106.3.e43

Moeller, MP, Carr, G, Seaver, L, Stredler-Brown, A & Holzinger, D 2013, 'Best practices in family-centered early intervention for children who are deaf or hard of hearing: An international consensus statement', *The Journal of Deaf Studies and Deaf Education*, vol. 18, no. 4, pp. 429–445. https://doi.org/10.1093/deafed/ent034

Moodley, S & Störbeck, C 2017, 'Data management for early hearing detection and intervention in South Africa', *South African Journal of Information Management*, vol. 19, no. 1, a779. https://doi.org/10.4102/sajim.v19i1.779

Mophosho, M 2018, 'Speech-language therapy consultation practices in multilingual and multicultural healthcare contexts: Current training in South Africa', *African Journal of*

Health Professions Education, vol. 10, no. 3, pp. 145–147. https://doi.org/10.7196/AJHPE.2018.v10i3.1045

Nkonki, LL, Chopra, M, Doherty, TM, Jackson, D & Robberstad, B 2011, 'Explaining household socio-economic related child health inequalities using multiple methods in three diverse settings in South Africa', *International Journal for Equity in Health*, vol. 13, no. 10, pp. 1–14. https://doi.org/10.1186/1475-9276-10-13

Noorbhai, K 2002, 'Early intervention services provided to families of deaf children', Master of Arts in Audiology, Department of Speech Pathology and Audiology, University of the Witwatersrand.

Olusanya, B 2005, 'Can the world's infants with hearing loss wait?', *International Journal of Pediatric Otorhinolaryngology*, vol. 69, no. 6, pp. 735–738. https://doi.org/10.1016/j.ijporl.2005.03.024

Olusanya, B 2006, 'Early hearing detection and intervention in developing countries: Current status and prospects', *Volta Review*, vol. 106, no. 3, pp. 381–418. https://doi.org/10.17955/tvr.106.3.m.575

Olusanya, B & Newton, V 2007, 'Global burden of childhood hearing impairment and disease control priorities for developing countries', *Lancet*, vol. 369, no. 9569, pp. 1314–1317. https://doi.org/10.1016/S0140-6736(07)60602-3

Olusanya, BO, Neumann, KJ & Saunders, JE 2014, 'The global burden of disabling hearing impairment: A call to action', *Bulletin of the World Health Organization*, vol. 92, no. 5, pp. 367–373. https://doi.org/10.2471/BLT.13.128728

Olusanya, BO, Swanepoel, DW, Chapchap, MJ, Castillo, S, Habib, H, Mukari, SZ, Martinez, NV, Lin, H-C & McPherson, B 2007, 'Progress towards early detection services for infants with hearing loss in developing countries', *BMC Health Services Research*, vol. 7, no. 1, pp. 1–15. https://doi.org/10.1186/1472-6963-7-14

Petrocchi-Bartal, L & Khoza-Shangase, K 2014, 'Hearing screening procedures and protocols in use at immunisation clinics in South Africa', *South African Journal of Communication Disorders*, vol. 61, no. 1, p. 9. https://doi.org/10.4102/sajcd.v61i1.66

Petrocchi-Bartal, L & Khoza-Shangase, K 2016, 'Infant hearing screening at primary health care immunization clinics in South Africa: The current status', *South African Journal of Child Health*, vol. 10, no. 2, pp. 139–143. https://doi.org/10.7196/SAJCH.2016.v10i2.1114

Petrocchi-Bartal, L, Khoza-Shangase, K & Kanji, A 2021, 'Implementing early hearing detection in the South African health care context', eds. K Khoza-Shangase & A Kanji, *Early detection and intervention in audiology: An African perspective*, Wits University Press, Johannesburg. https://doi.org/10.18772/22021026567

Pillay, D, Moonsamy, S & Khoza-Shangase, K 2010, 'Bridging the gap between early identification and intervention in the paediatric population with hearing impairments', *South African Journal of Child Health*, vol. 4, no. 4, pp. 92–94. https://doi.org/10.7196/SAJCH.294

Pillay, M, Tiwari, R, Kathard, H & Chikte, U 2020, 'Sustainable workforce: South African audiologists and speech therapists', *Human Resources for Health*, vol. 18, no. 1, pp. 1–13. https://doi.org/10.1186/s12960-020-00488-6

Popich, E, Louw, B & Eloff, I 2007, 'Caregiver education as a prevention strategy for communication disorders in South Africa', *Infants & Young Children*, vol. 20, no. 1, pp. 64–81. https://doi.org/10.1097/00001163-200701000-00007

Prendergast, SG, Lartz, MN & Fiedler, BC 2002, 'Ages of diagnosis, amplification, and early intervention of infants and young children with hearing loss: Findings from parent interviews', *American Annals of the Deaf*, vol. 147, no. 1, pp. 24–29. https://doi.org/10.1353/aad.2012.0198

Ranchod, S, Adams, C, Burger, R, Carvounes, A, Dreyer, K, Smith, A, Stewart, J & Biljon, CV 2017, 'South Africa's hospital sector: Old divisions and new developments', eds. A Padarath & P Barron, *South African Health Review 2017*, Health Systems Trust, Durban.

Ravi, R, Gunjawate, DR, Yerraguntla, K, Rajashekhar, B & Lewis, LE 2016, 'Knowledge and attitude of parents/caregivers towards hearing loss and screening in newborns – A systematic review', *International Journal of Audiology*, vol. 55, no. 12, pp. 715–722. https://doi.org/10.1080/14992027.2016.1215560

Rossetti, L 2004, *Communication intervention: Birth to three*, 2nd edn, Delmar Centage Learning, Clifton Park.

Russ, SA, Kuo, AA, Poulakis, Z, Barker, M, Rickards, F, Saunders, K, Jarman, FC, Wake, M & Oberklaid, F 2004, 'Qualitative analysis of parents' experience with early detection of hearing loss', *Archives of Disease in Childhood*, vol. 89, no. 4, pp. 353–358. https://doi.org/10.1136/adc.2002.024125

Samuels, A, Slemming, W & Balton, S 2012, 'Early childhood intervention in South Africa in relation to the developmental systems model', *Infants & Young Children*, vol. 25, no. 4, pp. 334–345. https://doi.org/10.1097/IYC.0b013e3182673e12

Sass-Lehrer, M 2004, 'Early detection of hearing loss: Maintaining a family-centered perspective', *Seminars in Hearing*, vol. 25, no. 4, pp. 295–307.

Sass-Lehrer, M 2015. *Early intervention for deaf and hard-of-hearing infants, toddlers, and their families: Interdisciplinary perspectives*, Oxford University Press, New York.

Say, L & Raineb, R 2007, 'A systematic review of inequalities in the use of maternal health care in developing countries: Examining the scale of the problem and the importance of context', *Bulletin of the World Health Organization*, vol. 85, no. 10, pp. 812–819. https://doi.org/10.2471/blt.06.035659

Scarinci, N, Erbasi, E, Moore, E, Ching, TYC & Marnane, V 2018a, 'The parents' perspective of the early diagnostic period of their child with hearing loss: Information and support', *International Journal of Audiology*, vol. 57, no. Suppl 2, pp. 3–14. https://doi.org/10.1080/14992027.2017.1301683

Scarinci, N, Gehrke, M, Ching, TYC, Marnane, V & Button, L 2018b, 'Factors influencing caregiver decision making to change the communication method of their child with hearing loss', *Deafness & Education International*, vol. 20, no. 3–4, pp. 123–153. https://doi.org/10.1080/14643154.2018.1511239

Scheepers, LJ, Swanepoel, DW & Le Roux, T 2014, 'Why parents refuse newborn hearing screening and default on follow-up rescreening – A South African perspective', *International Journal of Pediatric Otorhinolaryngology*, vol. 78, no. 4, pp. 652–658.

Schlebusch, L, Samuels, AE & Dada, S 2016, 'South African families raising children with autism spectrum disorders: Relationship between family routines, cognitive appraisal and family quality of life', *Journal of Intellectual Disability Research*, vol. 60, no. 5, pp. 412–423. https://doi.org/10.1111/jir.12292

Spivak, L, Sokol, H, Auerbach, C & Gershkovich, S 2009, 'Newborn hearing screening follow-up: Factors affecting hearing aid fitting by 6 months of age', *American Journal of Audiology*, vol. 18, no. 1, pp. 24–33. https://doi.org/10.1044/1059-0889(2008/08-0015)

Störbeck, C & Pittman, P 2008, 'Early intervention in South Africa: Moving beyond hearing screening', *International Journal of Audiology*, vol. 47, no. Suppl 1, pp. 36–43. https://doi.org/10.1080/14992020802294040

Störbeck, C & Young, A 2016, 'The HI HOPES data set of deaf children under the age of 6 in South Africa: Maternal suspicion, age of identification and newborn hearing screening', *BMC Pediatrics*, vol. 16, p. 45. https://doi.org/10.1186/s12887-016-0574-1

Swanepoel, DW & Almec, N 2008, 'Maternal views on infant hearing loss and early intervention in a South African community', *International Journal of Audiology*, vol. 47, no. Suppl 1, pp. 44–48. https://doi.org/10.1080/14992020802252279

Swanepoel, DW & Hall, JW 2010, 'A systematic review of telehealth applications in audiology', *Telemedicine and e-Health*, vol. 16, no. 2, pp. 181–200. https://doi.org/10.1089/tmj.2009.0111

Swanepoel, DW, Störbeck, C & Friedland, P 2009, 'Early hearing detection and intervention in South Africa', *International Journal of Pediatric Otorhinolaryngology*, vol. 73, no. 6, pp. 783–786. https://doi.org/10.1016/j.ijporl.2009.01.007

Thompson, M 1991, 'Early identification of hearing loss: Listen to parents', *Clinical Pediatrics*, vol. 30, no. 2, pp. 77–80. https://doi.org/10.1177/000992289103000202

Tsawe, M, Moto, A, Netshivhera, T, Ralesego, L, Nyathi, C & Susuman, AS 2015, 'Factors influencing the use of maternal healthcare services and childhood immunization in Swaziland', *International Journal for Equity in Health*, vol. 14, no. 32, pp. 1–11. https://doi.org/10.1186/s12939-015-0162-2

Van der Spuy, T & Pottas, L 2008, 'Infant hearing loss in South Africa: Age of intervention and parental needs for support', *International Journal of Audiology*, vol. 47, no. Suppl 1, pp. 30–35. https://doi.org/10.1080/14992020802286210

Vearey, J, Modisenyane, M & Hunter-Adams, J 2017, 'Towards a migration-aware health system in South Africa: A strategic opportunity to address health inequality', eds. A Padarath & P Barron, *South African Health Review 2017*, Health Systems Trust, Durban, pp. 89–98.

Wang, X, Wu, D, Zhao, Y, Li, D & He, D 2017, 'Knowledge and attitude of mothers regarding infant hearing loss in Changsha, Hunan province, China', *International Journal of Audiology*, vol. 56, no. 12, pp. 997–1002. https://doi.org/10.1080/14992027.2017.1366671

Watermeyer, J, Kanji, A & Cohen, A 2012, 'Caregiver recall and understanding of paediatric diagnostic information and assessment feedback', *International Journal of Audiology*, vol. 51, no. 12, pp. 864–869.

White, KR 2003, 'The current status of EHDI programs in the United States', *Mental Retardation and Developmental Disabilities Research Reviews*, vol. 9, no. 2, pp. 79–88. https://doi.org/10.1002/mrdd.10063

World Health Organization (WHO) 2008, *Task shifting: Global recommendations and guidelines*, World Health Organization, Geneva.

Woods, JJ, Wilcox, MJ, Friedman, M & Murch, T 2011, 'Collaborative consultations in natural environments: Strategies to enhance family-centered support services', *Language, Speech, and Hearing Services in Schools*, vol. 42, no. 3, pp. 379–392. https://doi.org/10.1044/0161-1461(2011/10-0016)

Wroblewska-Seniuk, KE, Dabrowski, P, Szyfter, W & Mazela, J 2017, 'Universal newborn hearing screening: Methods and results, obstacles, and benefits', *Pediatric Research*, vol. 81, no. 3, pp. 415–422. https://doi.org/10.1038/pr.2016.250

Yoshinaga-Itano, C 2004, 'Levels of evidence: Universal new-born hearing screening (UNHS) and early hearing detection and intervention systems (EHDI)', *Journal of Communication Disorders*, vol. 37, no. 5, pp. 451–465. https://doi.org/10.1016/j.jcomdis.2004.04.008

Yoshinaga-Itano, C 2014, 'Principles and guidelines for early intervention after confirmation that a child is deaf or hard of hearing', *Journal of Deaf Studies and Deaf Education*, vol. 19, no. 2, pp. 143–175. https://doi.org/10.1093/deafed/ent043

Yoshinaga-Itano, C, Sedey, AL, Wiggin, M & Chung, W 2017, 'Early hearing detection and vocabulary of children with hearing loss', *Pediatrics*, vol. 140, no. 2, a20162964. https://doi.org/10.1542/peds.2016-2964

Chapter 9

Anderson, RR 2009, 'Religious traditions and prenatal genetic counseling', *American Journal of Medical Genetics Part C: Seminars in Medical Genetics*, vol. 151, no. 1, pp. 52–61.

Anthony, TL 2016, 'Early identification of infants and toddlers with deafblindness', *American Annals of the Deaf*, vol. 161, no. 4, pp. 412–423. https://doi.org/10.1353/aad.2016.0034

Anthony, TL, Wiggin, MP, Yoshinaga-Itano, C & Raver, A 2015, *Strategies for infants and toddlers with sensory disabilities*, Brookes, Baltimore.

Batshaw, M, Pellegrino, L & Roizen, N 2007, *Children with disabilities*, Paul H. Brookes Publishing Co., Inc, Baltimore.

Biermann, J 2016, 'Approaches to inclusive education in Nigeria: The pivotal role of poverty and disability', *Zeitschrift Für Inklusion [Journal for Inclusion]*, viewed 10 May 2019, <https://www.inklusion-online.net/index.php/inklusion-online/article/view/338>

Blackburn, C, Read, J & Spencer, N 2012, *Children with neurodevelopmental disabilities*, viewed 10 May 2019, <https://assets.publishing.service.gov.uk/government/uploads/system/uploads/attachment_data/file/252659/33571_2901304_CMO_Chapter_9.pdf>

Boshoff, L & Tooke, L 2012, 'Congenital rubella – Is it nearly time to take action?', *South African Journal of Child Health*, vol. 6, no. 4, pp. 106–108. https://doi.org/10.7196/sajch.461

Burnett, RJ, Dlamini, NR, Meyer, JC, Fernandes, L, Motloung, BR, Ndlovu, TH, Simango, HA, Kibuuka, DK, Dochez, C, Montwedi, DN, Nkwinika, VV & Mphahlele, MJ 2019, 'Progress towards obtaining valid vaccination coverage data in South Africa', *South African Journal of Science*, vol. 115, no. 5–6, pp. 1–4. https://doi.org/10.17159/sajs.2019/6060

Cappagli, G, Finocchietti, S, Cocchi, E & Gori, M 2017, 'The impact of early visual deprivation on spatial hearing: a comparison between totally and partially visually deprived children', *Frontiers in Psychology*, vol. 8, p. 467. https://doi.org/10.3389/fpsyg.2017.00467

Dammeyer, J 2014, 'Deafblindness: A review of the literature', *Scandinavian Journal of Public Health*, vol. 42, no. 7, pp. 554–562. https://doi.org/10.1177/1403494814544399

Dammeyer, J 2015, 'Deafblindness and dual sensory loss research: Current status and future directions', *World Journal of Otorhinolaryngology*, vol. 5, no. 2, pp. 37–40. https://doi.org/10.5319/wjo.v5.i2.37

DB-LINK 2017, *Early interactions with children who are deaf-blind*, National Center on Deaf-Blindness, viewed 10 May 2020, <https://nationaldb.org/library/page/2062>

Department of Education 2001, *Education white paper 6. Special needs education: Building an inclusive education and training system*, viewed 03 February 2020, <https://www.vvob.org/files/publicaties/rsa_education_white_paper_6.pdf>

Department of Health 2015, *Framework and strategy for disability and rehabilitation services in South Africa 2015 – 2020*, viewed 10 September 2019, <https://view.officeapps.live.com/op/view.aspx?src=https%3A%2F%2Filifalabantwana.co.za%2Fwp-content%2Fuploads%2F2016%2F07%2FFramework-25-may_1_3.docx&wdOrigin=BROWSELINK>

Department of Social Development 2016, *White paper on the rights of persons with disabilities: Official publication and gazetting of the white paper on the rights of persons with disabilities*, viewed 10 September 2019, <https://www.gov.za/sites/default/files/gcis_document/201603/39792gon230.pdf>

De Vaan, G, Vervloed, MPJ, Knoors, H & Verhoeven, L 2013, *Autism spectrum disorders in people with sensory and intellectual disabilities symptom overlap and differentiating characteristics*, viewed 20 March 2019, <https://www.intechopen.com/books/recent-advances-in-autism-spectrum-disorders-volume-i/autism-spectrum-disorders-in-people-with-sensory-and-intellectual-disabilities-symptom-overlap-and-d>

Donohue, D & Bornman, J 2014, 'The challenges of realising inclusive education in South Africa', *South African Journal of Education*, vol. 34, no. 2, pp. 1–14. https://doi.org/10.15700/201412071114

Duplaga, M, Grysztar, M, Rodzinka, M & Kopec, A 2016, 'Scoping review of health promotion and disease prevention interventions addressed to elderly people', *BMC Health Services Research*, vol. 16, no. 5, p. 278. https://doi.org/10.1186/s12913-016-1521-4

Ehn, M, Anderzén-Carlsson, A, Möller, C & Wahlqvist, M 2019, 'Life strategies of people with deafblindness due to usher syndrome type 2a – A qualitative study', *International Journal of Qualitative Studies on Health and Well-Being*, vol. 14, no. 1, a1656790. https://doi.org/10.1080/17482631.2019.1656790

Fernandez Turienzo, C, Sandall, J & Peacock, JL 2016, 'Models of antenatal care to reduce and prevent preterm birth: A systematic review and meta-analysis', *BMJ Open*, vol. 6, no. 1, a009044. https://doi.org/10.1136/bmjopen-2015-009044

Gilsdorf, JR 2018, 'Into darkness and silence: What caused Helen Keller's deafblindness?', *Clinical Infectious Diseases*, vol. 67, no. 9, pp. 1445–1449. https://doi.org/10.1093/cid/ciy385

Global Research on Developmental Disabilities Collaborators 2018, 'Developmental disabilities among children younger than 5 years in 195 countries and territories, 1990–2016: A systematic analysis for the global burden of disease study', *The Lancet: Global Health*, vol. 6, no. 10, pp. 1100–1121. https://doi.org/10.1016/S2214-109X(18)30309-7

Greenberg, J, Kromberg, J, Loggenberg, K & Wessels, TM 2012, 'Genetic counseling in South Africa', ed. D Kumar, *Genomics and health in the developing world: Oxford mongraphs of medical genetics*, Oxford University Press, Oxford, pp. 531–546.

Groce, NE 2018, 'Global disability: An emerging issue', *The Lancet: Global Health*, vol. 6, no. 7, pp. 724–725. https://doi.org/10.1016/S2214-109X(18)30265-1

Hartshorne, TS & Schmittel, MC 2016, 'Social-emotional development in children and youth who are deafblind', *American Annals of the Deaf*, vol. 161, no. 4, pp. 444–453. https://doi.org/10.1353/aad.2016.0036

Hayes, AM & Bulat, J 2017, *Disabilities inclusive education systems and policies guide for low- and middle-income countries*, viewed 05 February 2019, <https://shared.rti.org/content/disabilities-inclusive-education-systems-and-policies-guide-low-and-middle-income-countries>

Hersh, M 2013, 'Deafblind people, communication, independence, and isolation', *The Journal of Deaf Studies and Deaf Education*, vol. 18, no. 4, pp. 446–463. https://doi.org/10.1093/deafed/ent022

Higuera, V 2016, *Premature birth complications*, viewed 05 February 2019, <https://www.healthline.com/health/pregnancy/premature-baby-complications>

Holte, L, Prickett, JG, Van Dyke, DC, Olson, RJ, Lubrica, P, Knutson, CL, Knutson, JF & Susan, B 2006, 'Issues in the evaluation of infants and young children who are suspected of or who are deaf-blind', *Infants & Young Children*, vol. 19, no. 3, pp. 213–227.

Hollowell, J, Oakley, L, Kurinczuk, JJ, Brocklehurst, P & Gray, R 2011, 'The effectiveness of antenatal care programmes to reduce infant mortality and preterm birth in socially disadvantaged and vulnerable women in high-income countries: A systematic review', *BMC Pregnancy and Childbirth*, vol. 11, no. 1, pp. 1–20. https://doi.org/10.1186/1471-2393-11-13

Jaiswal, A, Aldersey, H, Wittich, W, Mirza, M & Finlayson, M 2018, 'Participation experiences of people with deafblindness or dual sensory loss: A scoping review of global deafblind literature', *PLoS One*, vol. 13, no. 9, a0203772. https://doi.org/10.1371/journal.pone.0203772

Janssen, MJ, Riksen-Walraven, JM & Van Dijk, JPM 2002, 'Enhancing the quality of interaction between deafblind children and their educators', *Journal of Developmental and Physical Disabilities*, vol. 14, pp. 87–109. https://doi.org/10.1023/A:1013583312920

Joint Committee on Infant Hearing (JCIH) 2007, 'Year 2007 position statement: Principles and guidelines for early hearing detection and intervention programs', *Pediatrics*, vol. 120, no. 4, pp. 898–921. https://doi.org/10.1542/peds.2007-2333

Kanji, A & Khoza-Shangase, K 2012, 'The occurrence of high-risk factors for hearing loss in verylow-birth-weight neonates: A retrospective exploratory study of targeted hearing screening', *South African Journal of Communication Disorders*, vol. 59, no. 1, pp. 3–7. https://doi.org/10.4102/sajcd.v59i1.16

Kanji, A & Khoza-Shangase, K 2019, 'Early detection of hearing impairment in high-risk neonates: Let's talk about the high risk registry in the South African context', *South African Journal of Child Health*, vol. 13, no. 2, pp. 53–55.

Kanji, A & Khoza-Shangase, K 2021, 'Risk factors for hearing impairment in neonates in South Africa: Scoping the context for newborn hearing screening planning', *The Journal of Maternal-Fetal & Neonatal Medicine*, vol. 34, no. 13, pp. 2107–2116. https://doi.org/10.1080/14767058.2019.1658732

Khasnabis, C, Heinicke Motsch, K, Achu, K, Al Jubah, K, Brodtkorb, S, Chervin, P, Coleridge, P, Davies, M, Deepak, S, Eklindh, K, Goerdt, A, Greer, C, Heinicke-Motsch, K, Hooper, D, Ilagan, VB, Jessup, N, Khasnabis, C, Mulligan, D, Murray, B, Officer, A, Ortali, F, Ransom, B, Robert, A, Stubbs, S, Thomas, M, Balakrishna, V, Wabuge-Mwangi, R, Mattock, N & Lande, T 2010, *Community-based rehabilitation: CBR guidelines*, World Health Organization, Geneva.

Khoza-Shangase, K 2021a, 'Confronting realities to early hearing detection in South Africa', eds. K Khoza-Shangase & A Kanji, *Early detection and intervention in audiology: An African perspective*, Wits University Press, Johannesburg. https://doi.org/10.18772/22021026567

Khoza-Shangase, K 2021b, 'Continuity of care at school for the hearing-impaired child', eds. K Khoza-Shangase & A Kanji, *Early detection and intervention in audiology: An African perspective*, Wits University Press, Johannesburg. https://doi.org/10.18772/22021026567

Khoza-Shangase, K, Sebothoma, B & Moroe, NF 2021, 'Tele-audiology as part of efforts to enhance inclusivity and equality through ICT in South African schools: Some considerations', eds. M Maguvhe, RS Mphahlele & S Moonsamy, *Empowering students and maximising inclusiveness and equality through ICT*, Brill Sense, Boston, pp. 223–243.

Khumalo, S & Hodgson, TF 2001, *The right to basic education for children with disabilities: Basic education rights handbook-education rights in South Africa*, viewed 05 February 2019, <http://section27.org.za/wp-content/uploads/2017/02/Chapter-5.pdf>

Krahn, GL, Walker, DK & Correa-De-Araujo, R 2015, 'Persons with disabilities as an unrecognized health disparity population', *American Journal of Public Health*, vol. 1052, suppl. 2, pp. 198–206.

Maguvhe, MO 2014, 'Curriculum design, implementation and parental involvement in the education of the deafblind: South African teachers' perspectives', *Mediterranean Journal of Social Sciences*, vol. 5, no. 20, pp. 1186–1492. https://doi.org/10.5901/mjss.2014.v5n20p1486

Maluleke, NP, Chiwutsi, R & Khoza-Shangase, K 2021, 'Family-centred early hearing detection and intervention', eds. K Khoza-Shangase & A Kanji, *Early detection and intervention in audiology: An African perspective*, Wits University Press, Johannesburg. https://doi.org/10.18772/22021026567

Manga, T & Masuku, KP 2020, 'Challenges of teaching the deafblind learners: Experiences of educators and educator assistants in Johannesburg', *South African Journal of Communication Disorders*, vol. 67, no. 1, a649. https://doi.org/10.4102/sajcd.v67i1.649

Marschark, M & Hauser, PC 2012, *How deaf children learn: What parents and teachers need to know*, 1st edn, Oxford University Press, Oxford.

McLetchie, B & Riggio, M 2001, *Competencies for paraprofessionals working with learners who are deafblind in early intervention settings*, Hilton/Perkins, Watertown.

Mihigo, R, Okeibunor, J, Masresha, B, Mkanda, P, Poy, A, Zawaira, F & Cabore, J 2018, 'Immunization and vaccine development: Progress towards high and equitable immunization coverage in the Africa region', *Journal of Immunological Sciences*, no. 1, pp. 1–9. https://doi.org/10.29245/2578-3009/2018/si.1105

Minnesota Hands & Voices 2020, *Aural habilitation/rehabilitation*, viewed 03 February 2021, <https://www.mnhandsandvoices.org/resources-information/aural-habilitation-rehabilitation>

Moroe, NF 2021, 'Sensory impairments in early hearing detection and intervention', eds. K Khoza-Shangase & A Kanji, *Early detection and intervention in audiology: An African perspective*, Wits University Press, Johannesburg. https://doi.org/10.18772/22021026567

Moroe, NF & Hughes, K 2017, 'Parents are aware of the ototoxic effects of chemotherapy in paediatrics undergoing cancer treatment – Professional versus parental views: A pilot study', *South African Journal of Communication Disorders*, vol. 64, a183. https://doi.org/10.4102/sajcd.v64i1.183

Mpofu, B & Ndlovu-Gatsheni, J 2019, *Rethinking and unthinking development: Perspectives of inequality and poverty in South Africa and Zimbabwe*, Berghahn, Oxford.

National Disability Authority 2019, *Reasonable accommodations: Obstacles and opportunities to the employment of persons with a disability*, viewed 25 March 2020, <http://nda.ie/File-upload/Reasonable-Accommodation-Obstacles-and-Opportunities-to-the-Employment-of-Persons-with-Disabilities-pdf.pdf>

Nelson, C & Bruce, SM 2019, 'Children who are deaf/hard of hearing with disabilities: Paths to language and literacy', *Education Sciences*, vol. 9, no. 2, p. 134. https://doi.org/10.3390/educsci9020134

Newton, G & Moss, K 2001, 'Early identification of hearing and vision loss is critical to a child's development', *SEE/HEAR*, vol. 6, no. 3, pp. 27–30.

Ngxongo, TSP 2018, *Basic antenatal care approach to antenatal care service provision*, viewed 25 March 2020, <https://www.intechopen.com/books/selected-topics-in-midwifery-care/basic-antenatal-care-approach-to-antenatal-care-service-provision>

Olukemi, O 2019, *Best practices for social media marketing for health promotion*, viewed 25 March 2020, <http://www.engageafricafoundation.org/blog/view/best-practices-for-social-media-marketing-for-health-promotion>

Pandve, H 2014, 'Changing concept of disease prevention: From primordial to quaternary', *Archives of Medicine and Health Sciences*, vol. 2, no. 2, pp. 254–256. https://doi.org/10.4103/2321-4848.144366

Peters, DH, Garg, A, Bloom, G, Walker, DG, Brieger, WR & Rahman, MH 2008, 'Poverty and access to health in developing countries', *Annals of the New York Academy of Sciences*, vol. 1136, pp. 161–171. https://doi.org/10.1196/annals.1425.011

Ramaahlo, M, Tönsing, KM & Bornman, J 2018, 'Inclusive education policy provision in South African research universities', *Disability & Society*, vol. 33, no. 3, pp. 349–373. https://doi.org/10.1080/09687599.2018.1423954

Schuelka, MJ 2018, *Implementing inclusive education: The K4D research helpdesk*, viewed 25 March 2020, <https://assets.publishing.service.gov.uk/media/5c6eb77340f0b647b214c599/374_Implementing_Inclusive_Education.pdf>

Simcock, P 2017, 'One of society's most vulnerable groups? A systematically-conducted literature review exploring the vulnerability of deafblind people', *Health & Social Care in the Community*, vol. 25, no. 3, pp. 813–839. https://doi.org/10.1111/hsc.12317

Tomaševski, K 2001, *Human rights obligations: Making education available*, viewed 19 November 2017, <http://www.right-to-education.org/sites/right-to-education.org/files/resource-attachments/Tomasevski_Primer3.pdf>

UN Committee on the Rights of Persons with Disabilities 2016, *General comment No. 4 (2016), Article 24: Right to inclusive education*, viewed 02 April 2019, <https://www.refworld.org/docid/57c977e34.html>

United Nations (UN) 2006, *Convention on the Rights of Persons with Disabilities and Optional Protocol*, viewed 02 April 2019, <https://www.un.org/development/desa/disabilities/convention-on-the-rights-of-persons-with-disabilities.html>

Valente, D, Theurel, A & Gentaz, E 2018, 'The role of visual experience in the production of emotional facial expressions by blind people: A review', *Psychonomic Bulletin & Review*, vol. 25, no. 2, pp. 483–497. https://doi.org/10.3758/s13423-017-1338-0

Vesper, I 2019, *Facts and figures: Disabilities in developing countries*, viewed 03 February 2020, <https://www.scidev.net/global/features/facts-figures-disabilities-in-developing-countries/>

Wolford, M 2016, *A school psychologist's guide to deafblindness: Identifying & supporting students with combined hearing-vision loss*, viewed 06 June 2018, <https://ohiodeafblind.org/tools-and-resources/ocdbe-products/6-a-school-psychologist-s-guide-to-deafblindness-identifying-supporting-students-with-combined-hearing-vision-loss-2016/file>

World Federation of the Deafblind (WFDB) 2018, *At risk of exclusion from CRPD and SDGs implementation: Inequality and persons with deafblindness*, viewed 08 May 2020, <http://www.internationaldisabilityalliance.org/sites/default/files/wfdb_complete_initial_global_report_september_2018.pdf>

World Health Organization (WHO) 2010, *Community-based rehabilitation: CBR guidelines*, World Health Organization, Geneva.

World Health Organization (WHO) 2010. *The World Health Report: Health systems financing – the path to universal coverage*, World Health Organization, Geneva.

World Health Organization (WHO) 2018, *Disability and health*, World Health Organization, Geneva.

Zwanenburg, A & Tesni, S 2019, *Guidelines on best practice for persons living with deafblindness*, CBM inclusive education technical guideline, viewed 08 May 2020, <https://www.cbm.org/fileadmin/user_upload/Publications/Guidelines_on_best_practice_for_persons_living_with_deafblindness_EN.pdf>

Chapter 10

Ahmed, H, Shubina-Oleinik, O & Holt, JR 2017, 'Emerging gene therapies for genetic hearing loss', *JARO – Journal of the Association for Research in Otolaryngology*, vol. 18, no. 5, pp. 649–670. https://doi.org/10.1007/s10162-017-0634-8

Alfvén, T, Dahlstrand, J, Humphreys, D, Helldén, D, Hammarstrand, S, Hollander, AC, Målqvist, M, Nejat, S, Søgaard Jørgensen, P, Friberg, P & Tomson, G 2019, 'Placing children and adolescents at the centre of the sustainable development goals will deliver for current and future generations', *Global Health Action*, vol. 12, no. 1, a1670015. https://doi.org/10.1080/16549716.2019.1670015

Awoonor-Williams, JK, Tindana, P, Dalinjong, PA, Nartey, H & Akazili, J 2016, 'Does the operations of the national health insurance scheme (NHIS) in Ghana align with the goals of primary health care? Perspectives of key stakeholders in northern Ghana', *BMC International Health and Human Rights*, vol. 16, no. 1, pp. 1–11. https://doi.org/10.1186/s12914-016-0096-9

Bate, A, Donaldson, C & Murtagh, MJ 2007, 'Managing to manage healthcare resources in the English NHS? What can health economics teach? What can health economics learn?', *Health Policy*, vol. 84, no. 2–3, pp. 249–261. https://doi.org/10.1016/j.healthpol.2007.04.001

Bennett, S, Jessani, N, Glandon, D, Qiu, M, Scott, K, Meghani, A, El-Jardali, F, Maceira, D, Javadi, D & Ghaffar, A 2020, 'Understanding the implications of the sustainable development goals for health policy and systems research: Results of a research priority setting exercise', *Globalization and Health*, vol. 16, no. 1, pp. 1–13. https://doi.org/10.1186/s12992-019-0534-2

Blumenschein, K & Johannesson, M 1996, 'Economic evaluation in healthcare: A brief history and future directions', *Pharmaeconomics*, vol. 10, no. 2, pp. 114–122. https://doi.org/10.2165/00019053-199610020-00003

Bridges, JFP, Hauber, AB, Marshall, D, Lloyd, A, Prosser, LA, Regier, DA, Johnson, FR & Mauskopf, J 2011, 'Conjoint analysis applications in health – a checklist: A report of the ISPOR good research practices for conjoint analysis task force', *Value in Health*, vol. 14, no. 4, pp. 403–413. https://doi.org/10.1016/j.jval.2010.11.013

Cerf, ME 2020, 'Sustainable development goal integration, interdependence, and implementation: The environment–economic–health nexus and universal health coverage', *Global Challenges*, vol. 3, no. 9, a1900021. https://doi.org/10.1002/gch2.201900021

Chadha, S, Kamenov, K & Cieza, A 2019, 'Health system requirements for hearing care services', *Bulletin of the World Health Organization*, vol. 97, no. 10, pp. 647–647A. https://doi.org/10.2471/BLT.19.243683

Chorozoglou, M, Mahon, M, Pimperton, H, Worsfold, S & Kennedy, CR 2018, 'Societal costs of permanent childhood hearing loss at teen age: A cross-sectional cohort follow-up study of universal newborn hearing screening', *BMJ Paediatrics Open*, vol. 2, no. 1, pp. 1–11. https://doi.org/10.1136/bmjpo-2017-000228

Cookson, R, Mirelman, AJ, Griffin, S, Asaria, M, Dawkins, B, Norheim, OF, Verguet, S & Culyer, AJ 2017, 'Using cost-effectiveness analysis to address health equity concerns', *Value in Health*, vol. 20, no. 2, pp. 206–212. https://doi.org/10.1016/j.jval.2016.11.027

Culyer, AJ & Chalkidou, K 2019, 'Economic evaluation for health investments en-route to universal health coverage: Cost-benefit analysis or cost-effectiveness analysis?', *Value in Health*, vol. 22, no. 1, pp. 99–103. https://doi.org/10.1016/j.jval.2018.06.005

Cunningham, CE, Deal, K & Chen, Y 2010, 'Adaptive choice-based conjoint analysis: A new patient-centered approach to the assessment of health service preferences', *Patient*, vol. 3, no. 4, pp. 257–273. https://doi.org/10.2165/11537870-000000000-00000

Davies, L, Coyle, D, Drummond, M & The EC Network on the Methodology of Economic Appraisal of Health Technology 1994, 'Current status of economic appraisal of health technology in the European Community: Report of the network', *Social Science & Medicine*, vol. 38, no. 12, pp. 1601–1607. https://doi.org/10.1016/0277-9536(94)90060-4

Doshi, JA & Willke, RJ 2017, 'Advancing high-quality value assessments of health care interventions', *Value in Health*, vol. 20, no. 2, pp. 181–184. https://doi.org/10.1016/j.jval.2016.12.012

Dukhanin, V, Searle, A, Zwerling, A, Dowdy, DW, Taylor, HA & Merritt, MW 2018, 'Integrating social justice concerns into economic evaluation for healthcare and public health: A systematic review', *Social Science and Medicine*, vol. 198, pp. 27–35. https://doi.org/10.1016/j.socscimed.2017.12.012

Findlen, UM, Malhotra, PS & Adunka, OF 2019, 'Parent perspectives on multidisciplinary pediatric hearing healthcare', *International Journal of Pediatric Otorhinolaryngology*, vol. 116, pp. 141–146. https://doi.org/10.1016/j.ijporl.2018.10.044

Fitzpatrick, EM, Coyle, D, Gaboury, I, Durieux-Smith, A, Whittingham, JA, Grandpierre, V, Na, E & Salamatmanesh, M 2019, 'Service preferences of parents of children with mild bilateral or unilateral hearing loss: A conjoint analysis study', *Ear and Hearing: The Official Journal of the American Auditory Society*, vol. 40, no. 3, pp. 671–679. https://doi.org/10.1097/AUD.0000000000000651

Fortune, K, Becerra-posada, F, Buss, P, Galvão, AC, Contreras, A, Murphy, M, Rogger, C, Keahon, GE & Francisco, AD 2018, 'Health promotion and the agenda for sustainable development: WHO region of the Americas', *Bulletin of the World Health Organization*, vol. 96, no. 9, pp. 621–626. https://doi.org/10.2471/BLT.17.204404

Foteff, C, Kennedy, S, Milton, AH, Deger, M, Payk, F & Sanderson, G 2016, 'Cost-utility analysis of cochlear implantation in australian adults', *Otology and Neurotology*, vol. 37, no. 5, pp. 454–461. https://doi.org/10.1097/MAO.0000000000000999

Fusheini, A & Eyles, J 2016, 'Achieving universal health coverage in South Africa through a district health system approach: Conflicting ideologies of health care provision', *BMC Health Services Research*, vol. 16, no. 1, pp. 1–11. https://doi.org/10.1186/s12913-016-1797-4

Gage, H, Kaye, J, Owen, C, Trend, P & Wade, D 2006, 'Evaluating rehabilitation using cost-consequences analysis: An example in Parkinson's disease', *Clinical Rehabilitation*, vol. 20, no. 3, pp. 232–238. https://doi.org/10.1191/0269215506cr936oa

Ghebreyesus, TA 2017, 'All roads lead to universal health coverage', *The Lancet Global Health*, vol. 5, no. 9, pp. 839–840. https://doi.org/10.1016/S2214-109X(17)30295-4

Grosse, SD, Mason, CA, Gaffney, M, Vickie, T & White, KR 2018, 'What contribution did economic evidence make to the adoption of universal newborn hearing screening policies in the united states?', *International Journal of Neonatal Screening*, vol. 4, no. 3, pp. 139–148. https://doi.org/10.1016/j.physbeh.2017.03.040

Hartfiel, N & Edwards, RT 2019, 'Cost-consequence analysis in public health interventions', eds. RT Edwards & E McIntosh, *Applied health economics for public health practice and research*, Oxford University Press, Oxford, pp. 233–247.

Heidari, S, Manesh, AO, Rajabi, F & Moradi-Joo, M 2017, 'Cost-effectiveness analysis of automated auditory brainstem response and otoacoustic emission in universal neonatal hearing screening', *Iranian Journal of Pediatrics*, vol. 27, no. 2, pp. 1–8. https://doi.org/10.5812/ijp.5229

International Health Partnership 2018, *Health coverage advocacy guide*, viewed 15 April 2019, <https://www.uhc2030.org/fileadmin/uploads/uhc2030/Documents/Key_Issues/Advocacy/UHC_Advocacy_Guide_March_2018_final.pdf>

Jakovljevic, MM & Ogura, S 2016, 'Health economics at the crossroads of centuries – From the past to the future', *Frontiers in Public Health*, vol. 4, pp. 1–5. https://doi.org/10.3389/fpubh.2016.00115

Joint Committee on Infant Hearing (JCIH) 2019, 'Year 2019 position statement: Principles and guidelines for early hearing detection and intervention programs', *Journal of Early Hearing Detection and Intervention*, vol. 4, no. 2, pp. 1–44. https://doi.org/10.1542/peds.106.4.798

Kaur, P, Ng, C, Ling, W & Yin, LS 2020, 'Cost-utility analysis of hearing aid device for older adults in the community: A delayed start study', *Research Square*, vol. 20, p. 1112. https://doi.org/10.1186/s12913-020-05977-x

Kernick, D 2002, 'The impact of health economics on healthcare delivery: A health economist's perspective', *PharmacoEconomics*, vol. 20, no. 11, pp. 785–787. https://doi.org/10.2165/00019053-200220110-00007

Khoza-Shangase, K 2020, 'Pharmaco-audiology vigilance in the treatment of patients with HIV/AIDS: Ototoxicity monitoring protocol recommendation', *Infectious Diseases – Drug Targets*, vol. 20, no. 1, pp. 33–42. https://doi.org/10.2174/1871526518666181016102102

Khoza-Shangase, K & Michal, G 2014, 'Early intervention in audiology: Exploring the current status from a developing country context', *British Journal of Medicine and Medical Research*, vol. 4, no. 11, pp. 2238–2249. https://doi.org/10.9734/bjmmr/2014/7322

Lakdawalla, DN, Doshi, JA, Garrison, LP, Phelps, CE, Basu, A & Danzon, PM 2018, 'Defining elements of value in health care – A health economics approach: An ISPOR special task force report', *Value in Health*, vol. 21, no. 2, pp. 131–139. https://doi.org/10.1016/j.jval.2017.12.007

Lancsar, E & Louviere, J 2008, 'Conducting discrete choice experiments to inform healthcare decision making: A user's guide', *PharmacoEconomics*, vol. 26, no. 8, pp. 661–677. https://doi.org/10.2165/00019053-200826080-00004

Leclair, KL & Saunders, JE 2019, 'Meeting the educational needs of children with hearing loss', *Bulletin of the World Health Organization*, vol. 97, no. 10, pp. 722–724. https://doi.org/10.2471/BLT.18.227561

Maluleke, NP, Chiwutsi, R & Khoza-Shangase, K 2021a, 'Family-centered early hearing detection and intervention', eds. K Khoza-Shangase & A Kanji, *Early hearing detection and intervention in audiology: An African perspective*, Wits University Press, Johannesburg, pp. 196–218.

Maluleke, NP, Khoza-Shangase, K & Kanji, A 2019, 'Communication and school readiness abilities of children with hearing impairment in South Africa: A retrospective review of early intervention preschool record', *South African Journal of Communication Disorders*, vol. 66, no. 1, a604. https://doi.org/10.4102/sajcd.v66i1.604

Maluleke, NP, Khoza-shangase, K & Kanji, A 2021b, 'An integrative review of current practice models and/or process of family-centered early intervention for children who are deaf or hard of hearing', *Family and Community Health*, vol. 44, no. 1, pp. 59–71. https://doi.org/10.1097/FCH.0000000000000276

Maphumulo, WT & Bhengu, BR 2019, 'Challenges of quality improvement in the healthcare of South Africa post-apartheid: A critical review', *Curationis*, vol. 42, no. 1, a1901. https://doi.org/10.4102/curationis.v42i1.1901

Marshall, D, Bridges, JFP, Hauber, B, Cameron, R, Donnalley, L, Fyie, K & Johnson, FR 2010, 'Conjoint analysis applications in health – how are studies being designed and reported?: An update on current practice in the published literature between 2005 and 2008', *Patient*, vol. 3, no. 4, pp. 249–256. https://doi.org/10.2165/11539650-000000000-00000

Mauskopf, JA, Paul, JE, Grant, DM & Stergachis, A 1998, 'The role of cost-consequence analysis in healthcare decision-making', *PharmacoEconomics*, vol. 13, no. 3, pp. 277–288. https://doi.org/10.2165/00019053-199813030-00002

McGregor, M 2003, 'Cost-utility analysis: Use QALYs only with great caution', *Canadian Medical Association Journal*, vol. 168, no. 4, pp. 433–434.

McIntosh, E, Donaldson, C & Ryan, M 1999, 'Recent advances in the methods of cost-benefit analysis in healthcare', *PharmacoEconomics*, vol. 15, no. 4, pp. 357–367. https://doi.org/10.2165/00019053-199915040-00003

McNamee, P, Murray, E, Kelly, MP, Bojke, L, Chilcott, J, Fischer, A, West, R & Yardley, L 2016, 'Designing and undertaking a health economics study of digital health interventions', *American Journal of Preventive Medicine*, vol. 51, no. 5, pp. 852–860. https://doi.org/10.1016/j.amepre.2016.05.007

Meinzen-Derr, J, Wiley, S & Choo, D 2011, 'Impact of early intervention on expressive and receptive language development among young children with permanent hearing loss', *American Annals of the Deaf*, vol. 155, no. 5, pp. 580–591. <https://www.jstor.org/stable/26235114>.

National Academies of Sciences 2016, *Hearing health care for adults: Priorities for improving access and affordability*, The National Academies Press, Washington DC.

Neuman, PJ 2017, 'Improved CEAs could help optimise US spending on health', *PharmacoEconomics & Outcoms News*, vol. 726, no. 770, p. 1. https://doi.org/10.1007/s40274-017-3677-5

Olusanya, BO 2012, 'Neonatal hearing screening and intervention in resource-limited settings: An overview', *Archives of Disease in Childhood*, vol. 97, no. 7, pp. 654–659. https://doi.org/10.1136/archdischild-2012-301786

Peer, S 2015, 'Turning up the volume on hearing loss in South Africa', *South African Medical Journal*, vol. 105, no. 1, pp. 31–32. https://doi.org/10.7196/SAMJ.9218

Pribanikj, L & Milkovikj, M 2009, 'The benefit of early exposure to sign language', *Journal of Special Education & Rehabilitation*, vol. 10, pp. 28–39. https://doi.org/10.5281/zenodo.28532

Qiu, J, Yu, C, Ariyaratne, TV, Foteff, C, Ke, Z, Sun, Y, Zhang, L, Qin, F & Sanderson, G 2017, 'Cost-effectiveness of pediatric cochlear implantation in rural China', *Otology and Neurotology*, vol. 38, no. 6, pp. 75–84. https://doi.org/10.1097/MAO.0000000000001389

Ramkuma, V, Selvakumar, KRJ, Vanaja, CS, Nagarajam, R & Hall, J 2018, 'Cost and outcome of a community-based paediatric hearing screening programme in rural India with application of tele-audiology for follow-up diagnostic hearing assessment', *International Journal of Audiology*, vol. 57, no. 6, pp. 407–414. https://doi.org/10.1080/14992027.2018.1442592

Remme, M, Martínez-Alvarez, M & Vassall, A 2017, 'Cost-effectiveness thresholds in global health: Taking a multisectoral perspective', *Value in Health*, vol. 20, no. 4, pp. 699–704. https://doi.org/10.1016/j.jval.2016.11.009

Robertson, L, Skelly, C & Phillips, D 2019, 'Making hard choices in local public health spending with a cost-benefit analysis approach', *Frontiers in Public Health*, vol. 7, pp. 1–8. https://doi.org/10.3389/fpubh.2019.00147

Rognoni, C, Armeni, P, Tarricone, R & Donin, G 2020, 'Cost–benefit analysis in health care: The case of bariatric surgery compared with diet', *Clinical Therapeutics*, vol. 42, no. 1, pp. 60–75.E7. https://doi.org/10.1016/j.clinthera.2019.12.001

Russell, LB, Gold, MR, Siegel, JE, Daniels, N & Weinstein, MC 1996, 'The role of cost-effectiveness analysis in health and medicine', *Journal of the American Medical Association*, vol. 276, no. 14, pp. 1172–1177. https://doi.org/10.1001/jama.1996.03540140060028

Ryan, M & Farrar, S 2000, 'Using conjoint analysis to elicit preferences for health care', *British Medical Journal*, vol. 320, no. 7248, pp. 1530–1533. https://doi.org/10.1136/bmj.320.7248.1530

Saunders, JE, Barrs, DM, Gong, W, Wilson, BS, Mojica, K & Tucci, DL 2015, 'Cost effectiveness of childhood cochlear implantation and deaf education in Nicaragua: A disability adjusted life year model', *Otology and Neurotology*, vol. 36, no. 8, pp. 1349–1356. https://doi.org/10.1097/MAO.0000000000000809

Saunders, JE, Francis, HW & Skarzynski, PH 2016, 'Measuring success: Cost-effectiveness and expanding access to cochlear implantation', *Otology and Neurotology*, vol. 37, no. 2, pp. 135–140. https://doi.org/10.1097/MAO.0000000000000942

Sell, SK 2019, '21st-century capitalism: Structural challenges for universal health care', *Globalization and Health*, vol. 15, suppl. 1, pp. 1–9. https://doi.org/10.1186/s12992-019-0517-3

Sharma, R, Gu, Y, Ching, TYC, Marnane, V & Parkinson, B 2019, 'Economic evaluations of childhood hearing loss screening programmes: A systematic review and critique', *Applied Health Economics and Health Policy*, vol. 17, no. 3, pp. 331–357. https://doi.org/10.1007/s40258-018-00456-1

Shisana, O, Rehle, TM, Louw, J, Zungu-Dirwayi, N, Dana, P & Rispel, L 2006, 'Public perceptions on national health: Moving toward universal health coverage in South Africa', *South African Medical Journal*, vol. 96, no. 9, pp. 814–818. https://doi.org/10.7196/SAMJ.1255

Sørensen, CA, De Thurah, A, Lisby, M, Olesen, C, Sørensen, SB & Enemark, U 2020, 'Cost-consequence analysis of self-administration of medication during hospitalization: A pragmatic randomized controlled trial in a Danish hospital setting', *Therapeutic Advances in Drug Safety*, vol. 11, pp. 1–16. https://doi.org/10.1177/2042098620929921

Stafford-Smith, M, Griggs, D, Gaffney, O, Ullah, F, Reyers, B, Kanie, N, Stigson, B, Shrivastava, P, Leach, M & O'Connell, D 2017, 'Integration: The key to implementing the sustainable development goals', *Sustainability Science*, vol. 12, no. 6, pp. 911–919. https://doi.org/10.1007/s11625-016-0383-3

Steele, T, Pawaskar, M, Balkrishnan, R, Fleischer, A & Feldman, SR 2007, 'Does cost-effectiveness play a role in clinical trials?', *Dermatologic Therapy*, vol. 20, no. 2, pp. 110–119. https://doi.org/10.1111/j.1529-8019.2007.00119.x

Störbeck, C 2012, 'Childhood hearing loss in the developing world', *International Journal of Child Health and Nutrition*, vol. 1, no. 1, p. 59–65. https://doi.org/10.6000/1929-4247.2012.01.01.07

Swanepoel, D & Clark, JL 2018, 'Hearing healthcare in remote or resource-constrained environments', *Journal of Laryngology and Otology*, vol. 133, no. 1, pp. 11–17. https://doi.org/10.1017/S0022215118001159

Swanepoel, DW & Hall III JW 2010, 'A systematic review of telehealth applications in audiology', *Telemedicine and e-Health*, vol. 16, no. 2, pp. 181–200. https://doi.org/10.1089/tmj.2009.0111

Tangcharoensathien, V, Mills, A & Palu, T 2015, 'Accelerating health equity: The key role of universal health coverage in the sustainable development goals', *BMC Medicine*, vol. 13, no. 1, pp. 1–5. https://doi.org/10.1186/s12916-015-0342-3

Tobe, RG, Mori, R, Huang, L, Xu, L & Han, DSK 2013, 'Cost-effectiveness analysis of a national neonatal hearing screening program in China: Conditions for the scale-up', *PLoS One*, vol. 8, no. 1, a51990. https://doi.org/10.1371/journal.pone.0051990

Vas, V, Akeroyd, MA & Hall, DA 2017, 'A data-driven synthesis of research evidence for domains of hearing loss, as reported by adults with hearing loss and their communication partners', *Trends in Hearing*, vol. 21, pp. 1–25. https://doi.org/10.1177/2331216517734088

Verguet, S, Kim, JJ & Jamison, DT 2016, 'Extended cost-effectiveness analysis for health policy assessment: A tutorial', *PharmacoEconomics*, vol. 34, no. 9, pp. 913–923. https://doi.org/10.1007/s40273-016-0414-z

World Health Organization (WHO) 2014, *The case for investing in public health*, World Health Organization, Geneva.

World Health Organization (WHO) 2016, *Introduction to drug utilization research*: *Drug Utilization Research*, World Health Organization, Geneva.

World Health Organization (WHO) 2017, *Global costs of unaddressed hearing loss & cost-effectiveness of interventions: A WHO report, 2017*, World Health Organization, Geneva.

World Health Organization (WHO) 2020, *Deafness and hearing loss*, World Health Organization, Geneva.

Chapter 11

Al-Dayyeni, W, Sun, P & Qin, J 2018, 'Investigations of auditory filters based excitation patterns for assessment of noise-induced hearing loss', *Archives of Acoustics*, vol. 43, no. 3, pp. 477–486. https://doi.org/10.24425/123919

Aliabadi, M, Golmohammadi, R, Mansoorizadeh, M, Khotanlou, H & Hamadani, AO 2013, 'An empirical technique for predicting noise exposure level in the typical embroidery workrooms using artificial neural networks', *Applied Acoustics*, vol. 74, no. 3, pp. 364–374.

Aliabadi, M, Fereidan, M, Farhadian, M & Tajik, L 2015, 'Determining the effect of worker exposure conditions on the risk of hearing loss in noisy industrial workroom using Cox proportional hazard model', *International Journal of Occupational Safety and Ergonomics*, vol. 21, no. 2, pp. 201–206. https://doi.org/10.1080/10803548.2015.1029725

Ansari, H, Ansari-Moghaddam, A, Mohammadi, M, Tabatabaei, SM, Fazli, B & Pishevare-Mofrad, M 2016, 'Status of hearing loss and its related factors among drivers in Zahedan, South-Eastern Iran', *Global Journal of Health Science*, vol. 8, no. 8, p. 53097. https://doi.org/10.5539/gjhs.v8n8p66

Arenas, J & Suter, A 2014, 'Comparison of occupational noise legislation in the Americas: An overview and analysis', *Noise and Health*, vol. 16, no. 72, pp. 306–319. https://doi.org/10.4103/1463-1741.140511

Ashkezari, SJ, Namiranian, N, Rahmanian, M, Atighechi, S, Mohajeri-Tehrani, M-R & Gholami, S 2018, 'Is hearing impairment in diabetic patients correlated to other complications?', *Journal of Diabetes and Metabolic Disorders*, vol. 17, no. 2, pp. 173–179. https://doi.org/10.1007/s40200-018-0357-3

Badri, L 2010, 'Development of neural networks for noise reduction', *The International Arab Journal of Information Technology*, vol. 7, no. 3, pp. 289–294.

Bakay, WMH, Anderson, LA, García-Lazaro, JA, McAlpine, D & Schaette, R 2018, 'Hidden hearing loss selectively impairs neural adaptation to loud sound environments', *Nature Communications*, vol. 9, no. 1, p. 4298. https://doi.org/10.1038/s41467-018-06777

Basner, M, Babisch, W, Davis, AC, Brink, M, Clark, C, Janssen, S & Stansfeld, S 2014, 'Auditory and non-auditory effects of noise on health', *The Lancet*, vol. 383, no. 9925, pp. 1325–1332. https://doi.org/10.1016/S0140-6736(13)61613-X

Basu, S, Stuckler, D, Gonsalves, G & Lurie, M 2009, 'The production of consumption: Addressing the impact of mineral mining on tuberculosis in Southern Africa', *Globalization and Health*, vol. 5, no. 1, p. 11. https://doi.org/10.1186/1744-8603-5-11

Bauer, ER & Babich, DR 2006, 'Administrative controls for reducing worker noise exposures', in *Transactions of society for mining, metallurgy, and exploration, Inc.*, viewed 02 November 2022, <https://www.cdc.gov/niosh/mining/UserFiles/works/pdfs/acfrw.pdf>

Bayley, A, Woo, K & Wong, S 2013, *Wireless headset noise exposure dosimeter*, Plantronics, Booyen, Santa Cruz.

Beamer, B, McCleery, T & Hayden, C 2016, 'Buy quiet initiative in the USA', *Acoustics Australia*, vol. 44, no. 1, pp. 51–54. https://doi.org/10.1007/s40857-015-0036-1

Bhunu, CP, Mushayabasa, S & Smith, RJ 2012, 'Assessing the effects of poverty in tuberculosis transmission dynamics', *Applied Mathematical Modelling*, vol. 36, no. 9, pp. 4173–4185. https://doi.org/10.1016/j.apm.2011.11.046

Brauch, R 2017, 'Tech advances are reinventing hearing conservation programs: Open your ears', viewed 01 February 2017, <https://www.ishn.com/articles/105770-tech-advances-are-reinventing-hearing-conservation-programsilableonline>

Brereton, P & Patel, J 2016, 'Buy quiet as a means of reducing workplace noise', *Journal of Acoustics Australia*, vol. 44, no. 1, pp. 55–65. https://doi.org/10.1007/s40857-016-0051-x

Brodie, A, Smith, B & Ray, J 2018, 'The impact of rehabilitation on quality of life after hearing loss: A systematic review', *European Archives of Oto-Rhino-Laryngology*, vol. 275, no. 10, pp. 2435–2440. https://doi.org/10.1007/s00405-018-5100-7

Bronkhorst, JP & De Schutte, DW 2013, 'Reconstruction of percentage loss of hearing', *Occupational Health Southern*, vol. 19, no. 3, pp. 20–24.

Brown, AD, Beemer, BT, Greene, NT, Argo, TT, Meegan, GD & Tollin, DJ 2015, 'Effects of active and passive hearing protection devices on sound source localization, speech recognition, and tone detection', *PLoS One*, vol. 10, no. 8, a0136568. https://doi.org/10.1371/journal.pone.0136568

Bruce, RD & Wood, EW 2003, 'The USA needs a new national policy for occupational noise', *Noise Control Engineering*, vol. 51, no. 3, pp. 162–165.

Bruce, RD 2007, 'Engineering controls for reducing workplace noise', *National Academy of Engineering*, vol. 37, no. 3, pp. 33–39.

Brungart, DS, Barrett, ME, Schurman, J, Sheffield, B, Ramos, L, Martorana, R & Galloza, H 2019, 'Relationship between subjective reports of temporary threshold shift and the prevalence of hearing problems in military personnel', *Trends in Hearing*, vol. 23, a2331216519872601. https://doi.org/10.1177/2331216519872601

Byrne, DC 2005, 'A model hearing conservation program', paper presented at the Mining Hearing Loss Prevention Workshop, Pittsburgh Research Laboratory, Pittsburgh, 21–22 June.

Chadha, S & Cieza, A 2017, 'Promoting global action on hearing loss: World Hearing Day', *International Journal of Audiology*, vol. 56, no. 3, pp. 145–147. https://doi.org/10.1080/14992027.2017.1291264

Chaudhary, K 2017, *The hierarchy of hazard control*, LinkedIn, 08 July, viewed 03 November 2022, <https://www.linkedin.com/pulse/hierarchy-hazard-controls-kailash-chaudhary/>

Choi, CH, Du, X, Floyd, RA & Kopke, RD 2014, 'Therapeutic effects of orally administrated antioxidant drugs on acute noise-induced hearing loss', *Free Radical Research*, vol. 48, no. 3, pp. 264–272. https://doi.org/10.3109/10715762.2013.861599

Choi, SH & Choi, C-H 2015, 'Noise-induced neural degeneration and therapeutic effect of antioxidant drugs', *Journal of Audiology & Otology*, vol. 19, no. 3, pp. 111–119. https://doi.org/10.7874/jao.2015.19.3.111

Coco, L, Ingram, M & Marrone, N 2019, 'Qualitative research methods to investigate communication within a group aural rehabilitation intervention', *International Journal of Audiology*, vol. 58, no. 10, pp. 651–660. https://doi.org/10.1080/14992027.2019.1608377

Cullinan, K 2018, 'R1.4 billion settlement for miners with silicosis', *Health24*, 08 May 2019, viewed 02 November 2022, <https://www.news24.com/health24/news/public-health/r14-billion-settlement-for-miners-with-silicosis-tb-20180508>

Davis, RI, Qiu, W, Heyer, NJ, Zhao, Y, Qiuling Yang, MS, Li, N, Tao, L, Zhu, L, Zeng, L & Yao, D 2012, 'The use of the kurtosis metric in the evaluation of occupational hearing loss in workers in China: Implications for hearing risk assessment', *Noise Health*, vol. 14, no. 61, pp. 330–342. https://doi.org/10.4103/1463-1741.104903

Dale, LM, Goudreau, S, Perron, S, Ragettli, MS, Hatzopoulou, M & Smargiassi, A 2015, 'Socioeconomic status and environmental noise exposure in Montreal, Canada', *BMC Public Health*, vol. 15, no. 1, p. 205. https://doi.org/10.1186/s12889-015-1571-2

De Koker, E n.d., *Industrial audiology: Guidelines*, viewed 08 May 2019, <http://www.hpcsa.co.za/Uploads/editor/UserFiles/downloads/speech/draft_guidelines/indus_audi_draft.pdf>

Delecrode, CR, De Freitas, TD, Frizzo, ACF & Cardoso, ACV 2012, 'Prevalence of tinnitus in workers exposed to noise and organophosphates', *International Archives of Otorhinolaryngology*, vol. 16, no. 3, pp. 328–334. https://doi.org/10.7162/S1809-97772012000300005

De W Oosthuizen, S 2006, *Guidelines for hearing conservation programmes*, Provincial Occupational Health Unit, Bloemfontein, pp. 1–27.

Deng, WJ, Chen, W-C & Pei, W 2008, 'Back-propagation neural network based importance - Performance analysis for determining critical service attributes', *Expert Systems with Applications*, vol. 34, no. 2, pp. 1115–1125. https://doi.org/10.1016/j.eswa.2006.12.016

Ding, T, Yan, A & Liu, K 2019, 'What is noise-induced hearing loss?', *British Journal of Hospital Medicine*, vol. 80, no. 9, pp. 525–529. https://doi.org/10.12968/hmed.2019.80.9.525

Duplaga, M, Grysztar, M, Rodzinka, M & Kopec, A 2016, 'Scoping review of health promotion and disease prevention interventions addressed to elderly people', *BMC Health Services Research*, vol. 16, no. 5, pp. 455–465. https://doi.org/10.1186/s12913-016-1521-4

Edwards, AL & Kritzinger, D 2012, 'Noise-induced hearing loss milestones: Past and future', *The Journal of The Southern African Institute of Mining and Metallurgy*, vol. 112, pp. 865–869.

Elahi, N 2006, *Industrial safety management*, Kalpaz Publications, New Delhi.

Fabry, DA, Davila, EP, Arheart, KL, Serdar, B, Dietz, NA, Bandiera, FC & Lee, DJ 2011, 'Secondhand smoke exposure and the risk of hearing loss', *Tobacco Control*, vol. 20, no. 1, pp. 82–85. https://doi.org/10.1136/tc.2010.035832

Feder, K, Michaud, D, McNamee, J, Fitzpatrick, E, Davies, H & Leroux, T 2017, 'Prevalence of hazardous occupational noise exposure, hearing loss, and hearing protection usage among a representative sample of working Canadians', *Journal of Occupational and Environmental Medicine*, vol. 59, no. 1, pp. 92–113. https://doi.org/10.1097/JOM.0000000000000920

Fink, DJ 2017, 'What is a safe noise level for the public?', *American Journal of Public Health*, vol. 107, no. 1, pp. 44–45. https://doi.org/10.2105/AJPH.2016.303527

Gardner, F 2019, 'Are earlier interventions more effective? Pooling data from 15,000 families taking part in parenting interventions', viewed 20 July 2019, <https://www.acamh.org/app/uploads/2019/02/1330-Frances-Gardner-Are-early-interventions-more-effective.pdf>

Gumede, H 2018, 'The socio-economic effects of mechanising and/or modernising hard rock mines in South Africa', *South African Journal of Economic and Management Sciences*, vol. 21, no. 1, a848. https://doi.org/10.4102/sajems.v21i1.1848

Gumede, H, Blomerus, K, Coutts, D & De Beer, J 2014, 'Strategy towards a mining industry-wide buy-and-obtain quiet initiative to reduce noise-induced hearing loss', *The Journal of The Southern African Institute of Mining and Metallurgy*, vol. 114, pp. 923–928.

HearSafe Solutions 2018, *What is surveillance audiometry?*, viewed 13 May 2020, <https://hearsafe.solutions/index.php/blog/1-what-is-surveillance-audiometry>

Hind, SE, Haines-Bazrafshan, R, Benton, CL, Brassington, W, Towle, B & Moore, DR 2011, 'Prevalence of clinical referrals having hearing thresholds within normal limits', *International Journal of Audiology*, vol. 50, no. 10, pp. 708–716. https://doi.org/10.3109/14992027.2011.582049

Hong, O, Kerr, MJ, Poling, GL & Dhar, S 2013, 'Understanding and preventing noise-induced hearing loss', *Disease-a-Month*, vol. 59, no. 4, pp. 110–118. https://doi.org/10.1016/j.disamonth.2013.01.002

Jamir, L, Nongkynrih, B & Gupta, SK 2014, 'Community noise pollution in urban India: Need for public health action', *Indian Journal of Community Medicine*, vol. 39, no. 1, pp. 8–12. https://doi.org/10.4103/0970-0218.126342

Kardous, C 2016, *Understanding noise exposure limits: Occupational vs. general environmental noise*, viewed 15 November 2018, <https://www.ishn.com/articles/103315-understanding-noise-exposure-limits-occupational-vs-general-environmental-noise>

Keppler, H, Dhooge, I & Vinck, B 2015, 'Hearing in young adults. Part II: The effects of recreational noise exposure', *Noise and Health*, vol. 17, no. 78, pp. 245–252. https://doi.org/10.4103/1463-1741.165026

Kerketta, S, Gartia, R & Bagh, S 2012, 'Hearing threshold, loss, noise levels and worker's profiles of an open-cast chromite mines in Odisha, India', *The Malaysian Journal of Medical Sciences*, vol. 19, no. 4, pp. 63–71.

Khan, MW, Memon, MA, Khan, MN & Khan, MM 2010, 'Traffic noise pollution in Karachi, Pakistan', *Journal of Liaquat University of Medical and Health Sciences*, vol. 9, no. 3, pp. 114–120.

Khoza-Shangase, K 2010, 'Is there a need for ototoxicity monitoring in patients with HIV/AIDS?', *African Journal of Pharmacy and Pharmacology*, vol. 4, no. 9, pp. 574–579.

Khoza-Shangase, K 2020a, 'Hearing function of gold miners with and without a history of tuberculosis treatment: A retrospective data review', *Brazilian Journal of Otorhinolaryngology*, vol. 86, no. 3, pp. 294–299. https://doi.org/10.1016/j.bjorl.2018.12.003

Khoza-Shangase, K 2020b, 'Burden of disease: A scoping review of HIV/AIDS and TB in occupational noise-induced hearing loss', *South African Journal of Communication Disorders*, vol. 67, no. 2, a669. https://doi.org/10.4102/sajcd.v67i2.669

Khoza-Shangase, K & Moroe, NF 2020, 'Risk versus benefit: Should not audiologists assess this in the context of occupational noise-induced hearing loss in the mining industry?', *South African Journal of Communication Disorders*, vol. 67, no. 2, pp. 1–9. https://doi.org/10.4102/sajcd.v67i2.671

Khoza-Shangase, K, Ntlhakana, L & Nelson, G 2020, 'Estimating miners at risk for occupational noise-induced hearing loss: A review of data from a South African platinum mine', *South African Journal of Communication Disorders*, vol. 67, no. 2, pp. 1–8. https://doi.org/10.4102/sajcd.v67i2.677

Kirchner, DB, Evenson, E, Dobie, RA, Rabinowitz, P, Crawford, J, Kopke, R & Hudson, TW 2012, 'Occupational noise-induced hearing loss: ACOEM task force on occupational hearing loss', *Journal of Occupational and Environmental Medicine*, vol. 54, no. 1, pp. 106–108. https://doi.org/10.1097/JOM.0b013e318242677d

Kuang, D, Yu, Y & Tu, C 2019, 'Bilateral high-frequency hearing loss is associated with elevated blood pressure and increased hypertension risk in occupational noise-exposed workers', *PLoS One*, vol. 14, no. 9, a0222135. https://doi.org/10.1371/journal.pone.0222135

Le, TN, Straatman, LV, Lea, J & Westerberg, B 2017, 'Current insights in noise-induced hearing loss: A literature review of the underlying mechanism, pathophysiology, asymmetry, and management options', *Journal of Otolaryngology – Head & Neck Surgery*, vol. 46, no. 1, p. 41. https://doi.org/10.1186/s40463-017-0219-x

Leboea, ST 2017, 'The factors influencing SME failure in South Africa', MCom thesis, University of Cape Town.

Leshchinsky, A 2018, 'The impact of annual audiograms on employee's habits and awareness regarding hearing protection and noise induced hearing loss, on and off the job', *Workplace Health & Safety*, vol. 66, no. 4, pp. 201–206. https://doi.org/10.1177/2165079917743020

Li, X, Dong, Q, Wang, B, Song, H, Wang, S & Zhu, B 2019, 'The influence of occupational noise exposure on cardiovascular and hearing conditions among industrial workers', *Scientific Reports*, vol. 9, no. 1, p. 11524. https://doi.org/10.1038/s41598-019-47901-2

Liu, J, Xu, M, Ding, L, Zhang, H, Pan, L, Liu, Q, Ding, E, Zhao, Q, Wang, B, Han, L, Yang, D & Zhu, B 2016, 'Prevalence of hypertension and noise-induced hearing loss in Chinese coal miners', *Journal of Thoracic Disease*, vol. 8, no. 3, pp. 422–429. https://doi.org/10.21037/jtd.2016.02.59

Lobarinas, E, Spankovich, C & Le Prell, CG 2017, 'Evidence of "hidden hearing loss" following noise exposures that produce robust TTS and ABR wave-I amplitude reductions', *Hearing Research*, vol. 349, pp. 155–163. https://doi.org/10.1016/j.heares.2016.12.009

Lusk, SL, McCullagh, M, Dickson, VV & Xu, J 2016, 'Position statement: Harmful effects of environmental noise exposures', *Nursing Outlook*, vol. 64, no. 4, pp. 395–396. https://doi.org/10.1016/j.outlook.2016.06.001

McDaniel, M, Chinn, G, McCall, K & Stewart, A 2013, *Guidelines for audiometric baseline revision*, viewed 08 May 2019, <https://www.hearingconservation.org/assets/docs/Guidelines_for_Audiometric_B.pdf>

McTague, MF, Galusha, D, Dixon-Ernst, C, Kirsche, SR, Slade, MD, Cullen, MR & Rabinowitz, PM 2013, 'Impact of daily noise exposure monitoring on occupational noise exposures in manufacturing workers', *International Journal of Audiology*, vol. 52, suppl. 1, pp. 3–8. https://doi.org/10.3109/14992027.2012.743047

Michael, K, Tougaw, E & Wilkinson, R 2011, 'Role of continuous monitoring in a hearing conservation program', *Noise & Health*, vol. 13, no. 51, pp. 195–199. https://doi.org/10.4103/1463-1741.77204M

Mine Health and Safety Council (MHSC) 2014, *The health and safety summit: The road to zero harm – New milestones*, viewed 19 February 2016, <https://mhsc.org.za/sites/default/files/public/publications/Mr%20Msiza%202014%20Milestones_0.pdf>

Moroe, NF 2018, 'Occupational noise-induced hearing loss in South African large-scale mines: From policy formulation to implementation and monitoring', PhD thesis, University of the Witwatersrand.

Moroe, NF 2018, 'Occupational noise-induced hearing loss in South African large-scale mines: Exploring hearing conservation programmes as complex interventions embedded in a realist approach', *International Journal of Occupational Safety and Ergonomics*, vol. 2018, pp. 1–9. https://doi.org/10.1080/10803548.2018.1498183

Moroe, N, Khoza-Shangase, K, Madahana, M & Nyandoro, O 2019, 'A proposed preliminary model for monitoring hearing conservation programmes in the mining sector in South Africa', *The Journal of the Southern African Institute of Mining and Metallurgy*, vol. 119, no. 7, pp. 671–679. https://doi.org/10.17159/2411-9717/18/016/2019

Moroe, NF 2020a, 'Occupational noise-induced hearing loss in South African large-scale mines: Exploring hearing conservation programmes as complex interventions embedded in a realist approach', *International Journal of Occupational Safety and Ergonomics*, vol. 26, no. 4, pp. 753–761. https://doi.org/10.1080/10803548.2018.1498183

Moroe, NF 2020b, 'Occupational noise-induced hearing loss in the mining sector of South Africa: Perspectives of occupational health practitioners on how mineworkers are trained', *South African Journal of Communication Disorders*, vol. 67, no. 2, a676. https://doi.org/10.4102/sajcd.v67i2.676

Moroe, NF & Khoza-Shangase, K 2018, 'Management of occupational noise-induced hearing loss in the mining sector in South Africa: Where are the audiologists?', *Journal of Occupational Health*, vol. 60, no. 5, pp. 376–382. https://doi.org/10.1539/joh.2018-0020-OA

Moroe, NF & Khoza-Shangase, K 2020, 'Recent advances in hearing conservation programmes: A systematic review', *South African Journal of Communication Disorders*, vol. 67, no. 2, a675. https://doi.org/10.4102/sajcd.v67i2.675

Mostaghaci, M, Mirmohammadi, SJ, Mehrparvar, AH, Bahaloo, M, Mollasadeghi, A & Davari, MH 2013, 'Effect of workplace noise on hearing ability in tile and ceramic industry workers in Iran: A 2-year follow-up study', *The Scientific World Journal*, vol. 2013, a923731. https://doi.org/10.1155/2013/923731

Mukherjea, D, Rybak, LP, Sheehan, KE, Kaur, T, Ramkumar, V, Jajoo, S & Sheth, S 2011, 'The design and screening of drugs to prevent acquired sensorineural hearing loss', *Expert Opinion on Drug Discovery*, vol. 6, no. 5, pp. 491–505. https://doi.org/10.1517/17460441.2011.562887

Musiba, Z 2020, 'Classification of audiograms in the prevention of noise-induced hearing loss: A clinical perspective', *South African Journal of Communication Disorders*, vol. 67, no. 2, pp. 1–5. https://doi.org/10.4102/sajcd.v67i2.691

Ntlhakana, L, Kanji, A & Khoza-Shangase, K 2015, 'The use of hearing protection devices in South Africa: Exploring the current status in a gold and a non-ferrous mine', *Occupational Health Southern Africa*, vol. 21, no. 2, pp. 10–15.

Ntlhakana, L, Nelson, G, Khoza-Shangase, K & Dorkin, E 2022, 'Occupational hearing loss for platinum miners in South Africa: A case study of data sharing practices and ethical challenges in the mining industry', *International Journal of Environmental Research and Public Health*, vol. 19, no. 1, p. 1. https://doi.org/10.3390/ijerph19010001

Oguntunde, PE, Okagbue, HI, Oguntunde, OA & Odetunmibi, OO 2019, 'A study of noise pollution measurements and possible effects on public health in Ota Metropolis, Nigeria', *Open Access Macedonian Journal of Medical Sciences*, vol. 7, no. 8, pp. 1391–1395. https://doi.org/10.3889/oamjms.2019.234

Oishi, N & Schacht, J 2011, 'Emerging treatments for noise-induced hearing loss', *Expert opinion on emerging drugs*, vol. 16, no. 2, pp. 235–245. https://doi.org/10.1517/14728214.2011.552427

Olukemi, O 2019, *Best practices for social media marketing for health promotion*, viewed 03 March 2020, <http://www.engageafricafoundation.org/blog/view/best-practices-for-social-media-marketing-for-health-promotion>

Omer Ahmed, H 2012, 'Noise exposure, awareness, practice and noise-annoyance among steel workers in United Arab Emirates', *The Open Public Health Journal*, vol. 5, no. 1, pp. 28–35. https://doi.org/10.2174/1874944501205010028

Pandve, H 2014a, 'Changing concept of disease prevention: From primordial to quaternary', *Archives of Medicine and Health Sciences*, vol. 2, no. 2, pp. 254–256. https://doi.org/10.4103/2321-4848.144366

Pandve, HT 2014b, 'Quaternary prevention: Need of the hour', *Journal of Family Medicine and Primary Care*, vol. 3, no. 4, pp. 309–310.

Park, J, Chung, S, Lee, J, Sung, JH, Cho, SW & Sim, CS 2017, 'Noise sensitivity, rather than noise level, predicts the non-auditory effects of noise in community samples: A population-based survey', *BMC Public Health*, vol. 17, no. 1, pp. 1–9. https://doi.org/10.1186/s12889-017-4244-5

Patel, DS, Witte, K, Zuckerman, C, Murray-Johnson, L, Orrego, V, Maxfield, AM, Meadows-Hogan, S, Tisdale, J & Thimons, ED 2001, 'Understanding barriers to preventive health actions for occupational noise-induced hearing loss', *Journal of Health Communication*, vol. 6, no. 2, pp. 155–168. https://doi.org/10.1080/108107301750254484

Pienkowski, M 2017, 'On the etiology of listening difficulties in noise despite clinically normal audiograms', *Ear and Hearing: The Official Journal of the American Auditory Society*, vol. 38, no. 2, pp. 135–148. https://doi.org/10.1097/AUD.0000000000000388

Plack, CJ, Barker, D & Prendergast, G 2014, 'Perceptual consequences of "hidden" hearing loss', *Trends in Hearing*, vol. 18, a2331216514550621. https://doi.org/10.1177/2331216514550621

Plack, CJ, Léger, A, Prendergast, G, Kluk, K, Guest, H & Munro, KJ 2016, 'Toward a diagnostic test for hidden hearing loss', *Trends in Hearing*, vol. 20, a2331216516657466. https://doi.org/10.1177/2331216516657466

Pratt, SR, Kuller, L, Talbott, EO, McHugh-Pemu, K, Buhari, AM & Xu, X 2009, 'Prevalence of hearing loss in black and white elders: Results of the cardiovascular health study', *Journal of Speech, Language, and Hearing Research*, vol. 52, no. 4, pp. 973–989. https://doi.org/10.1044/1092-4388(2009/08-0026)

President's Office 1996, *Mine Health and Safety Act: No. 29 of 1996 (967)*, viewed 17 February 2019, <http://www.kznhealth.gov.za/occhealth/17242.pdf>

Pyykkö, I, Toppila, E, Zou, J & Kentala, E 2007, 'Individual susceptibility to noise-induced hearing loss', *Audiological Medicine*, vol. 5, no. 1, pp. 41–53. https://doi.org/10.1080/16513860601175998

Rabinowitz, PM, Galusha, D, Kirsche, SR, Cullen, MR, Slade, MD & Dixon-Ernst, C 2011, 'Effect of daily noise exposure monitoring on annual rates of hearing loss in industrial workers', *Occupational and Environmental Medicine*, vol. 68, no. 6, pp. 414–418. https://doi.org/10.1136/oem.2010.055905R

Rehman, M, Mohd Nawi, N & Ghazali, M 2012, 'Predicting noise-induced hearing loss (NIHL) and hearing deterioration index (HDI) in Malaysian industrial workers using GDAM algorithm', *Journal of Engineering and Technology (JET)*, vol. 3, pp. 179–197.

Ross, JAS, Macdiarmid, JI, Dick, FD & Watt, SJ 2010, 'Hearing symptoms and audiometry in professional divers and offshore workers', *Occupational Medicine*, vol. 60, no. 1, pp. 36–42. https://doi.org/10.1093/occmed/kqp152

Rutherford, C & Petersen, L 2019, 'Amplification and aural rehabilitation in resource-constrained environments', *The Journal of Laryngology & Otology*, vol. 133, no. 1, pp. 26–33. https://doi.org/10.1017/S0022215118001378

Ryan, AF, Kujawa, SG, Hammill, T, Le Prell, C & Kil, J 2016, 'Temporary and permanent noise-induced threshold shifts: A review of basic and clinical observations', *Otology & Neurotology*, vol. 37, no. 8, pp. 271–275. https://doi.org/10.1097/MAO.0000000000001071

Sabanci, K, Dilay, Y, Fahri, M & Özkan, A 2017, 'Noise source determination by using artificial neural network in a metal workshop', *Journal of Multidisciplinary Engineering Science and Technology*, vol. 4, no. 9, pp. 8084–8088.

Santaolalla, F, Salvador, C, Martínez, A, Sánchez, JM & Del Rey, AS 2013, 'Inner ear hair cell regeneration: A look from the past to the future', *Neural Regeneration Research*, vol. 8, no. 24, pp. 2284–2289. https://doi.org/10.3969/j.issn.1673-5374.2013.24.008

Schulz, T 2014, *Take 'em Home: Help workers protect their hearing off the clock*, viewed 06 June 2019, <https://ohsonline.com/Articles/2014/06/01/Take-Em-Home.aspx>

Shiell, A, Hawe, P & Gold, L 2008, 'Complex interventions or complex systems? Implications for health economic evaluation', *BMJ*, vol. 336, no. 7656, pp. 1281–1283. https://doi.org/10.1136/bmj.39569.510521.AD

Soares, MO, Oenning, NSX, Ziegelmann, PK & Goulart, BNG 2018, 'Association between self-reported hearing impairment and diabetes: A Brazilian population-based study', *Archives of Public Health*, vol. 76, no. 1, p. 62. https://doi.org/10.1186/s13690-018-0300-6

Strauss, S, Swanepoel, DW, Becker, P, Eloff, Z & Hall, JW III 2014, 'Noise and age-related hearing loss: A study of 40 123 gold miners in South Africa', *International Journal of Audiology*, vol. 53, no. 2, pp. 66–75.

Stuckler, D, Basu, S, McKee, M & Lurie, M 2011, 'Mining and risk of tuberculosis in sub-Saharan Africa', *American Journal of Public Health*, vol. 101, no. 3, pp. 524–530. https://doi.org/10.2105/AJPH.2009.175646

Stuckler, D, Steele, S, Lurie, M & Basu, S 2013, 'Introduction: "Dying for gold": The effects of mineral miningon HIV, tuberculosis, silicosis, and occupational diseases in Southern Africa', *International Journal of Health Services*, vol. 43, no. 4, pp. 639–649. https://doi.org/10.2190/HS.43.4.c

Sullivan, MJ, McDaniel, MF & Siegel, RD 2004, 'Using metrics to track progress of community outreach programs', *Chemical Engineering Progress*, vol. 100, no. 12, pp. 34–38.

Suter, AH 2012, 'Engineering controls for occupational noise exposure: The best way to save hearing', *Sound and Vibrations*, vol. 45, pp. 21–31.

Sweetow, RW 2018, 'Why and how should graduate students in audiology be taught and trained in counseling', *Seminars in Hearing*, vol. 39, no. 1, pp. 3–4. https://doi.org/10.1055/s-0037-1613699

The Georgia Tech 2019–2020, *Technical guide for: Noise control – Engineering controls, work practices, & administrative controls*, viewed 08 May 2020, <https://oshainfo.gatech.edu/wp-content/uploads/2019/03/Technical%20Guide%20for%20Noise%20Controls.pdf>

Tieu, C & Campbell, KC 2012, 'Current pharmacologic otoprotective agents in or approaching clinical trials: How they elucidate mechanisms of noise-induced hearing loss', *Otolaryngology*, vol. 3, no. 1, pp. 3–130. https://doi.org/10.4172/2161-119X.1000130

Tung, C-Y & Chao, K-P 2013, 'Effect of recreational noise exposure on hearing impairment among teenage students', *Research in Developmental Disabilities*, vol. 34, pp. 126–132. https://doi.org/10.1016/j.ridd.2012.07.015

Tye-Murray, N 2009, *Foundations of aural rehabilitation: Children, adults, and their family members*, 3rd edn, Delmar Cengage Learning, Clifton Park.

Verbeek, JH, Kateman, E, Morata, TC, Dreschler, WA & Mischke, C 2014, 'Interventions to prevent occupational noise-induced hearing loss: A cochrane systematic review', *International Journal of Audiology*, vol. 53, no. 2, pp. 84–96. https://doi.org/10.3109/14992027.2013.857436

Vijay, R, Sharma, A, Chakrabarti, T & Gupta, R 2015, 'Assessment of honking impact on traffic noise in urban traffic environment of Nagpur, India', *Journal of Environmental Health Science and Engineering*, vol. 13, no. 1, p. 10. https://doi.org/10.1186/s40201-015-0164-4

Wang, B, Han, L, Dai, S, Li, X, Cai, W, Yang, D, Chen, L, Wang, N, Zhu, B & Zhang, J 2018, 'Hearing loss characteristics of workers with hypertension exposed to occupational noise: A cross-sectional study of 270,033 participants', *BioMed Research International*, vol. 2018, a8541638. https://doi.org/10.1155/2018/8541638

Williams, CS & Rabinowitz, PM 2012, 'Usability of a daily noise exposure monitoring device for industrial workers', *The Annals of Occupational Hygiene*, vol. 56, no. 8, pp. 925–933.

World Health Organization (WHO) 2015, *Hearing loss due to recreational exposure to loud sounds: A review*, World Health Organization, Geneva.

Xua, D & Francis, AL 2019, 'Relationships among self-reported hearing problems, psychological distress, and cardiovascular disease in U.S. adults, national health interview survey 1997–2017', *Journal of Speech, Language, and Hearing Research*, vol. 62, no. 8, pp. 2872–2881. https://doi.org/10.1044/2019_JSLHR-H-18-0511

Yadav, MK & Yadav, KS 2018, 'Etiology of noise-induced hearing loss (NIHL) and its symptomatic correlation with audiometry observations in type II diabetes', *Indian Journal of Otolaryngology and Head & Neck Surgery*, vol. 70, no. 1, pp. 137–144. https://doi.org/10.1007/s12070-017-1188-0

Yongbing, S & Martin, W 2013, 'Noise-induced hearing loss in China: A potentially costly public health Issue', *Journal of Otology*, vol. 8, no. 1, pp. 51–56. https://doi.org/10.1016/S1672-2930(13)50007-9

Zheng, F & Zuo, J 2017, 'Cochlear hair cell regeneration after noise-induced hearing loss: Does regeneration follow development?', *Hearing Research*, vol. 349, pp. 182–196. https://doi.org/10.1016/j.heares.2016.12.011

Chapter 12

Aliabadi, M, Golmohammadi, R, Mansoorizadeh, M, Khotanlou, H & Ohadi Hamadani, A 2013, 'An empirical technique for predicting noise exposure level in the typical embroidery workrooms using artificial neural networks', *Applied Acoustics*, vol. 74, no. 3, pp. 364–374. https://doi.org/10.1016/J.APACOUST.2012.08.009

Amedofu, GK 2007, 'Effectiveness of hearing conservation program at a large surface gold mining company in Ghana', *African Journal of Health Sciences*, vol. 14, no. 1, pp. 49–53. https://doi.org/10.4314/ajhs.v14i1.30846

Amedofu, GK & Fuente, A 2008, 'Occupational hearing loss in developing countries', eds. B Mcpherson & R Brouillette, *Audiology in developing countries*, Nova Science Publishers, Inc, Hauppauge, pp. 189–221.

Australian Department of Finance 2016, *An overview of the risk management process: COMCOVER information sheet*, viewed 13 October 2019, <https://www.finance.gov.au/sites/default/files/Risk-Management-Process.pdf>

Berger, E, Franks, J & Lindgren, F 1996, *International review of field studies of hearing protector attenuation*, viewed 20 March 2019, <https://multimedia.3m.com.cn/mws/media/893203O/international-review-of-field-studies.pdf?fn=06%20International%20Review%20of%20Field>

Brink, LL, Talbott, EO, Burks, JA & Palmer, CV 2002, 'Changes over time in audiometric thresholds in a group of automobile stamping and assembly workers with a hearing conservation program', *AIHA Journal*, vol. 63, no. 4, pp. 482–487. https://doi.org/10.1080/15428110208984737

Bruce, RD 2007, 'Engineering controls for reducing workplace noise', *The National Academy of Engineering*, vol. 37, pp. 33–39.

Bruce, RD & Wood, EW 2003, 'The USA needs a new national policy for occupational noise', *Noise Control Engineering Journal*, vol. 51, pp. 162–165. https://doi.org/10.3397/1.2839711

Campbell, K, Claussen, A, Meech, R, Verhulst, S, Fox, D & Hughes, L 2011, 'D-methionine (D-met) significantly rescues noise-induced hearing loss: Timing studies', *Hearing Research*, vol. 282, no. 1–2, pp. 138–144. https://doi.org/10.1016/j.heares.2011.08.003

Datta, J & Petticrew, M 2013, 'Challenges to evaluating complex interventions: A content analysis of published papers', *BMC Public Health*, vol. 13, no. 568, pp. 1–18. https://doi.org/10.1186/1471-2458-13-568

Davies, H, Marion, S & Teschke, K 2008, 'The impact of hearing conservation programs on incidence of noise-induced hearing loss in Canadian workers', *American Journal of Industrial Medicine*, vol. 51, no. 12, pp. 923–931. https://doi.org/10.1002/ajim.20634

De Jong, MA, Luder, A & Gross, M 2019, 'Main aspects of peripheral and central hearing system involvement in unexplained HIV-related hearing complaints', *Frontiers in Neurology*, vol. 10, a845. https://doi.org/10.3389/fneur.2019.00845

Dekker, JJ, Edwards, AL, Franz, RM, Van Dyk, T & Banyini, A 2011, 'Meeting the milestones: Are South African small-to medium-scale mines up to the task?', *Journal of the Southern African Institute of Mining and Metallurgy*, vol. 111, no. 5, pp. 309–313.

Department of Minerals and Energy (DME) 2003, *Guideline for the compilation of a mandatory code of practice for an occupational health program for noise*, viewed 19 July 2019, <http://www.mmpa.org.za/wp-content/uploads/2019/10/NOISE-COP-PRESENTATION.pdf>

Edwards, AL 2013, *Ototoxicity in the South African Mining Industry: A position paper*, viewed 13 October 2019, <http://hdl.handle.net/10204/7068>

Edwards, AL, Dekker, JJ, Franz, RM, Van Dyk, T & Banyini, A 2011, 'Profiles of noise exposure levels in South African mining', *Journal of the Southern African Institute of Mining and Metallurgy*, vol. 111, no. 5, pp. 315–322.

Edwards, AL & Franz, RM 2009, *Macro and micromanagement of hearing conservation in the South African mining*, viewed 13 October 2019, <http://hdl.handle.net/10204/3895>

Edwards, A & Kritzinger, D 2012, 'Noise-induced hearing loss milestones: Past and future', *South African Institute of Mining and Metallurgy*, vol. 112, pp. 865–869.

Edwards, A, Milanzi, LA, Khoza, NN, Letsoalo, MS & Zungu, LI 2015, 'Evaluation of the current practices of noise-induced hearing loss (NIHL) awareness training in the South African mining industry', *Occupational Health Southern Africa*, vol. 21, no. 1, pp. 11–17.

Flood, D & Rohloff, P 2018, 'Indigenous languages and global health: Comment', *The Lancet*, vol. 6, no. 2, pp. e134–e135. https://doi.org/10.1016/S2214-109X(17)30493-X

Fuente, A & McPherson, B 2007, 'Central auditory processing effects induced by solvent exposure', *International Journal of Occupational Medicine and Environmental Health*, vol. 20, no. 3, pp. 271–279. https://doi.org/10.2478/v10001-007-0030-4

Fuente, A, McPherson, B & Hickson, L 2013, 'Auditory dysfunction associated with solvent exposure', *BMC Public Health*, vol. 13, no. 1, pp. 1–12. https://doi.org/10.1186/1471-2458-13-39

Gopal, KV 2008, 'Audiological findings in individuals exposed to organic solvents: Case studies', *Noise and Health*, vol. 10, no. 40, p. 74.

Grobler, LM, Swanepoel, DW, Strauss, S, Becker, P & Eloff, Z 2020, 'Occupational noise and age: A longitudinal study of hearing sensitivity as a function of noise exposure and age in South African gold mine workers', *South African Journal of Communication Disorders*, vol. 67, no. 2, a687. https://doi.org/10.4102/sajcd.v67i2.687

Henderson, D & Tanaka, C 2009, 'Advances in otoprotective drugs', *The ASHA Leader*, vol. 14, no. 4, pp. 5–6.

Hodgkinson, L & Prasher, D 2006, 'Effects of industrial solvents on hearing and balance: A review', *Noise and Health*, vol. 8, no. 32, p. 114. https://doi.org/10.4103/1463-1741.33952

Hong, O, Kerr, MJ, Poling, GL & Dhar, S 2013, 'Understanding and preventing noise-induced hearing loss', *Disease-a-Month*, vol. 59, no. 4, pp. 110–118. https://doi.org/10.1016/j.disamonth.2013.01.002

Khoza, K & Ross, E 2002, 'Auditory function in a group of adults infected with HIV/AIDS in Gauteng, South Africa', *South African Journal of Communication Disorders*, vol. 49, no. 1, pp. 17–27. https://doi.org/10.4102/sajcd.v49i1.214

Khoza-Shangase, K 2019, 'Best/next practice in speech-language and hearing professions: Being responsible and responsive to context', *HPCSA Bulletin*, viewed 02 March 2020, <https://www.hpcsa.co.za/Uploads/SLH/SLH%20newletter%20draft%202019.pdf>

Khoza-Shangase, K 2020a, 'Hearing function of gold miners with and without a history of tuberculosis treatment: A retrospective data review', *Brazilian Journal of Otorhinolaryngology*, vol. 86, no. 3, pp. 294–299. https://doi.org/10.1016/j.bjorl.2018.12.003

Khoza-Shangase, K 2020b, 'Burden of disease: A scoping review of HIV/AIDS and TB in occupational noise-induced hearing loss', *South African Journal of Communication Disorders*, vol. 67, no. 2, a669. https://doi.org/10.4102/sajcd.v67i2.669

Khoza-Shangase, K & Masondo, N 2020, 'What are the current audiological practices for ototoxicity assessment and management in the South African healthcare context?', *International Journal of Environmental Research and Public Health*, vol. 17, no. 7, a2613. https://doi.org/10.3390/ijerph17072613

Khoza-Shangase, K & Mophosho, M 2018, 'Language and culture in speech-language and hearing professions in South Africa: The dangers of a single story', *South African Journal of Communication Disorders*, vol. 65, no. 1, a594. https://doi.org/10.4102/sajcd.v65i1.594

Khoza-Shangase, K & Mophosho, M 2021, 'Language and culture in speech-language and hearing professions in South Africa: Re-imagining practice', *South African Journal of Communication Disorders*, vol. 68, no. 1, a793. https://doi.org/10.4102/sajcd.v68i1.793

Khoza-Shangase, K & Moroe, N 2020a, 'South African hearing conservation programmes in the context of tele-audiology: A scoping review', *South African Journal of Communication Disorders*, vol. 67, no. 2, a670. https://doi.org/10.4102/sajcd.v67i2.670

Khoza-Shangase, K & Moroe, N 2020b, 'Risk vs benefit: shouldn't audiologists assess this in the context of occupational noise induced hearing loss in the mining industry?', *South African Journal of Communication Disorders*, vol. 67, no. 2, a671. https://doi.org/10.4102/sajcd.v67i2.671

Khoza-Shangase, K, Moroe, N & Edwards, A 2020, 'Occupational hearing loss in Africa: an interdisciplinary view of the current status', *South African Journal of Communication Disorders*, vol. 67, no. 2, a700. https://doi.org/10.4102/sajcd.v67i2.700

Khoza-Shangase, K, Moroe, NF, Nyandoro, O & Madahana, M 2020, 'Feedback-based noise management matrix in action', *South African Journal of Communication Disorders*, vol. 67, no. 2, pp. 1–9.

Khoza-Shangase, K, Moroe, N & Neille, J 2021, 'Speech-language pathology and audiology in South Africa: Clinical training and service in the era of COVID-19', *International Journal of Telerehabilitation*, vol. 13, no. 1, a6376. https://doi.org/10.5195/ijt.2021.6376

Le Prell, CG, Hammill, TL & Murphy, WJ 2019, 'Noise-induced hearing loss: Translating risk from animal models to real-world environments', *The Journal of the Acoustical Society of America*, vol. 146, no. 5, pp. 3646–3651. https://doi.org/10.1121/1.5133385

Le, TN, Straatman, LV, Lea, J & Westerberg, B 2017, 'Current insights in noise-induced hearing loss: A literature review of the underlying mechanism, pathophysiology, asymmetry, and management options', *Journal of Otolaryngology – Head & Neck Surgery*, vol. 46, no. 1, p. 41. https://doi.org/10.1186/s40463-017-0219-x

Lobato, DCB, Lacerda, ABMD, Gonçalves, CGDO & Coifman, H 2014, 'Auditory effects of exposure to noise and solvents: A comparative study', *International Archives of Otorhinolaryngology*, vol. 18, pp. 136–141. https://doi.org/10.1055/s-0033-1361083

Madahana, MCI, Nyandoro, OTC & Moroe, NF 2020, 'Engineering noise control for mines: Lessons from the world', *South African Journal of Communication Disorders*, vol. 67, no. 2, a684. https://doi.org/10.4102/sajcd.v67i2.684

Mapuranga, M, Maziriri, ET & Letshaba, RK 2020, 'Does occupational noise matter among manufacturing SME workers? Empirical evidence from Magaba, Mbare, Zimbabwe', *South African Journal of Communication Disorders*, vol. 67, no. 2, a680. https://doi.org/10.4102/sajcd.v67i2.680

Medical Research Council 2000, *A framework for development and evaluation of RCTs for complex interventions to improve health*, viewed 10 December 2019, <https://mrc.ukri.org/documents/pdf/rcts-for-complex-interventions-to-improve-health>

Metidieri, MM, Rodrigues, HF, Filho, FJ, Ferraz, DP, Neto, AF & Torres, S 2013, 'Noise-induced hearing loss (NIHL): Literature review with a focus on occupational medicine', *International Archives of Otorhinolaryngology*, vol. 17, no. 2, pp. 208–212. https://doi.org/10.7162/S1809-97772013000200015

Mignolo, WD 2005, *The idea of Latin America*, Wiley-Blackwell Manifestos, London.

Mine Health and Safety Council (MHSC) 2016, *Home*, viewed 15 June 2019, <http://www.mhsc.org.za/>

Moore, GF, Audrey, S, Barker, M, Bond, L, Bonell, C, Hardeman, W, Moore, L, O'Cathain, A, Tinati, T, Wight, D & Baird, J 2015, 'Process evaluation of complex interventions: Medical Research Council guidance', *British Medical Journal*, vol. 350, a1258. https://doi.org/10.1136/bmj.h1258

Moroe, N 2020, 'Occupational noise induced hearing loss in the mining sector in South Africa: Perspectives from occupational health practitioners on how mineworkers are trained', *South African Journal of Communication Disorders*, vol. 67, no. 2, a676. https://doi.org/10.4102/sajcd.v67i2.676

Moroe, N & Khoza-Shangase, K 2018, 'Research into occupational noise induced hearing loss in South African large-scale mines: Access denied?', *AAS Open Research*, vol. 1, p. 4. https://doi.org/10.12688/aasopenres.12829.1

Moroe, N & Khoza-Shangase, K 2020, 'Recent advances in hearing conservation programmes: A systematic review', *South African Journal of Communication Disorders*, vol. 67, no. 2, a675. https://doi.org/10.4102/sajcd.v67i2.675

Moroe, NF 2018, 'Occupational noise-induced hearing loss in South African large-scale mines: Exploring hearing conservation programmes as complex interventions embedded in a realist approach', *International Journal of Occupational Safety and Ergonomics*, vol. 26, no. 4, pp. 753–761. https://doi.org/10.1080/10803548.2018.1498183

Moroe, NF, Khoza-Shangase, K, Kanji, A & Ntlhakana, L 2018, 'The management of occupational noise-induced hearing loss in the mining sector in Africa: A systematic review – 1994 to 2016', *Noise and Vibration Worldwide*, vol. 49, no. 5, pp. 181–191. https://doi.org/10.1177/0957456518781860

Moroe, NF, Khoza-Shangase, K, Madahana, MCI & Nyandoro, OTC 2019, 'A feedback-based noise monitoring model: A proposed model of managing occupational noise induced hearing loss in the mining sector in South Africa', *Journal of the Southern African Institute of Mining and Metallurgy*, vol. 119, pp. 671–679. https://doi.org/10.4102/sajcd.v67i2.678

Musiba, ZE 2015, 'The prevalence of noise-induced hearing loss among Tanzanian miners', *Occupational Medicine*, vol. 65, no. 5, pp. 386–390. https://doi.org/10.1093/occmed/kqv046

Musiba, ZE 2020, 'Classification of audiograms in the prevention of noise induced hearing loss', *South African Journal of Communication Disorders*, vol. 67, no. 2, a691. https://doi.org/10.10520/EJC169019

Ntlhakana, L, Kanji, A & Khoza-Shangase, K 2015, 'The use of hearing protection devices in South Africa: Exploring the current status in a gold and a non-ferrous mine', *Occupational Health Southern Africa*, vol. 21, pp. 10–15.

Ntlhakana, L, Khoza-Shangase, K & Nelson, G 2020a, 'Occupational noise-induced hearing loss in platinum miners: What do the data tell us?', *Occupational Health Southern Africa*, vol. 26, no. 1, pp. 8–14. https://doi.org/10.17159/2411-9717/1318/2021

Ntlhakana, L, Nelson, G & Khoza-Shangase, K 2020b, 'Estimating miners at risk for occupational noise-induced hearing loss: A review of data from a South African platinum mine', *South African Journal of Communication Disorders*, vol. 67, no. 2, pp. 1–8. https://doi.org/10.4102/sajcd.v67i2.677

Ntlhakana, L, Nelson, G, Khoza-Shangase, K & Dorkin, E 2022, 'Occupational hearing loss for platinum miners in South Africa: A case study of data sharing practices and ethical challenges in the mining industry', *International Journal of Environmental Research and Public Health*, vol. 19, no. 1, p. 1. https://doi.org/10.3390/ijerph19010001

Ntlhakana, L, Nelson, G, Khoza-Shangase, K & Maposa, I 2021, 'Predicting standard threshold shifts for occupational hearing loss among miners at a large-scale platinum mine in South Africa', *Journal of the Southern African Institute of Mining and Metallurgy*, vol. 121, no. 8, pp. 397–404.

Obasikene, G, Amadi, IF, Ibekwe, TS, Ezeanolue, BC & Ogisi, FO 2014, 'The effect of CD4 count level on the middle ear dynamics of HIV infected patients', *East African Medical Journal*, vol. 91, no. 1, pp. 29–32.

Ödkvist, LM, Bergholtz, LM, Ahlfeldt, H, Andersson, B, Edling, C & Strand, E 1982, 'Otoneurological and audiological findings in workers exposed to industrial solvents', *Acta Oto-Laryngologica*, vol. 93, no. Suppl 386, pp. 249–251. https://doi.org/10.3109/00016488209108532

Pawson, R, Greenhalgh, T, Harvey, G & Walshe, K 2005, 'Realist review – A new method of systematic review designed for complex policy interventions', *Journal of Health Services Research & Policy*, vol. 10, no. Suppl 1, pp. 21–34. https://doi.org/10.1258/1355819054308530

Pillay, M 2020, 'Chemicals, noise and occupational hearing health in South Africa: A mapping study', *South African Journal of Communication Disorders*, vol. 67, no. 2, a693. https://doi.org/10.4102/sajcd.v67i2.693

Pillay, M & Manning, WG 2020, 'A critical analysis of the current South African occupational health law and hearing loss', *South African Journal of Communication Disorders*, vol. 67, no. 2, a694. https://doi.org/10.4102/sajcd.v67i2.694

PoPIA n.d., *Protection of Personal Information Act (POPI Act)*, viewed 04 February 2020, <https://popia.co.za/>

Rabinowitz, PM, Galusha, D, Dixon-Ernst, C, Slade, M & Cullen, MR 2007, 'Do ambient noise exposure levels predict hearing loss in a modern industrial cohort?', *Occupational and Environmental Medicine*, vol. 64, pp. 53–59. https://doi.org/10.1136/oem.2005.025924

Rashaad Hansia, M & Dickinson, D 2010, 'Hearing protection device usage at a South African gold mine', *Occupational Medicine*, vol. 60, no. 1, pp. 72–74. https://doi.org/10.1093/occmed/kqp114

Sebothoma, B 2020, 'Middle ear pathologies in adults within the mining industry: A systematic review', *South African Journal of Communication Disorders*, vol. 67, no. 2, a679. https://doi.org/10.4102/sajcd.v67i2.679

Sebothoma, B & Khoza-Shangase, K 2018, 'A comparison between video otoscopic and standard tympanometry findings in adults living with human immunodeficiency virus (HIV) in South Africa', *South African Journal of Communication Disorders*, vol. 65, no. 1, a591. https://doi.org/10.4102/sajcd.v65i1.591

Sebothoma, B & Khoza-Shangase, K 2020, 'Middle ear pathologies in adults living with human immunodeficiency virus: A systematic review', *Annals of Otology, Rhinology & Laryngology*, vol. 129, no. 8, pp. 821–828. https://doi.org/10.1177/0003489420909847

Seixas, NS, Neitzel, R, Stover, B, Sheppard, L, Daniell, B, Edelson, J & Meischke, H 2011, 'A multi-component intervention to promote hearing protector use among construction workers', *International Journal of Audiology*, vol. 50, no. Suppl 1, pp. 46–56. https://doi.org/10.3109/14992027.2010.525754

Strauss, S, Swanepoel, DW, Becker, P, Eloff, Z & Hall, JW 3rd 2014, 'Noise and age-related hearing loss: A study of 40 123 gold miners in South Africa', *International Journal of Audiology*, vol. 53, no. 2, pp. 66–75. https://doi.org/10.3109/14992027.2013.865846

Suter, AH 2012, 'Engineering controls for occupational noise exposure: The best way to save hearing', *Sound & Vibrations*, vol. 45, pp. 24–31.

Tak, SW, Davis, RR & Calvert, GM 2009, 'Exposure to hazardous workplace noise and use of hearing protection devices among US workers – NHANES, 1999–2004', *American Journal of Industrial Medicine*, vol. 52, pp. 358–371. https://doi.org/10.1002/ajim.20690

Toivonen, M, Paakkonen, R, Savolainen, S & Lehtomäki, K 2002, 'Noise attenuation and proper insertion of earplugs into ear canals', *Annals in Occupational Hygiene*, vol. 46, no. 6, pp. 527–530. https://doi.org/10.1093/annhyg/mef065

Thorne, PR 2006, *Best practice in noise-induced hearing loss management and prevention: A review of literature, practices and policies for the New Zealand context*, viewed 03 March 2018, <https://dspace.nal.gov.au/xmlui/bitstream/handle/123456789/481/Best%20practice%20in%20noise%20-%20induced%20hearing%20loss%20management%20and%20prevention.pdf?sequence=1&isAllowed=y>

Workplace Safety Health Council (WSHC) 2014, *Workplace safety and health guidelines: Hearing conservation programme*, Workplace Safety Health Council, Singapore.

Yaakobi, E & Putter-Katz, H 2020, 'What best predicts the use of hearing protection devices?', *The American Journal of Psychology*, vol. 133, no. 3, pp. 313–327. https://doi.org/10.5406/amerjpsyc.133.3.0313

Chapter 13

Agarwal, G, Nagpure, PS, Pal, KS, Kaushal, AK & Kumar, M 2015, 'Audiometric notching at 4 kHz: Good screening test for assessment of early onset of occupational hearing loss', *Indian Journal of Otology*, vol. 21, no. 4, pp. 270–273. https://doi.org/10.4103/0971-7749.164552

Balfour-Kaipa, T 2014a, 'Occupational health milestones and Chamber's response to key health issues', viewed 10 January 2016, <https://slideplayer.com/slide/9226050/>

Balfour-Kaipa, T 2014b, 'Occupational health milestones and Chamber's response to key health issues', *Occupational Health Southern Africa*, vol. 20, no. 5, pp. 26–27.

Brits, J, Strauss, S, Eloff, Z, Becker, PJ & Swanepoel, DW 2012, 'Hearing profile of gold miners with and without tuberculosis', *Occupational and Environmental Medicine*, vol. 69, no. 4, pp. 243–249. https://doi.org/10.1136/oemed-2011-100106

Bronkorst, JP & Schutte, DW 2013, 'Reconstruction of percentage loss of hearing', *Occupational Health Southern Africa*, vol. 19, no. 3, pp. 20–24.

Chadambuka, A, Mususa, F & Muteti, S 2013, 'Prevalence of noise induced hearing loss among employees at a mining industry in Zimbabwe', *African Health Sciences*, vol. 13, no. 4, pp. 899–906. https://doi.org/10.4314/ahs.v13i4.6

Chamber of Mines 2016, *Noise team on the mine health and safety milestones*, Chamber of Mines, Johannesburg.

Chen Kou-Huang, Su Shih-Bin & Kow-Tong, C 2020, 'An overview of occupational noise-induced hearing loss among workers: Epidemiology, pathogenesis, and preventive measures', *Environmental Health and Preventive Medicine*, vol. 25, p. 65. https://doi.org/10.1186/s12199-020-00906-0

De Jager, M 2017, *Environmental noise impact assessment for Vlakvarkfontein extensions east of Delmas*, Enviro-Acoustic Research CC, Pretoria.

Department of Labour 2001, *The determination of permanent disablement resulting from hearing loss caused by exposure to excessive noise and trauma*, Department of Labour, Circular Instruction No. 171, 16 May, viewed 10 January 2017, <http://www.saflii.org/za/legis/consol_reg/cin171tdopdrfhlcbetenat1371.pdf>

Department of Mineral Resources 2016, *Guidance note for the implementation of standard threshold shift in the medical surveillance of noise induced hearing loss*, Department of Mineral Resources, 04 August, viewed 08 May 2019, <https://www.polity.org.za/print-version/mine-health-and-safety-act-regulations-guidance-note-for-implementation-of-standard-threshold-shift-in-medical-surveillance-of-noise-induced-hearing-loss-gazette-40142-notice-r839-2016-08-04>

Edwards, AL, Dekker, JJ, Franz, RM, Van Dyk, T & Banyini, A 2011, 'Profiles of noise exposure levels in South African mining', *Journal of the Southern African institute of Mining and Metallurgy*, vol. 111, no. 5, pp. 315–322.

Feuerstein, J & Chasin, M 2009, 'Noise exposure and issues in hearing conservation', ed. J Katz, *Handbook of clinical audiology*, 7th edn, Lippincott Williams & Wilkins, Philadelphia, pp. 678–698.

Franz, RM & Phillips, JJ 2001, 'Noise and vibration', eds. ER Guild, J Johnson & M Ross, *Handbook of occupational health practice in the South African mining industry*, The Safety in Mines Research Advisory Committee, Johannesburg, pp. 195–232.

Grobler, LM, Swanepoel, DW, Strauss, S, Becker, P & Eloff, Z 2020, 'Occupational noise and age: A longitudinal study of hearing sensitivity as a function of noise exposure and age in South African gold mine workers', *South African Journal of Communication Disorders*, vol. 67, no. 2, a687. https://doi.org/10.4102/sajcd.v67i2.687

Helm, JM, Swiergosz, AM, Haeberle, HS, Karnuta, JM, Schaffer, JL, Krebs, VE, Spitzer, AI & Ramkumar, PN 2020, 'Machine learning and artificial intelligence: Definitions, applications, and future directions', *Current Reviews in Musculoskeletal Medicine*, vol. 13, no. 1, pp. 69–76. https://doi.org/10.1007/s12178-020-09600-8

Hermanus, MA 2007, 'Occupational health and safety in mining-status, new developments, and concerns', *Journal of the Southern African Institute of Mining and Metallurgy*, vol. 107, no. 8, pp. 531–538.

Howard, J & Hoffman, MA 2017, *U.S. adults aged 20 to 69 years show signs of noise-induced hearing loss*, National Institute on Deafness and Other Communication Disorders (NIH), 07 February, viewed 08 May 2019, <https://www.nidcd.nih.gov/news/2017/us-adults-aged-20-69-years-show-signs-noise-induced-hearing-loss#:~:text=A%20new%20analysis%20from%20a,induced%20hearing%20loss%20(NIHL)>

Health Professionals Council of South Africa (HPCSA) 2016, *Guidelines for good practice in the health care professions confidentiality: protecting and providing information: Booklet 5*, Health Professionals Council of South Africa, Pretoria.

Katz, J, Medwetsky, L & Burkard, R 2009, 'Pure tone evaluation', ed. Katz, *Handbook of clinical audiology*, Lippincott Williams & Wilkins, Philadelphia, PA, pp. 30–49.

Khoza-Shangase, K 2020a, 'Hearing function of gold miners with and without a history of tuberculosis treatment: A retrospective data review', *Brazilian Journal of Otorhinolaryngology*, vol. 86, pp. 294–299. https://doi.org/10.1016/j.bjorl.2018.12.003

Khoza-Shangase, K 2020b, 'Burden of disease: A scoping review of HIV/AIDS and TB in occupational noise-induced hearing loss', *South African Journal of Communication Disorders*, vol. 67, no. 2, a669. https://doi.org/10.4102/sajcd.v67i2.669

Khoza-Shangase, K & Moroe, N 2020a, 'South African hearing conservation programmes in the context of tele-audiology: A scoping review', *South African Journal of Communication Disorders*, vol. 67, no. 2, a670. https://doi.org/10.4102/sajcd.v67i2.670

Khoza-Shangase, K & Moroe, N 2020b, 'Risk vs benefit: Shouldn't audiologists assess this in the context of occupational noise induced hearing loss in the mining industry?', *South African Journal of Communication Disorders*, vol. 67, no. 2, a671. https://doi.org/10.4102/sajcd.v67i2.671

Khoza-Shangase, K, Moroe, N & Edwards, A 2020, 'Occupational hearing loss in Africa: An interdisciplinary view of the current status', *South African Journal of Communications Disorders*, vol. 67, no. 2, a700. https://doi.org/10.4102/sajcd.v67i2.700

Kitcher, ED, Ocansey, G, Abaidoo, B & Atule, A 2014, 'Occupational hearing loss of market mill workers in the city of Accra, Ghana', *Noise and Health*, vol. 16, no. 70, p. 183.

Kuang, D, Yu, YY & Tu, C 2019, 'Bilateral high-frequency hearing loss is associated with elevated blood pressure and increased hypertension risk in occupational noise exposed workers', *PLoS One*, vol. 14, no. 9, a0222135. https://doi.org/10.1371/journal.pone.0222135

Masaka, E 2009, 'The prevalence of noise induced hearing loss at a nickel mine in Zimbabwe', MA thesis, University of Witwatersrand.

Masterson, EA, Bushnell, PT, Themann, CL & Morata, TC 2016a, 'Hearing impairment among noise-exposed workers – United States, 2003–2012', *Morbidity and Mortality Weekly Report*, vol. 65, no. 15, pp. 389–394. https://doi.org/10.15585/mmwr.mm6515a2

Masterson, EA, Themann, CL, Luckhaupt, SE, Li, J & Calvert, GM 2016b, 'Hearing difficulty and tinnitus among US workers and non-workers in 2007', *American Journal of Industrial Medicine*, vol. 59, no. 4, pp. 290–300. https://doi.org/10.1002/ajim.22565

Mazlan, AN & Yahya, K 2015, 'Compensation process for noise induced hearing loss', *Jurnal Teknologi*, vol. 74, no. 4, pp. 13–17. https://doi.org/10.11113/jt.v74.4603

Mine Health & Safety Inspectorate (MHSI) 2017, *Department of mineral resources annual report*, viewed 08 May 2019, <https://www.mineralscouncil.org.za/work/health-and-safety>

Moroe, N 2020, 'Occupational noise induced hearing loss in the mining sector in South Africa: Perspectives from occupational health practitioners on how mineworkers are trained', *South African Journal of Communication Disorders*, vol. 67, no. 2, a676. https://doi.org/10.4102/sajcd.v67i2.676

Moroe, N & Khoza-Shangase, K 2018a, 'Management of occupational noise induced hearing loss in the mining sector in South Africa: Where are the audiologists?', *Journal of Occupational Health*, vol. 60, pp. 376–382. https://doi.org/10.1539/joh.2018-0020-OA

Moroe, N & Khoza-Shangase, K 2018b, 'Research into occupational noise induced hearing loss in South African large-scale mines: Access denied?', *AAS Open Research*, vol. 1, p. 4. https://doi.org/10.12688/aasopenres.12829.1

Moroe, N & Khoza-Shangase, K 2020, 'Recent advances in hearing conservation programmes: A systematic review', *South African Journal of Communication Disorders*, vol. 67, no. 2, a675. https://doi.org/10.4102/sajcd.v67i2.675

Moroe, N, Khoza-Shangase, K, Kanji, A & Ntlhakana, L 2018, 'The management of occupational noise-induced hearing loss in the mining sector in Africa: A systematic review - 1994 to 2016', *Noise & Vibration Worldwide*, vol. 49, no. 5, pp. 181–190. https://doi.org/10.1177/0957456518781860

Moroe, NF 2018, 'Occupational noise-induced hearing loss in South African large-scale mines: Exploring hearing conservation programmes as complex interventions embedded in a realist approach', *International Journal of Occupational Safety and Ergonomics*, vol. 26, no. 4, pp. 753–761. https://doi.org/10.1080/10803548.2018.1498183

Moroe, NF, Khoza-Shangase, K, Madahana, MCI & Nyandoro, OTC 2019, 'A feedback-based noise monitoring model: A proposed model of managing occupational noise induced hearing loss in the mining sector in South Africa', *Journal of the Southern African Institute of Mining and Metallurgy*, vol. 119, pp. 671–679. https://doi.org/10.17159/24119717/18/016/2019

Moroe, NF, Khoza-Shangase, K, Nyandoro, O & Madahana, M 2020, 'Feedback-based noise management matrix in action', *South African Journal of Communication Disorders*, vol. 67, no. 2, a678. https://doi.org/10.4102/sajcd.v67i2.678

Musiba, Z 2015, 'The prevalence of noise induced hearing loss among Tanzanian miners', *Occupational Medicine*, vol. 65, no. 5, pp. 386–390. https://doi.org/10.1093/occmed/kqv046

Naylor, CD 2018, 'On the prospects for a (deep) learning health care system', *JAMA*, vol. 320, no. 11, pp. 1099–1100. https://doi.org/10.1001/jama.2018.11103

Nelson, DI, Nelson, RY, Concha-Barrientos, M & Fingerhut, M 2005, 'The global burden of occupational noise-induced hearing loss', *American Journal of Industrial Medicine*, vol. 48, no. 6, pp. 446–458. https://doi.org/10.1002/ajim.20223

Ntlhakana, L, Khoza-Shangase, K & Nelson, G 2020a, 'Occupational noise-induced hearing loss in platinum miners: What do the data tell us?', *Occupational Health Southern Africa*, vol. 26, no. 1, pp. 8–14. https://doi.org/10.17159/2411-9717/1318/2021

Ntlhakana, L, Nelson, G & Khoza-Shangase, K 2020b, 'Estimating miners at risk for occupational noise-induced hearing loss: A review of data from a South African platinum mine', *South African Journal of Communication Disorders*, vol. 67, no. 2, a677. https://doi.org/10.4102/sajcd.v67i2.677

Ntlhakana, L, Nelson, G, Khoza-Shangase, K & Dorkin, E 2022, 'Occupational hearing loss for platinum miners in South Africa: A case study of data sharing practices and ethical challenges in the mining industry', *International Journal of Environmental Research and Public Health*, vol. 19, no. 1, p. 1. https://doi.org/10.3390/ijerph19010001

Pillay, M 2020, 'Chemicals, noise and occupational hearing health in South Africa: A mapping study', *South African Journal of Communication Disorders*, vol. 67, no. 2, pp. 1–11. https://doi.org/10.4102/sajcd.v67i2.693

Pillay, M, Tiwari, R, Kathard, H & Chikte, U 2020, 'Sustainable workforce: South African audiologists and speech therapists', *Human Resources for Health*, vol. 18, no. 1, pp. 1–13. https://doi.org/10.1186/s12960-020-00488-6

Rehman, MZ, Nawi, NM & Ghazali, MI 2012, 'Predicting noise-induced hearing loss (NIHL) and hearing deterioration index (HDI) in Malaysian industrial workers using GDAM algorithm', *Journal of Engineering and Technology (JET)*, vol. 3, pp. 179–197.

Republic of South Africa Government Gazette 1993, *Compensation for occupational injuries and diseases Act of 1993*, Republic of South Africa, 06 October, viewed 02 February 2018, <https://www.gov.za/sites/default/files/gcis_document/201409/act130of1993.pdf>

Sebothoma, B 2020, 'Middle ear pathologies in adults within the mining industry: A systematic review', *South African Journal of Communication Disorders*, vol. 67, no. 2, a679. https://doi.org/10.4102/sajcd.v67i2.679

Seixas, NS, Neitzel, R, Stover, B, Sheppard, L, Feeney, P, Mills, D & Kujawa, S 2012, '10-year prospective study of noise exposure and hearing damage among construction workers', *Occupational and Environmental Medicine*, vol. 69, no. 9, pp. 643–650. https://doi.org/10.1136/oemed-2011-100578

Selig, J 2022, *What is machine learning?: A Definition*, Expert AI, 14 March, viewed 03 November 2022, <https://www.expert.ai/blog/machine-learning-definition/>

South Africa 2001, *Circular instruction no. 171. (2001): The determination of permanent disablement resulting from hearing loss caused by exposure to excessive noise and trauma*, viewed 22 April 2019, <http://www.saflii.org/za/legis/consol_reg/cin171tdopdrfhlcbetenat1371/>

South Africa 2013, *Protection of Personal Information Act No. 4 of 2013*, viewed 22 April 2019, <https://www.gov.za/documents/protection-personal-information-act>

South African National & Standards 2013, *The measurement and assessment of occupational noise for hearing conservation purposes*, vol. 10083:2013, South African National Standards, Pretoria.

Strauss, S, Swanepoel, DW, Becker, P, Eloff, Z & Hall III JW 2014, 'Noise and age-related hearing loss: A study of 40 123 gold miners in South Africa', *International Journal of Audiology*, vol. 53, suppl. 2, pp. 66–75. https://doi.org/10.3109/14992027.2013.865846

Strauss, S, Swanepoel, DW, Becker, P, Hall, JI & Eloff, Z 2012, 'Prevalence and degree of noise-induced hearing loss in South African gold miners', *Occupational Health Southern Africa*, vol. 18, no. 6, pp. 20–25.

World Health Organization (WHO) 2010, *Burden of disease from environmental noise*, World Health Organization, Geneva.

World Health Organization (WHO) 2020, *Ear health*, World Health Organization, Geneva.

Zhao, Y, Li, J, Zhang, M, Lu, Y, Xie, H, Tian, Y & Qiu, W 2019, 'Machine learning models for the hearing impairment prediction in workers exposed to complex industrial noise: A pilot study', *Ear and Hearing: The Official Journal of the American Auditory Society*, vol. 40, no. 3, p. 690. https://doi.org/10.1097/AUD.0000000000000649

Zhou, H, Zhou, Y, Zhang, H, Yu, A, Zhu, B & Zhang, L 2021, 'Socio-economic disparity in the global burden of occupational noise-induced hearing loss: An analysis for 2017 and the trend since 1990', *Occupational and Environmental Medicine,* vol. 78, no. 2, pp. 125–128. https://doi.org/10.1136/oemed-2020-106556

Index

E

F

H

I

L

M

N

O

Made in United States
Troutdale, OR
11/03/2026

56844637R00215